Springer Series in Statistics

Series editors
Peter Bickel, CA, USA
Peter Diggle, Lancaster, UK
Stephen E. Fienberg, Pittsburgh, PA, USA
Ursula Gather, Dortmund, Germany
Ingram Olkin, Stanford, CA, USA
Scott Zeger, Baltimore, MD, USA

More information about this series at http://www.springer.com/series/692

Gerhard Tutz • Matthias Schmid

Modeling Discrete Time-to-Event Data

Springer

Gerhard Tutz
LMU Munich
Munich, Germany

Matthias Schmid
University of Bonn
Bonn, Germany

ISSN 0172-7397 ISSN 2197-568X (electronic)
Springer Series in Statistics
ISBN 978-3-319-80285-5 ISBN 978-3-319-28158-2 (eBook)
DOI 10.1007/978-3-319-28158-2

Printed on acid-free paper

This Springer imprint is published by Springer Nature
The registered company is Springer International Publishing AG Switzerland

Preface

In recent years, a large variety of textbooks dealing with time-to-event analysis has been published. Most of these books focus on the statistical analysis of observations in *continuous* time. In practice, however, one often observes *discrete* event times—either because of grouping effects or because event times are intrinsically measured on a discrete scale. Statistical methodology for discrete event times has been mainly presented in journal articles and a few book chapters. In this book we introduce basic concepts and give several extensions that allow to model discrete time data adequately. In particular, modeling discrete time-to-event data strongly profits from the smoothing and regularization methods that have been developed in recent decades. The presented approaches include methods that allow to find much more flexible models than in the early times of survival modeling.

The book is aimed at applied statisticians, students of statistics and researchers from areas like biometrics, social sciences and econometrics. The mathematical level is moderate, instead we focus on basic concepts and data analysis.

Objectives

The main aims of the book are

- to provide a thorough introduction to basic and advanced concepts of discrete hazard modelling,
- to exploit the relationship between hazard models and generalized linear models,
- to demonstrate how existing statistical software can be used to fit discrete time-to-event models, and
- to illustrate the statistical methodology for discrete time-to-event models by considering applications from the social sciences, economics and biomedical sciences.

Special Topics

This book provides a comprehensive treatment of statistical methodology for discrete time-to-event models. Special topics include

- non-parametric modeling of survival (e.g., by using smooth baseline hazards and/or smooth predictor effects),
- methods for the evaluation of model fit and prediction accuracy of discrete time-to-event models,
- regularized estimation techniques for predictor selection in high-dimensional covariate spaces, and
- tree-based methods for discrete time-to-event analysis.

In addition, each section of the book contains a set of exercises on the respective topics.

Implementation and Software

- All numerical results presented in this book were obtained by using the R System for Statistical Computing (R Core Team 2015). Hence readers are able to reproduce all the results by using freely available software.
- Various functions and tools for the analysis of discrete time-to-event data are collected in the R package *discSurv* (Welchowski and Schmid 2015).

We are grateful to many colleagues for valuable discussions and suggestions, in particular to Kaveh Bashiri, Moritz Berger, Jutta Gampe, Andreas Groll, Wolfgang Hess, Stephanie Möst, Vito M. R. Mugeo, Margret Oelker, Hein Putter, Micha Schneider and Steffen Unkel. Silke Janitza carefully read preliminary versions of the book and helped to reduce the number of mistakes. We also thank Helmut Küchenhoff for late but substantial suggestions.

Special thanks go to Thomas Welchowski for his excellent programming work and to Pia Oberschmidt for assisting us in compiling the subject index.

München, Germany — Gerhard Tutz
Bonn, Germany — Matthias Schmid
April 2015

Contents

Chapter 1
Introduction

1.1 Survival and Time-to-Event Data

Survival analysis consists of a body of methods that are known under different names. In biostatistics, where one often examines the time to death, survival analysis is the most often used name. In the social sciences one often speaks of *event history data*, in technical applications of *reliability methods*. In all of these areas one wants to model *time-to-event data*. The focus is on the modeling of the time it takes until a specific event occurs. More generally, one has mutually exclusive states that can be taken over time. For example, in the analysis of unemployment the states can refer to unemployment, part-time employment, full-time employment or retirement. One wants to model the course of an individual between these states over time. An event occurs if an individual moves from one state to another. In a *single spell* analysis, which is the most extensively treated case in this book, one considers just one time period between two events, for example, how long it takes until unemployment ends.

Since one models the transition between states, one also uses the name *transition models*. More general names for the type of data to be modeled, which do not refer to a specific area of applications, are *duration data*, *sojourn data* or *failure time data*, and the corresponding models are called *duration models* or *failure time models*. We will most often use the term survival data and survival models but, depending on the context, also use alternative names.

What makes survival data special? In a regression model, if one wants to investigate how predictors determine a specific survival time T, time takes the role of the response variable. Thus one has a response variable with a restricted support because $T \geq 0$ has to hold. Nevertheless, by using some transformation, for example, $\log(T)$, such that all values can occur, one might be tempted to consider it as a common regression problem of the form $\log(T) = \boldsymbol{x}^T\boldsymbol{\gamma} + \epsilon$, where $\boldsymbol{x}$ denotes the predictors, $\boldsymbol{\gamma}$ is a vector of coefficients, and ϵ is a noise variable. Although models like that can be used in simple cases they do not work in more general settings. There are in particular two issues that are important in the modeling of survival

G. Tutz, M. Schmid, *Modeling Discrete Time-to-Event Data*,
Springer Series in Statistics, DOI 10.1007/978-3-319-28158-2_1

data, namely the modeling of the underlying *dynamics* of the process, which can be captured in the form of a risk or hazard function, and *censoring*, which means that in some cases the exact time is not available. In the following these two aspects are briefly sketched.

The Hazard Rate

In time-to-event data one often considers the so-called *hazard function*. In the case of discrete time (e.g., if time is given in months), it has the simple form of a conditional probability. Then the *hazard* or *intensity function* for a given vector of predictors $\boldsymbol{x}$ is defined by

$$\lambda(t|\boldsymbol{x}) = P(T = t \,|\, T \geq t, \boldsymbol{x}), \quad t = 1, 2, \ldots$$

It represents the conditional probability that the time period T ends at time t, given $T \geq t$ (and $\boldsymbol{x}$). In survival analysis, for example, the hazard is the current risk of dying at time t given the individual has survived until then. When considering duration of unemployment it can be the probability that unemployment ends in month t given the person was unemployed until then. In the latter case a positive event ends the spell, and the hazard represents an opportunity rather than a risk. But the important point is that the hazard function is a current (local on the time scale) measure for the strength of the tendency to move from one state to the other. It measures at each time point the tendency that a transition takes place. In this sense it measures the underlying dynamics of survival. Typically one is interested in studying the dynamics behind the time under investigation. The hazard rate becomes even more important when covariates vary over time, for example, if treatment in a clinical study is modified over time. Then a simple regression model with (transformed) time as response will not work, because in a regression model one has to consider covariates that are fixed at the beginning of the time under investigation. However, time-varying covariates can be considered within the hazard function framework by specifying

$$\lambda(t|\boldsymbol{x}_t) = P(T = t \,|\, T \geq t, \boldsymbol{x}_t), \quad t = 1, 2, \ldots,$$

where $\boldsymbol{x}_t$ can include the available information on covariates up until time t. Then the hazard function measures the current risk given the covariate values up until time t, so that $\lambda(t|\boldsymbol{x}_t)$ represents the dynamics of the underlying process given any value of the covariates at or before t. More formally the phenomenon to be modeled is a stochastic process, that is, a collection of random variables indexed by time with values that correspond to the states. The modeling as a stochastic process (more concisely, a counting process) is extensively treated in Andersen et al. (1993) and Fleming and Harrington (2011).

Even without using the counting process framework one way to handle survival data is to specify a parametric or non-parametric model for the hazard function. If the hazard given $\boldsymbol{x}$ or $\boldsymbol{x}_t$ is specified, the behavior of the survival time is implicitly defined. In fact, most of the models considered in this book are *hazard rate models*.

Censoring and Truncation

The second issue that makes survival data special is *censoring*. An observation is called "censored" if its survival time has not been fully observed, that is, the exact time within one state is not known. Censoring may, for example, occur if observations in a study drop out early (so that they are lost before the event of interest occurs), or if the event of an observation occurs after the study has been finished. These situations are illustrated in Fig. 1.1. For observation 1 a spell started at $t = 0$, and the observation remained in the study until its event occurred. The black dot indicates that the event of observation 1 has actually been observed. In contrast, for observation 2 the spell started later than for observation 1, but it was right censored because it dropped out of the study before its event occurred. Similarly, for observation 4 the exact survival time is not known because it has not occurred before the end of the study (indicated by the dashed line). It should be noted that in Fig. 1.1 time refers to calendar time. What is actually modeled in survival is the spell length, that is, the time from entry time until transition to another state.

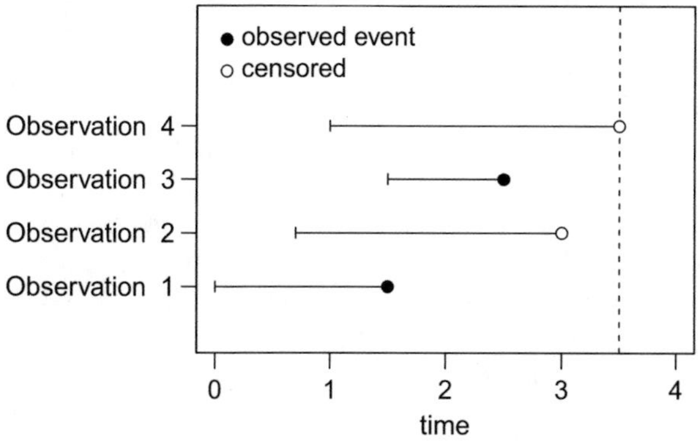

Fig. 1.1 Four observations for which spells start at different times. Exact survival time is observed for observations 1 and 3 (*black dots*); for observations 2 and 4 the end of the spell is not observed (*circles*), since observation 2 drops out early and observation 4 is still alive at the end of the study, which is shown as a *dashed line*

The most common types of censoring are

- *right censoring:* In this case the beginning of a spell is known but the exact exit time, that is, the time when a transition takes place, is not observed. At the observed time it is only known that the transition to another state has not yet occurred. Thus it is only known that the spell length is larger than the observed time. For observation i one knows $T_i > t_i$, where t_i is the observed time.
- *left censoring:* Here the entry to the relevant state is not known but the end of the spell is observed. A consequence is that again the spell length is not observed exactly.

A phenomenon that should be distinguished from censoring is *truncation*. Truncation occurs if survival times are systematically excluded from the sample and the exclusion depends on the survival time. As an example, Klein and Moeschberger (2003) consider the survival of residents of a retirement center. Because residents must survive to a specific age to enter the center, all individuals who died earlier will not be in the sample. Observed survival times are thus left truncated. Right truncation occurs if individuals that tend to have longer spells are systematically excluded from the sample. If, for example, mortality is investigated by recorded deaths, longer lifetimes tend to be excluded. In summary, one may distinguish between

- *right truncation:* longer spells are systematically excluded from the sample.
- *left truncation:* short spells are excluded, in particular, when survival times below some threshold are not observed.

Jenkins (2004) makes the connection between left truncation and econometric concepts as *stock sampling with follow-up* and *delayed entry*. Stock sampling occurs if one samples, for example, from a stock of persons that are unemployed at some fixed time and interviews them later. Then, persons with short unemployment time will tend to be excluded from the sample. More details on censoring and truncation and alternative forms of censoring are found in Lawless (1982) and Klein and Moeschberger (2003).

We will most often assume that the survival time is independent of the censoring time. Then the observed time is given as the minimum $\min\{T_i, C_i\}$, where T_i is the survival time of individual i and C_i is the censoring time of individual i. Censoring time refers to the time an individual is under observation. It is itself a duration time which can be modeled separately.

1.2 Continuous Versus Discrete Survival

Most textbooks on survival analysis assume that the survival time is continuous and the event to be modeled may occur at any particular time point. Several books are available that treat continuous survival data extensively, for example, Lawless (1982), Lancaster (1992), Kalbfleisch and Prentice (2002) and Klein and

Moeschberger (2003). What in these books is often considered very briefly, if at all, is the case of *discrete survival*, which is the topic of the present book.

Although we imagine time as a continuum, in practice measurement of time is always discrete. In particular in the medical sciences, economics and the social sciences duration is usually measured, for example, in days, years or months. Thus, even though the transition between states takes place at a specific time point, the exact time points are usually not known. What is available are the data that summarize what was happening during a specific interval. One can use positive integers, $1, 2, 3, \ldots$ to denote time. More formally, continuous time is divided into intervals

$$[0, a_1), [a_1, a_2), \ldots, [a_{q-1}, a_q), [a_q, \infty).$$

In this book discrete event times are denoted by T, where $T = t$ means that the event has occurred in the interval $[a_{t-1}, a_t)$, also called "time period t". One also speaks of *grouped survival data* or *interval censoring*. In grouped survival data there are typically some observations that have the same survival time. This phenomenon is usually referred to as "ties". In continuous time, ties ideally should not occur. In fact, some models and estimation methods for continuous time even assume that there are no ties in the data. Nevertheless, in practical applications with continuous event times ties occur, which might be taken as a hint for underlying grouping. In some areas, for example in demography, discrete data are quite natural. For example, life tables traditionally use years as a measure for life span.

In some cases the underlying transition process is what Jenkins (2004) calls *intrinsically discrete*. Consider, for example, time to pregnancy. A natural measure for the time it takes a couple to conceive is the number of menstrual cycles, which is a truly discrete response, see also Scheike and Jensen (1997) for an application of discrete survival models to model fertility. Genuinely discrete measurements may also result from surveys that are taken every month or year. For example, the IFO Business Climate for Germany (http://www.cesifo-group.de/ifoHome), is based on a survey in which firms from Germany are asked each month if "Production has decreased", "Production has remained unchanged", or "Production has increased". Consequently, when investigating the factors that determine how long the answer of a firm remains the same, one obtains time-discrete measurements. Also, when considering the important problem of panel mortality, where one investigates for how long a firm or an individual is in a panel, the response is the number of times the questionnaire was sent back and is therefore genuinely discrete.

In summary, discrete time-to-event data occur as

- *intrinsically discrete measurements*, where the measurements represent natural numbers, or
- *grouped data*, which represent events in underlying time intervals, and the response refers to an interval.

The basic modeling approaches are the same for both types of data, in particular when the intervals in grouped data have the same length (e.g., if they represent months or years). In the following sections, we will therefore distinguish between the two types of data only if necessary.

In principle, traditional modeling approaches for continuous time-to-event data can be applied to discrete time-to-event data as well (at least if the discrete event times are equally spaced). However, statistical methods that are specially designed for discrete event times have a number of advantages in this case:

- Considering discrete time-to-event models has the advantage that hazards can be formulated as conditional probabilities. Hence they are much more accessible for interpretation than continuous hazard functions.
- In practice, many event times are intrinsically discrete or are observed on a discrete scale. Consequently, using discrete time-to-event models is more exact (and therefore more appropriate) than the approximation of the observed data by a continuous survival model.
- In contrast to survival models for continuous time, models for discrete event times do not cause problems with ties.
- Discrete time-to-event models can be embedded into the generalized linear model (GLM) framework. Consequently, estimation is easily accomplished by using standard software for the estimation of GLMs.
- The embedding into the framework of GLMs allows to use the methodology also for advanced models, for example, when including subject-specific parameters in so-called frailty models.

1.3 Overview

The remainder of this book is organized as follows: In the rest of Chap. 1 we introduce several example data sets, which represent typical situations in which (discrete) survival modeling is important. These applications will be used throughout the book to illustrate and explain statistical methodology. In Chap. 2 we will consider *life tables*, which are a frequently used statistical technique in demography to analyze discrete survival data (that are usually measured in years). Because life table estimates usually do not involve covariates, they represent the most basic form of a discrete-time survival model. In Chap. 3, the life table framework is extended to *regression models* for discrete survival data. More specifically, the models considered in Chap. 3 belong to the group of "discrete hazard models", as they regress the discrete hazard function on a set of covariates. In addition to defining and characterizing the most common types of discrete hazard models, the chapter also covers methods for estimation and model fitting. Also continuous time survival and the connection to discrete time data is briefly considered. In Chap. 4, various diagnostic tools for the models considered in Chap. 3 are considered. These tools include statistical hypothesis tests that evaluate the significance of predictors, as well as goodness-of-fit tests, residuals, and measures of prediction accuracy. While the regression models considered in Chaps. 3 and 4 follow the "classical" assumption of linear covariate effects of the form $\boldsymbol{x}^\top\boldsymbol{\gamma}$, Chap. 5 extends this approach by considering *smooth* hazard and survival functions. Moreover, the linear discrete hazard models of Chap. 3 are extended by smooth nonlinear covariate effects (modeled, e.g., via kernel smoothers or splines). The underlying methodology closely follows the Generalized Additive Model (GAM) framework introduced by Hastie and Tibshirani (1990) for regression models with uncensored response. Chapter 6 deals with *discrete-time survival trees*, which are a convenient nonparametric approach to model discrete survival data in situations where the GAM framework is not appropriate or where complex (non-additive) interaction patterns between the covariates exist. Chapter 7 deals with *techniques for variable selection and model choice*, which are important in situations where the set of available covariates is large. In these situations one is often interested in fitting a "sparse" survival model that contains a small subset of highly informative predictors. To identify these predictors, statistical methods such as penalized regression and gradient boosting (presented in Chap. 7) can be applied. In Chap. 8, the focus is on *competing risks models*, which are needed to model discrete survival data with several "competing" target events. For example, when modeling duration of unemployment, these target events might be defined by full-time or part-time jobs that end the unemployment spell. In Chap. 9 methods to deal with *unobserved heterogeneity* are presented. They are important when some relevant covariates that affect survival behavior have not been observed. This missing information may cause severe artefacts when not accounted for in statistical analysis. Regression techniques such as the class of "frailty models" covered in Chap. 9 can be used to address this issue. The final chapter (Chap. 10) provides a brief overview of multiple spell analysis.

At the end of each chapter subsections on software and on references for further reading are found. Data sets and additional program code is contained in the R add-on package *discSurv* (Welchowski and Schmid 2015), which accompanies the book.

1.4 Examples

This section introduces some example data sets that serve as typical applications of discrete-time survival modeling. The data will be analyzed in later chapters. Additional data sets will also be described and analyzed in later chapters, see page 236 for a complete list of examples considered in this book.

Example 1.1 Duration of Unemployment
This data set was originally analyzed by McCall (1996) and Cameron and Trivedi (2005). It contains information about the duration of unemployment spells of $n = 3343$ U.S. citizens. Data were derived from the January Current Population Survey's Displaced Workers Supplements (DWS) in the years 1986, 1988, 1990 and 1992. The events of interest are the re-employment of a person in a part-time job or a full-time job. Unemployment duration was measured in 2-week intervals; observed event times ranged from one interval (2 weeks) to 28 intervals (56 weeks).

Table 1.1 Explanatory variables that are used to model the time to re-employment (`UnempDur` data set, as contained in the R add-on package *Ecdat*, Croissant 2015)

Variable	Categories/unit	Sample proportion/median (range)
Age	Years	34 (20–61)
Filed unemployment claim?	Yes/no	55 %/45 %
Eligible replacement rate		0.50 (0.07–2.06)
Eligible disregard rate		0.10 (0.00–1.02)
Log weekly earnings in lost job	$	5.68 (2.71–7.60)
Tenure in lost job	Years	2 (0–40)

Unemployment spells were measured in 2-week intervals. The replacement rate is defined as the weekly benefit amount divided by the amount of weekly earnings in the lost job (cf. Cameron and Trivedi 2005, p. 604). The disregard rate is defined as the disregard (i.e., the amount up to which recipients of unemployment insurance who accept part-time work can earn without any reduction in unemployment benefits) divided by the weekly earnings in the lost job

In this book we analyze a publicly available version of the data that is part of the R add-on package *Ecdat* (Croissant 2015). The list of explanatory variables that will be used for modeling unemployment duration is presented in Table 1.1. □

Example 1.2 Munich Founder Study
In the German Munich Founder Study data were collected on business founders who registered their new companies at the local chambers of commerce in Munich and surrounding administrative districts. From a total of 28,646 business registrations during the years 1985 and 1986 a stratified random sample of about 6000 firms was drawn. In the spring of 1990, 1849 firm founders were interviewed. Data were collected in a stratified manner with bankrupt businesses being over-represented. The first part of the interview concerned start-up characteristics of the firm and its development; the second part dealt with attributes of the founder. The data of the Munich Founder Study, which are described in detail in Brüderl et al. (1992), are available at the Central Archive for Empirical Social Research, University of Cologne, Germany (http://www.gesis.org/ZA). We restrict our analysis to the 1124 complete cases of firms that were newly founded. The dependent variable for our analyses is the failure time measured in months. Observed failure times ranged from 1 month to 66 months (median 46 months). For those firms that were still in business at the interview, the failure time is censored; the censoring rate was 71 %. As risk factors we include variables that have been shown to be important predictors in previous analyses of the data (see for example Brüderl et al. 1992). These include the initial size of the firm (legal form, amount of capital invested and number of employees), the business strategy (i.e., the market aimed for at founding) and the human capital of the founder. These covariates were measured at the time point of foundation. Thus we include the following variables; see also Table 1.2: (a) The economic sector (industry, commerce or service). (b) Legal form of the business: on the basis of German law we classify the business as either a small business or a partnership. (c) Financing of the business: we classify companies according to their seed capital, equity capital and debt capital. (d) Number of employees: we distinguish between single- or two-person businesses and companies with two or more employees. Note that the number of employees includes the founder. (e) Target market of business: founders were asked a series of questions regarding their business strategy at the time of founding. We record whether the founder aimed for a local or national market, and whether he aimed at a special clientele (or even at a single client) or at a widespread clientele. (f) Human capital of the founder: we include two human capital indicators—one indicator measures professional experience ($<$10 years vs. $\geq$10 years), the other indicator refers to general human capital (which is measured by the school degree: secondary school/O-level vs. A-level). □

Table 1.2 Explanatory variables for the Munich Founder Study

Variable	Categories	Number	Sample proportion (%)
Economic sector	Industry	201	16.42
	Commerce	507	41.42
	Service	516	42.16
Legal form	Small trade	575	46.98
	Partnership	649	53.02
Seed capital	Less than/equal to 25,000 DM	454	37.09
	Larger than 25000 DM	770	62.91
Equity capital	0 DM	110	8.99
	More than 0 DM	1114	91.01
Debt capital	0	794	64.87
	More than 0	430	35.13
Target market	Local	642	52.45
	National	582	47.55
Clientele	Widespread	868	70.92
	One/few important customer(s)	356	29.08
Degree	Sec. school/O-level	755	61.68
	A-level	469	38.32
Gender	female	953	77.86
	male	271	22.14
Professional experience	Less than 10 years	437	35.70
	10 or more years	787	64.30
Number of employees	0 or 1	497	40.60
	2 or more	727	59.40

Example 1.3 Copenhagen Stroke Study
From 1991 to 1993, the Copenhagen Stroke Study enrolled 1197 stroke patients in the City of Copenhagen, Denmark (Joergensen et al. 1996). All patients included in the study were admitted to a hospital with acute stroke and were treated on a single stroke unit from the time of admission to the end of rehabilitation regardless of their age and health condition. During a 10-year follow-up, the time from admission to death was recorded for each patient. In addition, minimum survival times were recorded for patients that were lost during the follow-up period.

We analyze the effect of various demographic and medical factors on survival time after admission to hospital. Risk factors include age and sex of the patients, diabetes, alcohol consumption, and stroke history (see Table 1.3).

A subset of the study data ($n = 518$) is publicly available as part of the R add-on package *pec* (Gerds 2015). Observed survival times range from 1 day to 4262 days, with 22 % of the survival times being censored. In this book we will use various grouped versions of the data (e.g., a data set where survival times have been rounded to years) to investigate the efficiency and appropriateness of discrete-time survival modeling. □

Example 1.4 Congressional Careers
This data set reflects careers of incumbent members of the U.S. Congress. It is available online at http://psfaculty.ucdavis.edu/bsjjones/eventhistory.html. A congressman can end his legislative career in four different ways: He might retire (*retirement*), he might be ambitious and seek an alternative office (*ambition*), he might lose a primary election (*primary*), or he might lose a general

Table 1.3 Explanatory variables for the Copenhagen Stroke Study (data set `cost` in R package *pec*)

Variable	Categories/unit	Sample proportion/median (range)
Sex	Female/male	53 %/47 %
Hypertension	Yes/no	33 %/67 %
Ischemic heart disease	Yes/no	20 %/80 %
Previous stroke	Yes/no	18 %/82 %
Other disabling disease	Yes/no	16 %/84 %
Alcohol intake	Yes/no	32 %/68 %
Diabetes	Yes/no	14 %/86 %
Smoking status	Yes/no	46 %/54 %
Atrial fibrillation	Yes/no	13 %/87 %
Hemorrhage (stroke subtype)	Yes/no	5 %/95 %
Age	Years	75 (25–95)
Scandinavian stroke score	0 (worst)–58 (best)	46 (0–58)
Cholesterol level	mmol/L	5.9 (1.5–11.6)

election (*general*). The dependent variable is defined by the transition process of a Congressman from his first election up to one of the competing events *general, primary, retirement* or *ambition*. The duration until the occurrence of one of the competing events is measured as terms served, where a maximum of 16 terms can be reached. Career path data were collected on every member of the House of Representatives from each freshman class elected from 1950 to 1976. Each incumbent in the data set was tracked from the first re-election bid until the last term served in office. A member initially elected in 1950 does not enter the risk set until the election cycle of 1952, as the members of the House of Representatives serve two-year terms. At each subsequent election, a terminating event or re-election is observed. Once a terminating event is experienced, the incumbent is no longer observed. The data set covers all election cycles from 1952 up to 1992. A detailed description can be found in the book by Box-Steffensmeier and Jones (2004) and in Jones (1994).

Originally, up to 20 terms occurred, however, only for very few Congressmen. Hence, due to stability reasons, durations that exceed 15 terms have been aggregated. Furthermore, only complete cases, that is, observations with no missing values for any covariate, have been incorporated in the analysis. The data set considered in this book contains the career paths of 860 Congressmen. Several covariates are available: The covariate *age* gives the incumbent's age at each election cycle and, to improve interpretability, is centered around 51 years. The incumbent's margin of victory in his or her previous election is collected in the variable *priorm*, which is centered around a margin of 35. The covariate *redistricting* indicates if the incumbent's district was substantially redistricted. The covariate *scandal* captures if an incumbent was involved in an ethical or sexual misconduct scandal or if the incumbent was under criminal investigation. The covariates *openGub* and *openSen* indicate if there is an open gubernatorial and/or open senatorial seat available in the incumbent's state. The data set considers members of the Republican and the Democratic party. Whether the Congressman is a member of the Republican party is gathered in the variable *republican*. Finally, *leadership* describes if a member is in the House leadership and/or is a chair of a standing House committee. With the exception of the predictor *republican* all covariates are time-varying, that is, the covariate values per object may vary over the duration time. Further details and descriptive statistics are presented in Tables 1.4 and 1.5. □

Table 1.4 Description of variables for the Congressional Careers data; response (top) and covariates (bottom)

Variable	Description
surv	Duration of time (measured in terms served) the incumbent has spent in Congress prior to the election cycle
general	Terminating event ($\in \{0, 1\}$), coded 1 if incumbent lost the general election and 0 if he won the general election
primary	Terminating event ($\in \{0, 1\}$), coded 1 if incumbent lost the primary election and 0 if he won the primary election
retirement	Terminating event ($\in \{0, 1\}$), coded 1 if incumbent retires from work and 0 otherwise
ambition	Terminating event ($\in \{0, 1\}$), coded 1 if incumbent has a higher ambition than re-election and 0 otherwise. The baseline event for the binary indicator variables above (general=0 & primary=0 & retirement=0 & ambition=0) occurred when the incumbent candidated for re-election and won it
age	Incumbent's age measured in years at each election cycle
district	Reciprocal of the number of Congressional districts in the state; measures the proportion of the state the incumbent's district encompasses
leader	Indicator of prestige position ($\in \{0, 1\}$), coded 1 if a member is in the House leadership and/or is a chair of a standing House committee and 0 otherwise
opengub	Dummy variable ($\in \{0, 1\}$), coded 1 if there is an open gubernatorial seat available in the incumbent's state and 0 if not
opensen	Dummy variable ($\in \{0, 1\}$), coded 1 if there is an open senatorial seat available in the incumbent's state and 0 if not
prespart	Dummy variable ($\in \{0, 1\}$), coded 1 if the incumbent's party affiliation is the same as the president's
priorm	The incumbent's margin of victory in his or her previous election
redist	Dummy variable ($\in \{0, 1\}$), coded 1 if incumbent's district was substantially redistricted and 0 otherwise
reform	Coded 1 for the election cycles 1968, 1970 and 1972 (because there was a house reform) and 0 otherwise
republican	Dummy variable ($\in \{0, 1\}$), coded 1 if incumbent is Republican and 0 otherwise
scandal	Dummy variable ($\in \{0, 1\}$), coded 1 if incumbent was involved in an ethical or sexual misconduct scandal or when incumbent was under criminal investigation and 0 if not

Table 1.5 Descriptive statistics of covariates for the Congressional Careers data

Variable	Categories/unit	Sample proportion/median (range)
age	Years	51 (27–83)
district	Proportion	7 % (0–100 %)
leader	Prestige position	3 %
	Otherwise	97 %
opengub	Gubernatorial seat available	20 %
	Otherwise	80 %
opensen	Senatorial seat available	13 %
	Otherwise	87 %
prespart	Same party as president	48 %
	Otherwise	52 %
priorm	Margin of victory in percent	29 % (0–100 %)
redist	Incumbent's district was substantially redistricted	2 %
	Otherwise	98 %
reform	Era of house reform	17 %
	Otherwise	83 %
republican	Republican	42 %
	Otherwise	58 %
scandal	Ethical, sexual misconduct scandal or incumbent under criminal investigation	1 %
	Otherwise	99 %

Example 1.5 Family Dynamics
The Pairfam study is devoted to the analysis of intimate relationships and family dynamics. Data are collected in the form of a panel, see release 4.0 (Nauck et al. 2013). The panel was started in 2008 and contains about 12,000 randomly chosen respondents belonging to the birth cohorts 1971–1973, 1981–1983 and 1991–1993. Pairfam follows the cohort approach, i.e. the main focus is on an anchor person of a certain birth cohort who provides detailed information, orientations and attitudes (mainly with regard to their family plans) of both partners. Interviews are conducted yearly; a detailed description of the study can be found in Huinink et al. (2011). Here we use a subsample of the data that consists of 1237 observations corresponding to 690 anchor women with available birth dates living in Germany. Each of the women has participated in at least two of the first four Pairfam waves. The covariates that were available are given in Table 1.6. □

Table 1.6 Description of covariates for the Pairfam data: response (top), control (middle) and leisure variables (bottom)

Variable	Description
child	A dummy ($\in \{0, 1\}$) indicating if the woman gave birth to her first child within the regarded interval (or is currently pregnant)
age	Age (in years) of the anchor woman
page	Age (in years) of the male partner
sat6	Degree of life satisfaction ($\in \{0, 1, \ldots, 10\}$) of the anchor woman
reldur	Duration of the relationship (in months)
relstat	Status of relationship (categorical with three levels: "living apart together", "cohabitation", "married")
yeduc	Years of education ($\in [8, 20]$) of the anchor woman
pyeduc	Years of education ($\in [8, 20]$) of the male partner
casprim	Employment status of the anchor woman (categorical with five levels: "in education", "full-time employed", "part-time employed", "non-working", "other")
pcasprim	Employment status of the male partner (categorical—see *casprim*)
siblings	Number of siblings of the anchor woman
hlt7	Average sleep length of the anchor woman (in hours)
leisure	(Approx.) yearly leisure time of the anchor woman (in hours) spent for the following five major categories: (1) bar/cafe/restaurant; (2) sport; (3) internet/tv; (4) meet friends; (5) discotheque
leisure.partner	Relative proportion ($\in [0, 1]$) of *leisure* that the partner spends together with the anchor woman
holiday	Time of the anchor woman (in weeks) spent on holiday

Chapter 2
The Life Table

The life table is one of the oldest tools to analyze survival in homogeneous populations. In classical applications in demography and actuarial science it was used to estimate the probability of death for each age given an interval or year of birth. In the following it serves as a model for all kinds of observed times. Time can refer to survival time, waiting time, lifetime, duration of marriage, duration of unemployment, or any other time-to-event. It is assumed that individuals or, more general, statistical units are at risk of experiencing a single target event.

We will assume that time is recorded in discrete intervals. Consequently, continuous time is subdivided into intervals $[0, a_1), [a_1, a_2), \ldots, [a_{q-1}, a_q), [a_q, \infty)$. In many applications the first q intervals are equally spaced (representing years, months, or weeks) and time is measured in these units. Discrete time-to-event is denoted by T, where $T = t$ means that the event has occurred in the interval $[a_{t-1}, a_t)$, which is also called *time period t*.

In most empirical studies the occurrence of the event under consideration is not observed for all observations. Rather for part of the observations it is only known that the time-to-event exceeds a certain value. This phenomenon is called *censoring*, more specific *right censoring*, since it is known that survival time is larger than or equal to the time the individual has been observed for the last time. Censoring is denoted by C, where $C = t$ means that an observation has been censored in time period t.

2.1 Life Table Estimates

In life tables one assumes that the population is homogeneous. The probability that for a randomly drawn individual the target event occurs in period t is denoted by

$$\pi_t = P(T = t).$$

G. Tutz, M. Schmid, *Modeling Discrete Time-to-Event Data*,
Springer Series in Statistics, DOI 10.1007/978-3-319-28158-2_2

The probabilities $\pi_1, \pi_2, \dots$ represent the discrete density of the random variable $T \in \{1, 2, \dots, \}$. It is often useful to consider the conditional probability that the target event occurs in time period t given it has not yet occurred. The corresponding conditional function

$$\lambda_t = P(T = t \,|\, T \geq t), \quad t = 1, \dots, q,$$

is called *hazard function*. It can be seen as a current indicator of the dynamics of the underlying process. For instance, in survival it may represent the probability of death at age t given that age t is reached. Therefore it measures the risk at age t, which always requires that t has to be reached. For individuals the hazard function is more informative than the unconditional probability of death at age t, because the latter only represents the survival probability given the individual has been born. Given a specific age the conditional probability is much more relevant. Moreover, focussing on the conditional risk instead of the unconditional survival probability turns out to be useful for estimation if censoring occurs. A related measure is the *cumulative hazard* $\Lambda_t := \sum_{s=1}^{t} \lambda_s$, which is the sum of the hazards up to time t.

The life table explicitly uses estimates of the hazards and is based on the following simple links between probabilities and hazards. It is straightforward to derive

$$S(t) = P(T > t) = \prod_{s=1}^{t} (1 - \lambda_s), \tag{2.1}$$

which is the probability of surviving interval t, also called *survival function* (see Exercise 2.1). The probability of an event in interval t is determined by

$$\pi_t = P(T = t) = \lambda_t \prod_{s=1}^{t-1} (1 - \lambda_s) = \lambda_t S(t - 1).$$

If survival times for all individuals are observed, it is straightforward to estimate the probability of an event in interval t as the number of deaths within the interval divided by the number of individuals. Estimates of the hazard rate can be obtained in a similar way as relative frequencies conditional on survival until interval t. But in most applications one has to expect censoring, that is, for part of the observations one knows only that they lived up to a specific time point. In this situation one observes for a random sample of n individuals either the survival time or the censoring time.

Let us assume that the observations of discrete time-to-event are given in the following form:

- n_t, which denotes the number of individuals at risk in interval $[a_{t-1}, a_t)$ (still under observation at time a_{t-1}),
- d_t, which denotes the number of observed target events in interval $[a_{t-1}, a_t)$ (*d* referring to *d*eaths), and
- w_t, which denotes the numbers of censored observations in interval $[a_{t-1}, a_t)$ (*w* referring to *w*ithdrawals).

Thus the number of observations at risk in the first, second, or, more generally, the rth interval are given by

$$n_1 = n,\ n_2 = n_1 - d_1 - w_1, \ldots, n_r = n_{r-1} - d_{r-1} - w_{r-1}, \tag{2.2}$$

respectively. Without censoring, a natural estimate of $\lambda_t = P(T = t \mid T \geq t)$ is the proportion of observed events to the number of individuals at risk

$$\hat{\lambda}_t = \frac{d_t}{n_t}. \tag{2.3}$$

If censoring occurs, that is, $w_t > 0$, the estimator is appropriate only if censoring occurs at the end of the interval. If censoring is assumed to occur at the beginning of the interval $[a_{t-1}, a_t)$, a better choice is $\hat{\lambda}_t = d_t/(n_t - w_t)$.

The *standard life table estimator* takes the withdrawals into account by using

$$\hat{\lambda}_t = \frac{d_t}{n_t - w_t/2}. \tag{2.4}$$

Hence the estimator implicitly assumes that withdrawals are at risk during half the interval. It is a compromise between censoring at the beginning and the end of the interval. Based on (2.1) the probability of surviving beyond a_t can be estimated by

$$\hat{S}(t) = \prod_{s=1}^{t} (1 - \hat{\lambda}_s) \tag{2.5}$$

for $t = 1, \ldots, q$. Consequently, the estimated probability of failure in interval $[a_{t-1}, a_t)$ is obtained as

$$\hat{P}(T = t) = \hat{\lambda}_t \prod_{i=1}^{t-1} (1 - \hat{\lambda}_i)$$

for $t = 1, \ldots, q$.

It should be noted that the life table estimator and the corresponding probabilities are computed for the q intervals $[0, a_1), [a_1, a_2), \ldots, [a_{q-1}, a_q)$ only. The probability $P(T = q + 1)$, which corresponds to the interval $[a_q, \infty)$, is then implicitly given. This is because if a random variable T can take values $\{1, \ldots, q + 1\}$, the probabilities $\pi_t = P(T = t)$ sum up to 1, that is, $\sum_{t=1}^{q+1} \pi_t = 1$. For the hazards one obtains $\lambda_t = P(T = t \mid T \geq t)$, in particular $\lambda_{q+1} = 1$ since $P(T = q + 1 \mid T \geq q + 1) = 1$. If the life table estimator is used to estimate mortality, $\lambda_{q+1} = 1$ is quite natural because any human being is mortal. In other cases, for example, if life tables are used to model the duration of unemployment,

$\lambda_{q+1} = 1$ does not mean that unemployment ends in the last category. But the last hazard λ_{q+1} can be used to compute $P(T = q+1) = \hat{\lambda}_{q+1} \prod_{i=1}^{q}(1 - \hat{\lambda}_i)$, which is the probability that the duration of unemployment is beyond a_q. Table 2.1 shows the estimates of the hazard in an unemployment study considered by Fahrmeir et al.

Table 2.1 Life table estimates obtained from the German unemployment data (Example 2.1)

$[a_{t-1}, a_t)$ months	n_t	w_t	$n_t - w_t/2$	d_t	$\hat{\lambda}_t$	$\hat{P}(T \geq t)$	$\hat{P}(T = t)$
[1, 2)	1669	131	1603.5	197	0.1229	0.8771	0.1229
[2, 3)	1341	7	1337.5	178	0.1331	0.7604	0.1167
[3, 4)	1156	12	1150.0	159	0.1383	0.6553	0.1051
[4, 5)	985	3	983.5	89	0.0905	0.5960	0.0593
[5, 6)	893	9	888.5	86	0.0968	0.5383	0.0577
[6, 7)	798	6	795.0	81	0.1019	0.4834	0.0548
[7, 8)	711	4	709.0	53	0.0748	0.4473	0.0361
[8, 9)	654	5	651.5	58	0.0890	0.4075	0.0398
[9, 10)	591	7	587.5	45	0.0766	0.3763	0.0312
[10, 11)	539	0	539.0	20	0.0371	0.3626	0.0140
[11, 12)	519	4	517.0	25	0.0484	0.3448	0.0175
[12, 13)	490	21	479.5	188	0.3921	0.2096	0.1352
[13, 14)	281	2	280.0	30	0.1071	0.1871	0.0225
[14, 15)	249	3	247.5	22	0.0889	0.1705	0.0166
[15, 16)	224	2	223.0	26	0.1166	0.1506	0.0199
[16, 17)	196	1	195.5	16	0.0818	0.1383	0.0123
[17, 18)	179	2	178.0	15	0.0843	0.1267	0.0117
[18, 19)	162	2	161.0	18	0.1118	0.1125	0.0142
[19, 20)	142	3	140.5	7	0.0498	0.1069	0.0056
[20, 21)	132	3	130.5	8	0.0613	0.1003	0.0066
[21, 22)	121	6	118.0	12	0.1017	0.0901	0.0102
[22, 23)	103	1	102.5	6	0.0585	0.0849	0.0053
[23, 24)	96	0	96.0	4	0.0417	0.0813	0.0035
[24, 25)	92	8	88.0	16	0.1818	0.0665	0.0148
[25, 26)	68	0	68.0	3	0.0441	0.0636	0.0029
[26, 27)	65	1	64.5	2	0.0310	0.0616	0.0020
[27, 28)	62	1	61.5	3	0.0488	0.0586	0.0030
[28, 29)	58	1	57.5	4	0.0696	0.0545	0.0041
[29, 30)	53	0	53.0	0	0.0000	0.0545	0.0000
[30, 31)	53	2	52.0	3	0.0577	0.0514	0.0032
[31, 32)	48	2	47.0	3	0.0638	0.0481	0.0033
[32, 33)	43	0	43.0	1	0.0233	0.0470	0.0011
[33, 34)	42	2	41.0	2	0.0488	0.0447	0.0023
[34, 35)	38	0	38.0	3	0.0789	0.0412	0.0035
[35, 36)	35	0	35.0	0	0.0000	0.0412	0.0000

(1996). It starts with 1669 unemployed persons; 36 were still unemployed after 36 months. It is discussed in detail in Example 2.1.

2.1.1 Distributional Aspects

Without censoring (i.e., $w_t = 0$) the number of deaths is multinomially distributed with $(d_1, \dots, d_q) \sim M(n, (\pi_1, \dots, \pi_q))$, where $\pi_t = P(T = t)$. Using (2.2) and (2.5) yields the simple estimate

$$\hat{S}(t) = \frac{n - d_1 - \dots - d_t}{n},$$

which is the number of individuals surviving beyond a_t divided by the sample size. Since $n - d_1 - \dots - d_t \sim B(n, S(t))$, expectation and variance of $\hat{S}(t)$ are given by

$$\begin{aligned} \mathrm{E}(\hat{S}(t)) &= S(t), \\ \mathrm{var}(\hat{S}(t)) &= S(t)(1 - S(t))/n, \end{aligned}$$

respectively, and the covariance for $t_1 < t_2$ is given by

$$\mathrm{cov}(\hat{S}(t_1), \hat{S}(t_2)) = \frac{(1 - S(t_1))S(t_2)}{n}.$$

For $\hat{\lambda}_t = d_t/n_t$ one obtains

$$\begin{aligned} \mathrm{E}(\hat{\lambda}_t) &= \lambda(t), \\ \mathrm{var}(\hat{\lambda}_t) &= \lambda(t)(1 - \lambda(t))\, \mathrm{E}(1/n_t), \end{aligned}$$

where it is assumed that $n_t > 0$.

In the censored case ($w_t > 0$) we have a multinomial distribution $(d_1, w_1, \dots, d_q, w_q) \sim M(n, (\pi_1^d, \pi_1^w, \dots, \pi_q^d, \pi_q^w))$. Considering continuous survival time T and censoring time C, the probabilities are given by

$$\pi_r^d = P(T \in [a_{r-1}, a_r), T \le C) \quad \text{and} \quad \pi_r^w = P(C \in [a_{r-1}, a_r), C < T).$$

Since the frequencies $(d_1/n, w_1/n, \dots, w_q/n)$ are asymptotically normally distributed, the standard life table estimate $\hat{\lambda}_t = d_t/(n_t - w_t/2)$ is also asymptotically normal with expectation

$$\lambda_t^* = \frac{\pi_t^d}{\pi_t^0 + \pi_t^w/2},$$

where $\pi_t^0 = \mathrm{E}(n_t/n)$. However, only in the case without withdrawals it holds that $\lambda_t^* = \lambda(t)$. Thus, the standard life table estimator is not a consistent estimator. Concerning the asymptotic variance of $\hat{\lambda}_t$ in the random censorship model, Lawless (1982) derives

$$\widehat{\mathrm{var}}(\hat{\lambda}_t) = \frac{1}{n}\,(\lambda_t^* - \lambda_t^{*2})\,\frac{\pi_t^0 - \pi_t^w/4}{(\pi_t^0 - \pi_t^w/2)(\pi_t^0 - \pi_t^w/2)}.$$

For the covariance $\mathrm{cov}(\hat{\lambda}_{t_1}, \hat{\lambda}_{t_2}) = 0$ holds asymptotically. Since $(n_t - w_t/2)/n$ converges to $\pi_t^0 - \pi_t^w/2$, the usual estimate

$$\widehat{\mathrm{var}}(\hat{\lambda}_t) = \frac{\hat{\lambda}_t - \hat{\lambda}_t^2}{n_t - w_t/2}$$

will overestimate $\mathrm{var}(\hat{\lambda}_t)$ if λ_t and λ_t^* are not too different. For $\hat{S}(t)$, Lawless (1982) derives

$$\mathrm{var}(\hat{S}(t)) = S^*(t)^2 \sum_{i=1}^{t} \frac{\mathrm{var}(1 - \hat{\lambda}_t)}{(1 - \lambda_t^*)^2}$$

for large sample sizes, where $S^*(t) = \prod_{i=1}^{t}(1 - \lambda_i^*)$. Approximating $\mathrm{var}(1 - \hat{\lambda}_t)$ by $\hat{\lambda}_t(1 - \hat{\lambda}_t)/(n_t - w_t/2)$ and $S^*(t), \lambda_t^*$ by $\hat{S}(t), \hat{\lambda}_t$, respectively, yields Greenwood's (1926) often used formula

$$\mathrm{var}(\hat{S}(t)) = \hat{S}(t)^2 \sum_{i=1}^{t} \frac{\hat{\lambda}_t}{(1 - \hat{\lambda}_t)(n_t - w_t/2)}.$$

2.1.2 *Smooth Life Table Estimators*

The life table estimate of the hazards, which in the simplest case without withdrawals has the form $\hat{\lambda}_t = d_t/n_t$, can be very volatile. In particular for large t, typically only few observations are at risk and estimates become unstable. The result are jumps in the estimated function that occur when the hazards $\hat{\lambda}_t$ are plotted against time. This problem can be addressed by applying smoothing techniques to $\hat{\lambda}_t$. For example, one might use smoothing techniques like averaging over neighborhood estimates or spline fitting. Note that one should be careful to take the local sample size into account, which for the estimate in interval t is $n_t = n_{t-1} - d_{t-1} - w_{t-1}$.

As an example, consider *local smoothing*, which in its simplest form borrows information from the neighborhood of t by computing

$$\tilde{\lambda}_t = \sum_{s=1}^{q} \hat{\lambda}_s n_s w_\gamma(s,t),$$

where $w_\gamma(s,t)$ is a weight function that gives observations that are close to t large weights and observations that are far away from t small weights. It should be standardized such that $\sum_s n_s w_\gamma = 1$. Often one uses weight functions that are based on *kernels*. A kernel is a continuous symmetric function that fulfills $\int K(u)du = 1$, where the corresponding kernel weight is given by

$$w_\gamma(s,t) \propto K\left(\frac{s-t}{\gamma}\right),$$

and where γ is a tuning parameter. Candidates for the choice of K are the Gaussian kernel, which uses the standard Gaussian density for K, and kernels with finite support like the Epanechnikov kernel $K(u) = \frac{3}{4}(1-u^2)$ for $|u| \leq 1$ and zero otherwise. If γ is small, the weights decrease fast with increasing distance $|s-t|$, and estimates are based solely on observations from the close neighborhood of x. For large γ estimates from a wide range of neighbors are included. More refined local smoothers are local polynomial regression smoothers, see, for example, Hastie and Loader (1993) and Loader (1999). In Chap. 5 more details are given, and an alternative smooth estimator that is based on an expansion in basis functions ("penalized regression spline") is considered in more detail.

Example 2.1 German Unemployment Data (Socio-Economic Panel)
Table 2.1 shows the life table for the socio-economic panel data considered in Fahrmeir et al. (1996). Figure 2.1 visualizes the corresponding estimated hazard rates of transition from unemployment to employment. Inspection of the estimate shows that the hazard of the transition to employment has a peak at approximately 13 months and another peak at approximately 25 months after beginning of the unemployment spell. These effects should be seen in connection with the collection of data: In the socio-economic panel people are asked in intervals of 1 year, and the unemployment status is established retrospectively. Therefore, it is likely that the effects are due to *heaping*, which means that respondents tend to remember that they were unemployed for a year or two when the exact times were close to 1 or 2 years. Because the raw estimates of the hazard rates are relatively volatile, Fig. 2.1 also shows a smoothed hazard rate (gray line) that was obtained by applying a penalized regression spline estimator (as implemented in the R package *mgcv*, Wood 2015). It is seen that smoothed estimation ameliorates the heaping bias in the estimates. Short-term unemployment is captured by the peak of the smoothed hazard rate at 4 months after beginning of the unemployment spell. Note that the spline estimate has been weighted by the observations at risk (given by $n_t - w_t/2$), thereby imposing large weights on time points with a large number of individuals at risk. In addition to presenting point estimates, Fig. 2.1 also contains 95 % confidence bands for the estimated hazards. The bands were obtained by addition and subtraction of 1.96 times the estimated standard deviation of the hazard estimates.

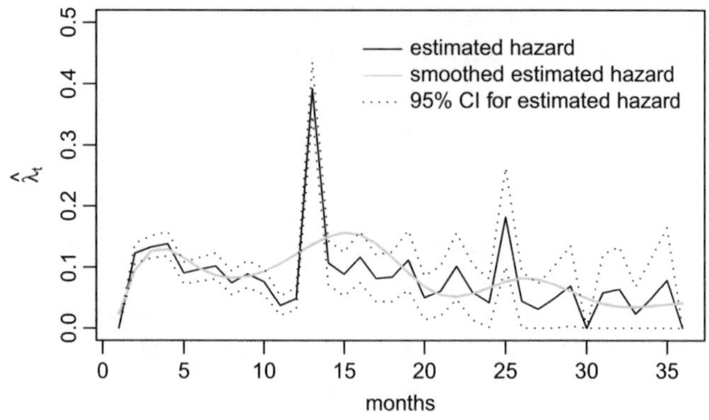

Fig. 2.1 Hazard estimates obtained from the German unemployment data (Example 2.1)

Figure 2.2 shows the estimated survival function obtained from the German unemployment data. For each time point t, this function corresponds to the estimated probability of still being unemployed after t months. It is seen that heaping effects in the estimated hazards (for example, at 13 months after beginning of the unemployment spell) lead to a relatively large decrease in the estimated survival function at the respective time points. The 95 % confidence bands shown in the upper panel of Fig. 2.2 were obtained by addition and subtraction of 1.96 times the estimated standard deviation of the estimated survival function. The lower panel of Fig. 2.2 shows the smoothed estimated survival function that is based on the smoothed hazard estimates presented in Fig. 2.1. Similar to the hazard estimates in Fig. 2.1, heaping effects in the estimated survival function have become much smaller in size. □

Example 2.2 Duration of Unemployment of U.S. Citizens
Using the unemployment data from Example 1.1, we analyzed the time to re-employment (regardless of whether re-employment was at a full-time job or at a part-time job). Unemployment spells were measured in 2-week intervals; 39 % of the observations were censored. Raw and smoothed life table estimates were calculated separately for the group of people who filed an unemployment insurance (UI) claim and the group of people who did not file a UI claim. The hazard estimates are visualized in Fig. 2.3. Obviously, the raw hazard estimates are quite volatile, whereas the smoothed hazard estimates clearly show that people who filed a UI claim tend to have a smaller chance of getting re-employed than people who did not file a UI claim. This is especially true for the first 20 weeks. One might speculate that among the people who filed a UI claim is a group of unemployed persons who—due to benefits from the state-funded unemployment compensation program—might have less motivation to search for a new job within the first weeks of their unemployment spell. Both hazard curves start to increase after 20 weeks and have a peak after 26 weeks. This could be due to the fact that in many U.S. states workers are eligible for up to 26 weeks of benefits from the state-funded unemployment compensation program. The smoothed survival curves for the two subpopulations are shown in Fig. 2.4. □

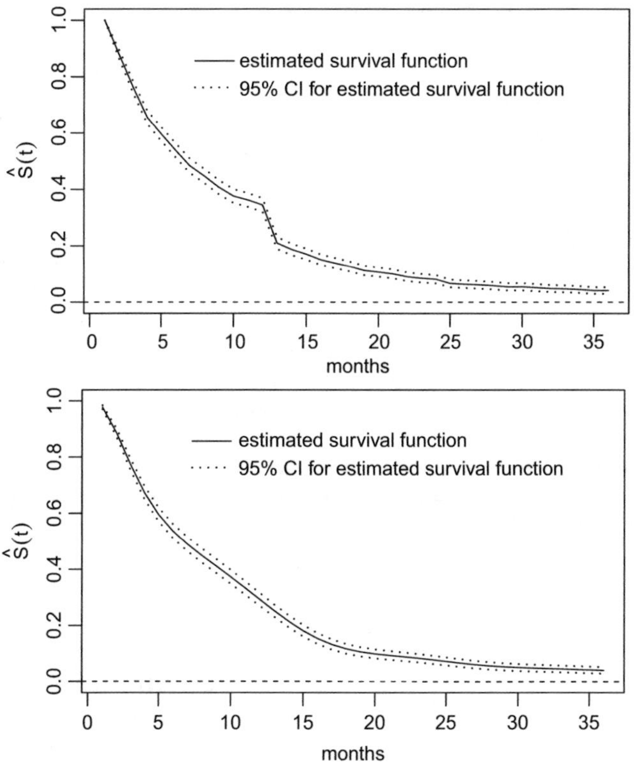

Fig. 2.2 Estimates of the survival function obtained from the German unemployment data (Example 2.1). Life table estimates are shown in the *upper panel*, smoothed estimates are shown in the *lower panel*

2.1.3 Heterogeneous Intervals

The life table estimates considered so far determine the risk of survival for fixed t, with t denoting the tth interval. This strategy works fine as long as the intervals are equally spaced, for example when t is measured in months or years. If, however, the intervals $[0, a_1), [a_1, a_2), \ldots \ldots, [a_{q-1}, a_q)$ have varying length, some care should be taken when presenting and interpreting estimates.

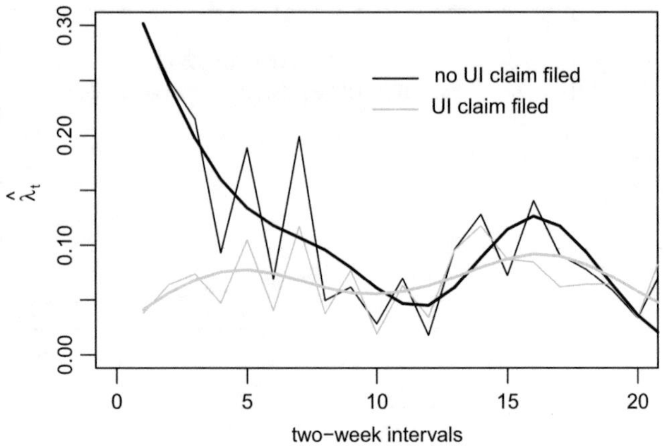

Fig. 2.3 Raw and smoothed hazard estimates obtained from the U.S. unemployment data (Example 2.2). Smoothed estimates were obtained by applying a penalized regression spline estimator (as implemented in the R package *mgcv*)

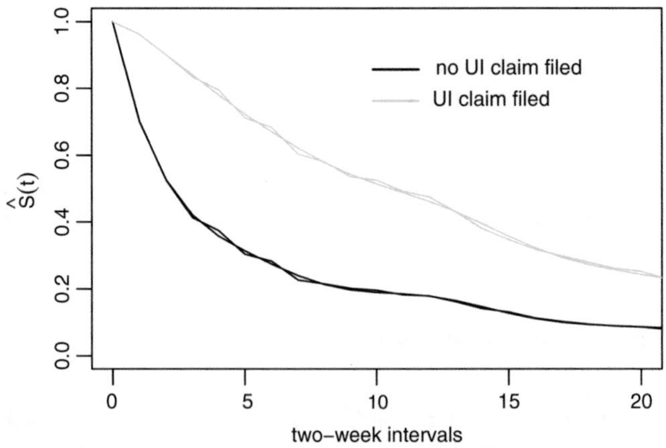

Fig. 2.4 Raw and smoothed estimated survival functions obtained from the U.S. unemployment data (Example 2.2). Smoothed estimates were obtained by applying a penalized regression spline estimator (as implemented in the R package *mgcv*). It is seen that people who filed a UI claim have lower probabilities of getting re-employed than people who did not file a UI claim

To derive life table estimators in situations where time intervals are of varying length, we assume that there is an underlying continuous time (denoted by T_c). It should be noted that T_c itself is not observed. What is observed are data in intervals, that means, $T = t$ if $T_c \in [a_{t-1}, a_t)$. In this case one also refers to *interval-censored* data. In particular, discrete survival transforms into continuous time by

$$S(t) = P(T > t) = P(T_c > a_t) = S_c(a_t),$$

where $S_c(a_t)$ denotes survival on the continuous time scale. The life table estimator provides an estimate of $\hat{P}(T = t)$ in the tth interval, which is also an estimator of the probability $P(T_c \in [a_{t-1}, a_t))$. If one assumes that the density is constant over fixed intervals, one obtains the estimator for the density of the continuous time (denoted by $f(x)$) by

$$\hat{f}(x) = \frac{\hat{S}(t) - \hat{S}(t-1)}{a_t - a_{t-1}} \quad \text{for} \quad x \in [a_{t-1}, a_t).$$

With $\Delta_t := a_t - a_{t-1}$ denoting the length of the interval and $c_t := (\hat{S}(t) - \hat{S}(t-1))/(a_t - a_{t-1})$ denoting the estimated value of the density within the interval $[a_{t-1}, a_t)$ one obtains the estimated cumulative distribution function for continuous time as a polygon

$$\hat{F}(x) := \hat{P}(T_c \le x) = \sum_{s=1}^{t-1} c_s \Delta_s + c_t x \quad \text{for} \quad x \in [a_{t-1}, a_t).$$

The corresponding continuous survival function

$$\hat{P}(T_c > x) = 1 - \hat{F}(x)$$

is again a polygon that connects estimates at the boundaries of the intervals linearly.

2.2 Kaplan–Meier Estimator

In the following an estimator is considered that is strongly related to the life table estimator, although it assumes that time is observed on a continuous scale. It is also used in applications to compare estimates based on grouped data to estimates that use the exact lifetime when available.

Let $t_{(1)} < \ldots < t_{(m)}$ denote the observed *continuous* lifetimes, which, for simplicity, are assumed to be distinct. Thus the data contain no ties. Based on the observations one constructs the intervals

$$[0, t_{(1)}), [t_{(1)}, t_{(2)}), \ldots, [t_{(m)}, \infty).$$

Then estimates of the probability of surviving the interval $[t_{(j-1)}, t_{(j)})$, $p_j = P(T_c > t_{(j)} \mid T_c \geq t_{(j-1)})$, and the hazard in the interval, $\lambda_j = P(T_c \in [t_{(j-1)}, t_{(j)}) \mid T_c \geq t_{(j-1)})$ are given by

$$\hat{p}_j = 1 - \hat{\lambda}_j = 1 - \frac{1}{|R_j|}, \quad j = 2, 3, \ldots,$$

where $|R_j|$ denotes the number of individuals at risk ("risk set") in the interval $[t_{(j-1)}, t_{(j)})$.

The *Kaplan–Meier estimator* (Kaplan and Meier 1958), also called *product-limit estimator*, is defined in analogy to the survival function in life table estimates (Eq. (2.1)) by

$$\hat{S}(t) = \begin{cases} 1 & \text{if } t < t_{(1)}, \\ \prod_{j: t_{(j)} < t}(1 - \frac{1}{|R_j|}) & \text{if } t > t_{(1)}. \end{cases}$$

It is a step function that decreases by $1/m$ just after each observed lifetime. If ties occur, the factor $1 - 1/|R_j|$ is replaced by $1 - d_j/|R_j|$, where d_j is the number of observations with value $t_{(j)}$. Censored observations that do not coincide with times of deaths automatically reduce the risk set in the next interval. If observations coincide with observed values $t_{(j)}$, it is customary to assume that the censoring time is infinitesimally larger than the observed lifetime to obtain the size of the risk set.

The Kaplan–Meier estimator can also be derived as a maximum likelihood estimator, see Lawless (1982) or Kalbfleisch and Prentice (2002). Under the random censorship model, Breslow and Crowley (1974) showed that the random function $\sqrt{n}(\hat{S}(t) - S(t))$ converges weakly to a mean zero Gaussian process. An asymptotically motivated estimator of the variance (Kaplan and Meier 1958) is given by

$$\widehat{\text{var}}(\hat{S}(t)) = \hat{S}(t)^2 \sum_{t_{(j)} < t} \frac{d_j}{|R_j|(|R_j| - d_j)}.$$

Example 2.3 Copenhagen Stroke Study

Figure 2.5 shows the Kaplan–Meier estimates (black lines) for patients with diabetes and without diabetes, as obtained from the Copenhagen Stroke Study. It is seen that survival is considerably smaller if patients suffer from diabetes at the time of admission to hospital. For example, the estimated 5-year survival rate in the diabetes group is only 38.4 % (95 % CI: [27.2 %, 49.5 %]) whereas it is 50.8 % (95 % CI: [46.1 %, 55.4 %]) in the group of patients without diabetes.

In addition to the Kaplan–Meier estimates, Fig. 2.5 shows the life table estimates of the diabetes and non-diabetes groups. Life table estimates were computed from grouped data: While the original data were measured in days, life table estimates were based on 12-month intervals. It is seen that even at this relatively coarse 1-year level, the life table estimates are a close approximation to the Kaplan–Meier estimates. □

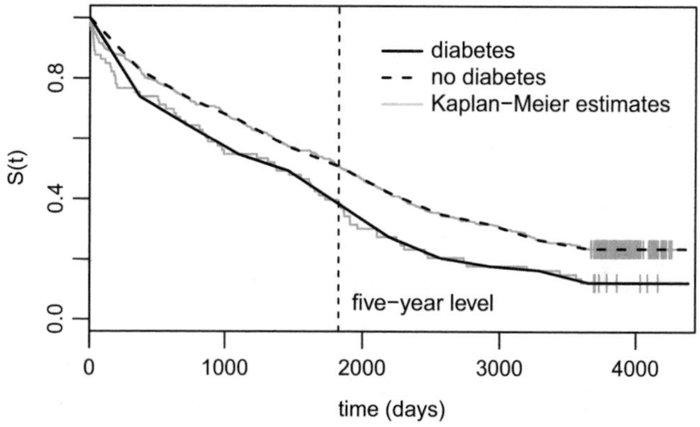

Fig. 2.5 Kaplan–Meier and life table estimates obtained from the Copenhagen Stroke Study. The *black lines* correspond to life table estimates based on 12-month time intervals. Gray step functions correspond to Kaplan–Meier estimates. The *vertical dashes* indicate censored survival times

2.3 Life Tables in Demography

Life tables in demography are a special presentation of discrete survival data that involve some specific notation. In demography there are in particular two forms of life tables: the *cohort life table* and the *current life table*. The cohort life table reflects the mortality of a specific group of individuals, the so-called cohort. It is constructed for this group of people from birth to death of the last member of the group. The methods considered in Sect. 2.1 refer to this type of data; one assumes that the population is homogeneous and that a random sample from the population is available. In contrast, current life tables contain the mortality of a population during a current time interval, for example, a year. They represent a cross-sectional view on survival. The observed mortality aims at measuring survival that is to be expected if the same mortality pattern that holds for the current year holds throughout life. Complete life tables are computed for each year whereas so-called abridged life tables deal with greater time intervals. We consider the principal structure of life tables following closely (Chiang 1984). As an example we consider the life tables given in Tables 2.2 and 2.3, which refer to Swedish citizens that were born in 1920.

Example 2.4 Swedish Life Table Data
The data set was extracted from the Human Mortality Database at www.mortality.org. It contains the mortality numbers of a virtual population of 100,000 Swedish men and 100,000 Swedish woman born in 1920. Excerpts of the data are presented in Tables 2.2 and 2.3. □

Table 2.2 Excerpt from the Swedish life table data (male population)

Age	m_x	q_x	a_x	l_x	d_x	L_x	T_x	$\hat{e}_x$
0	0.07886	0.07450	0.26	100,000	7450	94,463	6,568,254	65.68
1	0.01259	0.01251	0.48	92,550	1158	91,951	6,473,792	69.95
2	0.00495	0.00494	0.49	91,393	451	91,160	6,381,840	69.83
3	0.00346	0.00346	0.51	90,941	314	90,786	6,290,680	69.17
4	0.00310	0.00309	0.49	90,627	280	90,484	6,199,894	68.41
5	0.00225	0.00224	0.48	90,346	203	90,240	6,109,410	67.62
⋮	⋮	⋮	⋮	⋮	⋮	⋮	⋮	⋮
104	0.56391	0.43103	0.45	32	14	24	47	1.45
105	0.90000	0.60000	0.44	18	11	12	22	1.21
106	0.46875	0.38462	0.53	7	3	6	10	1.36
107	0.70588	0.50000	0.42	4	2	3	4	0.88
108	3.00000	1.00000	0.33	2	2	1	1	0.33

Table 2.3 Excerpt from the Swedish life table data (female population)

Age	m_x	q_x	a_x	l_x	d_x	L_x	T_x	$\hat{e}_x$
0	0.05943	0.05680	0.22	100,000	5680	95,567	7,269,901	72.70
1	0.01069	0.01063	0.48	94,320	1003	93,796	7,174,334	76.06
2	0.00474	0.00473	0.47	93,318	442	93,085	7,080,538	75.88
3	0.00265	0.00265	0.51	92,876	246	92,755	6,987,453	75.23
4	0.00250	0.00249	0.48	92,630	231	92,510	6,894,698	74.43
5	0.00211	0.00211	0.49	92,399	195	92,300	6,802,188	73.62
⋮	⋮	⋮	⋮	⋮	⋮	⋮	⋮	⋮
104	0.54815	0.42775	0.49	200	86	156	328	1.64
105	0.66443	0.49500	0.48	115	57	85	172	1.50
106	0.73585	0.53061	0.47	58	31	42	86	1.49
107	0.64706	0.48889	0.50	27	13	21	44	1.64
108	0.67925	0.52174	0.56	14	7	11	24	1.72
109	0.33333	0.28571	0.50	7	2	6	13	2.00
.	0.62500	1.00000	1.60	5	5	8	8	1.60

In the following we consider the discrete table for intervals of length 1, $[x, x+1)$. The first interval is $[0, 1)$, the second $[1, 2)$, etc. The last interval, $[q, \infty)$ is open-ended. The entries in the table are:

l_x: Number alive at age x. The first number, l_0 is an arbitrary figure called the *radix*. Typically one assigns the value 100,000. Thus the successive figures represent the number of survivors at the age x from a group of size l_0. Slightly misleading it is sometimes called the "probability" of survival from birth to age x (multiplied by 100,000).

d_x: Number of deaths within the age interval $[x, x + 1)$. Of course it is not the number of actually observed deaths but has meaning only in conjunction with the radix, 100,000.

q_x: Proportion of those alive at age x dying in the interval $[x, x + 1)$. It represents an estimate of the probability that an individual still alive at the exact age x will die in the interval $[x, x + 1)$; it is given by $q_x = d_x/l_x$.

m_x: Mortality or death rate at age x (see below).

a_x: Fraction of the interval $[x, x + 1)$ lived by persons who die in the interval. If $a_x = 0.5$, it is assumed that they live on average during half of the interval.

L_x: Total number of years lived within the age interval $[x, x + 1)$ for all persons. With the fraction a_x it is given by $L_x = (l_x - d_x) + a_x d_x$. As a sum over the years lived by all the persons it represents the so-called *person-years*.

T_x: Total number of years lived beyond age x, given by $T_x = L_x + L_{x+1} + \cdots + L_q$.

$\hat{e}_x$: Expected number of years yet to be lived by a person of age x, given by $\hat{e}_x = T_x/l_x$.

Typically life tables are given for $x \in \{0, 1, \ldots\}$. Thus l_0 refers to the number of persons with which the life table starts, l_1 is the number of persons who reach age 1, etc. The number of deaths is the difference for successive ages, $d_x = l_x - l_{x+1}$, and the proportion of deaths within the age interval $[x, x + 1)$ is given by $q_x = d_x/l_x$. It can be seen as a probability estimate and is a pure number as all probabilities. Life table analysis in demography customarily also uses the age-specific death rate, which should be distinguished from the probability of dying in the interval. Let us consider more generally the interval $[x, x + \Delta_x)$. Then the age-specific death rate or mortality rate is defined by

$$m_x = \frac{\text{number of individuals dying in interval } [x, x + \Delta_x)}{\text{number of years lived in the interval } [x, x + \Delta_x) \text{ by those alive at } x}.$$

It can be seen as the proportion of the number of occurrences and the exposure time. Formally it is given by

$$m_x = \frac{d_x}{\Delta_x(l_x - d_x) + \Delta_x a_x d_x} = \frac{q_x}{\Delta_x - q_x \Delta_x(1 - a_x)},$$

where a_x denotes the fraction of the interval $[x, x + \Delta_x)$ lived by persons who die in the interval, d_x is the corresponding number of deaths, and $q_x = d_x/l_x$. The death rate is a rate, and its units are death per person-year. It is considered as a measure of mortality which should not be confused with the probability of death in an interval. In general it is not the same as q_x. Formally the relation is

$$q_x = \frac{m_x \Delta_x}{1 + (1 - a_x) m_x \Delta_x}.$$

Let us consider the case where the length of the interval is one. Then the estimate of the probability $q_x = d_x/l_x$ simply uses the number of deaths in the interval and the number of individuals entering the interval. It makes no assumptions on the time lived during the interval. In contrast, the death rate given by $m_x = d_x/(l_x - d_x + a_x d_x)$ includes the fraction a_x. If one assumes that on average the persons dying in interval $[x, x+1)$ live through half of the interval, that is, the fraction a_x equals 0.5, one obtains $m_x = d_x/(l_x - d_x/2)$, which has the same form as the standard life table estimator (2.4) considered in Sect. 2.1. Apart from notation, the only difference is that withdrawals are replaced by deaths. But withdrawals refer to all individuals that get lost, for example, during a treatment study. The correction by $d_x/2$ in the denominator aims at correcting for the distribution of deaths within the interval.

In general, the correction factors in life tables can be determined empirically if exact lifetimes (not rounded to years) are available. It has been shown that, in particular for the first entries, the fractions differ from 0.5. For example, Chiang (1972) showed that for the 1960 California mortality data, the values $a_0 = 0.09$, $a_1 = 0.43$, $a_2 = 0.45$, $a_3 = 0.47$, $a_4 = 0.49$ are more appropriate to account for the large proportion of infant deaths.

For an extensive discussion of all forms of life tables, see Chiang (1984). Formal concepts are also given by Chiang (1972).

Lee Carter Models

It is of particular interest to study the dynamics of mortality over time. For example, life expectancy in the USA rose from 47 to 75 years from 1900 to 1988 (Lee and Carter 1992). Especially for the social security systems the decline of mortality over time raises problems. In their seminal paper, Lee and Carter (1992) proposed a bilinear model for age-specific mortality that has been widely used and extended. For the death rate at age x in year t, in the following denoted by $m_x(t)$, they consider the model

$$\log(m_x(t)) = \alpha_x + \beta_x \kappa_t + \varepsilon_x(t).$$

The parameters α_x and β_x are age-specific while κ_t is time-varying. The error term with mean 0 and variance σ_ε^2 reflects particular age-specific historical influences. Following Brouhns et al. (2002) one can interpret the parameters in the following way:

α_x represents the basic effect of age; $\exp(\alpha_x)$ determines the general shape of the mortality pattern.

β_x represents the age-specific change of mortality. It indicates the sensitivity of mortality at age x to variations in the time effect κ_t.

κ_t represents the variation over time. The actual mortality is modulated by the age-specific response β_x.

For a fixed number of time points and ages the constraints $\sum_x \beta_x = 0$ and $\sum_t \kappa_t = 0$ are used to obtain identifiability. The model is typically fit to historical data and the resulting estimates are used to model and forecast future mortality as a stochastic time series.

Lee and Carter (1992) estimated the parameters by using least squares methods. However, special fitting procedures are necessary; one cannot use ordinary least squares methods here because there are no regressors, only the bilinear form that contains parameters. Various extensions and modifications have been proposed, for example, Brouhns et al. (2002) proposed a Poisson regression approach. Currie et al. (2004) obtain smooth mortality surfaces by penalized estimation methods using splines.

2.4 Literature and Further Reading

Life Table Estimators. Properties of estimates of cohort life tables are extensively discussed in Lawless (1982). Current life tables and concepts used in demography are found in Chiang (1984) and Preston et al. (2000). Smoothing procedures for life table estimates by localizing techniques were considered by Tutz and Pritscher (1996) and Patil and Bagkavos (2012).

Lee Carter Models. The basic approach is outlined in Lee and Carter (1992). Lee (2000) gives an overview on extensions and various applications. Smoothing procedures were proposed by Currie et al. (2004) and Delwarde et al. (2007).

2.5 Software

The life table estimators $\hat{\lambda}_t$ and $\hat{S}(t)$ are implemented in the R function *lifeTable*, which is part of the package *discSurv* (Welchowski and Schmid 2015) that accompanies this book. In addition to the point estimates of λ_t and $S(t)$, *lifeTable* also provides estimates of the standard deviations of $\hat{\lambda}_t$ and $\hat{S}(t)$. A smoothed version of the estimated hazard rate can be obtained by considering $\hat{\lambda}_t$ as outcome variable of an additive model with covariate vector $(1, 2, \ldots)$ and by applying the *gam* function in R package *mgcv* (Wood 2015). For example, the penalized regression spline estimate presented in Fig. 2.2 was obtained by specifying $s(x, bs = \text{"}ps\text{"})$ in the formula argument of *gam*. A weighted estimate of the hazard can be obtained by setting the *weights* argument of *gam* equal to the values of $n_t - w_t/2$. Kaplan–Meier estimates can be calculated by using the *survfit* function in the R add-on package *survival*.

2.6 Exercises

2.1 Consider the hazard function $\lambda_t = P(T = t \mid T \geq t)$ and the survival function $S(t) = P(T > t)$ for $t = 1, \ldots, q$. Show that the following links between these functions hold:

(a) $S(t) = P(T > t) = \prod_{s=1}^{t}(1 - \lambda_s)$,
(b) $P(T = t) = \lambda_t \prod_{s=1}^{t-1}(1 - \lambda_s) = \lambda_t\, S(t - 1)$.

2.2 Consider the multinomial distribution $(Y_1, \ldots, Y_k) \sim M(n, (\pi_1, \ldots, \pi_k))$, which has the mass function

$$P(Y_1 = y_1, \ldots, Y_q = y_q)$$
$$= \frac{n!}{y_1! \ldots y_q!(n - y_1 - \cdots - y_q)!}\, \pi_1^{y_1} \ldots \pi_q^{y_q}\, (1 - \pi_1 - \cdots - \pi_q)^{n - y_1 - \cdots - y_q}. \tag{2.6}$$

Let conditional probabilities be defined by

$$\lambda_i := P(Y = i \mid Y \geq i) = \pi_i/(1 - \pi_1 - \cdots - \pi_{i-1}), \quad i = 1, \ldots, q = k - 1.$$

(a) Show that

$$\pi_i = \lambda_i \prod_{j=1}^{i-1}(1 - \lambda_j).$$

(b) Show that the multinomial distribution can be represented as a product of binomial distributions

$$P(Y_1 = y_1, \ldots, Y_q = y_q)$$
$$= \prod_{i=1}^{q} \frac{(n - y_1 - \cdots - y_{i-1})!}{y_i!(n - y_1 - \cdots - y_i)!}\, \lambda_i^{y_i}(1 - \lambda_i)^{n - y_1 - \cdots - y_{i-1}}. \tag{2.7}$$

(c) Does this mean that the binomial distributions are independent?

2.3 Show that the discrete time hazard

$$\lambda_t = P(T = t \mid T \geq t) = P(T_c \in [a_{t-1}, a_t) \mid T_c > a_{t-1})$$

can be computed from the continuous time hazard by

$$\lambda_t = 1 - \exp\left(-\int_{a_{t-1}}^{a_t} \lambda_c(t)dt\right).$$

If the hazard function does not depend on time, that is, $\lambda_c(t) = \lambda_c$ for $t \in [0, \infty)$, one obtains

$$\lambda_t = 1 - \exp(-\lambda_c(a_{t-1} - a_t)).$$

Interpret this relation with reference to the exponential distribution.

2.4 We consider a data set of $n = 423$ couples that took part in a Danish study on fertility (Bonde et al. 1998). The outcome variable of interest is time to pregnancy (TTP), which is defined as the "duration that a couple waits from initiating attempts to conceive until conception occurs" (Scheike and Keiding 2006, http://publicifsv.sund.ku.dk/~ts/survival/sas/ttp.txt). It is measured by the number of menstrual cycles until conception and is therefore an intrinsically discrete time variable. The aim is to analyze the effects of various environmental and lifestyle factors on TTP (cf. Table 2.4). Among the inclusion criteria of the study were "no use of contraception to conceive," as well as "prior knowledge of fertility." The median number of observed menstrual cycles was four; 39 % of the observations were censored.

(a) Convert the data into life table format by considering the number of menstrual cycles as discrete time variable.
(b) Estimate the discrete hazard rate, its standard deviation, and a weighted smooth version of the discrete hazard rate.
(c) Plot the estimated hazard rates and their 95 % CIs.

2.5 Again consider the TTP data. The aim is now to analyze the effects of various covariates on TTP.

Table 2.4 Explanatory variables for the analysis of time to pregnancy (TTP)

Variable	Categories/unit	Sample proportion/median (range)
Intake of caffeine for the male	mg per day	378.55 (0.00–3661.42)
Intake of caffeine for the female	mg per day	250 (0–1,100)
Number of drinks for the male	Counts	7 (0–84)
Number of drinks for the female	Counts	2 (0–39)
Smoking status of the male	Yes	31 %
	No	69 %
Smoking status of the female	Yes	29 %
	No	71 %
Smoking status of the male's mother	Yes	36 %
	No	54 %
	Not available	10 %
Smoking status of the female's mother	Yes	38 %
	No	53 %
	Not available	9 %

(a) Split the data into cohorts of non-smoking and smoking females. Convert the data into life table format, in the same way as in Exercise 2.4.
(b) Estimate the survival function in both cohorts. In addition, compute the standard deviations of the survival function estimates and illustrate the results. Is there an effect of smoking on the time to pregnancy?
(c) Repeat the above analysis for couples where both partners smoke and compare the results to those obtained from couples where neither partner smokes.

2.6 Verify the formulas for m_x and q_x in Sect. 2.3.

Chapter 3
Basic Regression Models

Life tables as considered in the previous chapter yield estimates of discrete hazard rates and survival functions without relating them to covariates such as age, sex, etc. If covariates are available one can estimate separate life tables for specific combinations of covariate values. The so-obtained life tables allow to investigate the effect of covariates on survival. The method is, however, restricted to cases with not too many combinations of covariate values.

This chapter extends the life table methodology by introducing statistical models that directly link the hazard rate to an additive combination of multiple covariates. As explained in Chap. 1, many applications involve survival times that are measured on a discrete scale, for example, in days, months, or weeks. One can consider the measurement as a discretized version of the underlying continuous time, but discrete time often is the natural way how observations are collected. In the following let time take values in $\{1,\ldots,k\}$. If time results from intervals one has k underlying intervals $[a_0,a_1), [a_1,a_2), \ldots\ldots, [a_{q-1},a_q), [a_q,\infty)$, where $q=k-1$. Often for the first interval $a_0=0$ is assumed, and a_q denotes the final follow-up. Discrete time $T\in\{1,\ldots,k\}$ means that $T=t$ is observed if failure occurs within the interval $[a_{t-1},a_t)$. In the following we will consider the response T for given covariates $\boldsymbol{x}=(x_1,\ldots,x_p)^T$, which are assumed to have an impact on the survival time.

3.1 The Discrete Hazard Function

The stochastic behavior of the discrete random variable T given $\boldsymbol{x}$ can be described in the usual way by specifying the probability density function $P(T=t\,|\,\boldsymbol{x})$, $t=1,\ldots,k$, or the cumulative density function, which is equivalent to the distribution function $F(t|\boldsymbol{x})=P(T\le t\,|\,\boldsymbol{x})$. As already mentioned before in survival analysis often one uses an alternative representation that captures the dynamic aspect of time

G. Tutz, M. Schmid, *Modeling Discrete Time-to-Event Data*,
Springer Series in Statistics, DOI 10.1007/978-3-319-28158-2_3

as a response. The main tool is the *hazard function*, which for given vector of explanatory variables $\boldsymbol{x}$ has the form

$$\lambda(t|\boldsymbol{x}) = P(T = t \,|\, T \geq t, \boldsymbol{x}), \quad t = 1, \ldots, q. \tag{3.1}$$

It is the conditional probability for failure in interval $[a_{t-1}, a_t)$ given the interval is reached and describes the instantaneous rate of death at time t given that the individual survives until t.

The corresponding *discrete survival function* is given by

$$S(t|\boldsymbol{x}) = P(T > t \,|\, \boldsymbol{x}) = \prod_{i=1}^{t} (1 - \lambda(i|\boldsymbol{x})). \tag{3.2}$$

The survival function describes the probability that failure occurs later than at time t. In other words, if one considers the underlying intervals, it represents the probability of surviving interval $[a_{t-1}, a_t)$. The survival function is directly linked to the more conventional cumulative density function by $F(t|\boldsymbol{x}) = P(T \leq t|\boldsymbol{x}) = 1 - P(T > t|\boldsymbol{x}) = 1 - S(t|\boldsymbol{x})$.

Alternatively, one can also consider the probability of reaching period t or interval $[a_{t-1}, a_t)$, which is given by an alternative definition of the survival function:

$$\tilde{S}(t|\boldsymbol{x}) := P(T \geq t \,|\, \boldsymbol{x}) = \prod_{i=1}^{t-1} (1 - \lambda(i|\boldsymbol{x})). \tag{3.3}$$

The only difference to $S(t|\boldsymbol{x})$ is that now period t is included. The link between the alternative survival functions is given by $\tilde{S}(t|\boldsymbol{x}) = S(t-1|\boldsymbol{x})$.

The unconditional probability of failure at time t (i.e., of an event in interval $[a_{t-1}, a_t)$) is simply computed as

$$P(T = t \,|\, \boldsymbol{x}) = \lambda(t|\boldsymbol{x}) \prod_{s=1}^{t-1} (1 - \lambda(s|\boldsymbol{x})) = \lambda(t|\boldsymbol{x})\, \tilde{S}(t|\boldsymbol{x}). \tag{3.4}$$

This expression has a simple interpretation: The probability of failure at time t is composed of the conditional probabilities of surviving the first $t-1$ intervals, where each transition to the next category is given by $1 - \lambda(s|\boldsymbol{x})$, and the probability of failure at time t, given all previous intervals were survived. A summary of basic concepts is presented in Fig. 3.1.

Basic Concepts

Discrete hazard:

$$\lambda(t|\boldsymbol{x}) = P(T = t \,|\, T \geq t, \boldsymbol{x}), \quad t = 1, \dots, q$$

Unconditional probability of failure at time t:

$$P(T = t \,|\, \boldsymbol{x}) = \lambda(t|\boldsymbol{x}) \prod_{s=1}^{t-1} (1 - \lambda(s|\boldsymbol{x}))$$

Survival function:

$$S(t|\boldsymbol{x}) = P(T > t \,|\, \boldsymbol{x}) = \prod_{i=1}^{t} (1 - \lambda(i|\boldsymbol{x}))$$

Fig. 3.1 Summary of basic concepts for discrete-time survival analysis

3.2 Parametric Regression Models

A common way to specify a model for time-to-event data is to choose a parametrization of the hazard function. For fixed t the hazard function $\lambda(t|\boldsymbol{x}) = P(T = t \,|\, T \geq t, \boldsymbol{x})$ essentially models a binary response that distinguishes between the event taking place in category t or not (always given $T \geq t$). In other words, it distinguishes between category $\{t\}$ and categories $\{t+1, \dots, k\}$ given $T \geq t$. Nowadays a wide range of models is available for binary data, in particular in the generalized linear modeling framework (see, for example, McCullagh and Nelder 1989, Tutz 2012, or Agresti 2013). For binary response $Y \in \{0, 1\}$ with given covariates $\boldsymbol{x}$ an important class of models has the form

$$P(Y = 1|\boldsymbol{x}) = h(\gamma_0 + \boldsymbol{x}^T \boldsymbol{\gamma}), \tag{3.5}$$

where $h(\cdot)$ is a fixed *response function*, which is assumed to be strictly monotonically increasing. It links the response probability and the linear predictor $\gamma_0 + \boldsymbol{x}^T \boldsymbol{\gamma}$, which contains the effects of covariates. Since probabilities are restricted to the interval $[0, 1]$ natural candidates for the response function $h(\cdot)$ are distribution functions. By using the binary model for the decision between $\{t\}$ and categories $\{t+1, \dots, k\}$ given $T \geq t$ one obtains the discrete hazard model

$$\lambda(t|\boldsymbol{x}) = h(\gamma_{0t} + \boldsymbol{x}^T \boldsymbol{\gamma}). \tag{3.6}$$

The main extension (compared to (3.5)) is that the intercept γ_{0t} now depends on time. Since the response function $h(\cdot)$ is strictly monotonically increasing, one can construct the inverse function $g = h^{-1}$, and the model has the form

$$g(\lambda(t|\boldsymbol{x})) = \gamma_{0t} + \boldsymbol{x}^T\boldsymbol{\gamma}. \tag{3.7}$$

In generalized linear model (GLM) terminology $g(\cdot)$ is called the *link function*. The two models, (3.6) and (3.7), are equivalent, but reveal different aspects of the model.

In the following sections we will first consider simple models of the form (3.6). We will introduce several popular versions and discuss properties of the model and the interpretation of parameters, which depend on the chosen response function.

3.2.1 Logistic Discrete Hazards: The Proportional Continuation Ratio Model

The most widely used binary regression model is the logit model, which uses the logistic distribution function $h(\eta) = \exp(\eta)/(1 + \exp(\eta))$. The corresponding *logistic discrete hazard model* has the form

$$\lambda(t|\boldsymbol{x}) = \frac{\exp(\gamma_{0t} + \boldsymbol{x}^T\boldsymbol{\gamma})}{1 + \exp(\gamma_{0t} + \boldsymbol{x}^T\boldsymbol{\gamma})},$$

which models the occurrence of the event at time t (given it is reached) as a logistic model. An alternative version is

$$\log\left(\frac{\lambda(t|\boldsymbol{x})}{1 - \lambda(t|\boldsymbol{x})}\right) = \gamma_{0t} + \boldsymbol{x}^T\boldsymbol{\gamma}. \tag{3.8}$$

It is easily derived that the model can also be written as

$$\log\left(\frac{P(T = t\,|\,\boldsymbol{x})}{P(T > t\,|\,\boldsymbol{x})}\right) = \gamma_{0t} + \boldsymbol{x}^T\boldsymbol{\gamma}. \tag{3.9}$$

The ratio $P(Y = t\,|\,\boldsymbol{x})/P(Y > t\,|\,\boldsymbol{x})$ is known as *continuation ratio*, to which the model owes its name *continuation ratio model* (Agresti 2013). It compares the probability of an event at t to the probability of an event later than t. It also represents conditional odds because it is equivalent to $P(T = t\,|\,T \geq t, \boldsymbol{x})/(1 - P(T = t\,|\,T \geq t, \boldsymbol{x}))$, which compares the conditional probability of an event at time t to the conditional probability of an event later than t, both under the condition $T \geq t$. This representation is particularly useful for the interpretation of parameters.

In model (3.8) it is assumed that the intercepts γ_{0t} vary over time whereas the parameter $\boldsymbol{\gamma}$ is fixed. This separation of time variation and covariate effects makes interpretation of parameters easy. The intercepts, which vary over time, can be interpreted as a *baseline hazard*, that is, the hazard that is always present for any given set of covariates. Specifically, γ_{0t} is the log continuation ratio for the covariate vector $\boldsymbol{x}^T = (0, \ldots, 0)$. Alternatively one can consider the exponential form of model (3.8), which is given by

$$\psi(t|\boldsymbol{x}) := \frac{P(T = t\,|\,\boldsymbol{x})}{P(T > t\,|\,\boldsymbol{x})} = e^{\gamma_{0t}}(e^{\gamma_1})^{x_1} \ldots (e^{\gamma_p})^{x_p},$$

where $\psi(t|\boldsymbol{x})$ denotes the continuation ratio at value t. It follows that the exponential of the intercept is given by

$$\exp(\gamma_{0t}) = \psi(t|\boldsymbol{0}) = \frac{P(T = t\,|\,\boldsymbol{0})}{P(T > t\,|\,\boldsymbol{0})}$$

and can be directly interpreted as the continuation ratio for covariate values $\boldsymbol{x}^T = \boldsymbol{0}^T = (0, \ldots, 0)$. The presence of the baseline hazard for all values of covariates can be illustrated by considering the ratio of continuation ratios at two time periods, t and s. From

$$\frac{\psi(t|\boldsymbol{x})}{\psi(s|\boldsymbol{x})} = \exp(\gamma_{0t} - \gamma_{0s}) \tag{3.10}$$

it is seen that the ratio of the continuation ratios of two periods does not depend on the value of the covariate vector. Therefore the basic shape of the continuation ratios is the same for all values of the predictor.

The interpretation of the coefficients $\boldsymbol{\gamma}$ is easily obtained from (3.9) and (3.10). The parameter γ_j represents the change in the log continuation ratios (or the conditional log odds ratios) if x_j increases by one unit. Correspondingly,

$$\exp(\gamma_j) = \frac{\psi(t\,|\,x_1, \ldots, x_j + 1, \ldots, x_p)}{\psi(t\,|\,x_1, \ldots, x_j, \ldots, x_p)}$$

is the factor by which the continuation ratio changes if x_j is increased by one unit. It is important to note that the change does not depend on time. It is the same for all periods, allowing for a simple interpretation of effects: If a predictor increases the continuation ratio, the increase is the same for all periods, and, of course, the same relationship holds for a decrease. An alternative view on this strong property of the model is obtained by considering two populations characterized by the values of the predictor $\boldsymbol{x}$ and $\tilde{\boldsymbol{x}}$. One sees from

$$\frac{\psi(t|\boldsymbol{x})}{\psi(t|\tilde{\boldsymbol{x}})} = \exp((\boldsymbol{x} - \tilde{\boldsymbol{x}})^T\boldsymbol{\gamma}) \tag{3.11}$$

that the comparison of these subpopulations in terms of the continuation ratio does not depend on time. If one compares, for example, two therapies, represented by $x = 1$ and $x = 0$, one obtains $\psi(t \mid x = 1)/\psi(t \mid x = 0) = \exp(\gamma)$. If the modeled event is death and γ is positive, this means that the therapy coded as $x = 0$ is to be preferred over the therapy coded as $x = 1$ because the continuation ratio of the latter therapy is higher at all time points. Property (3.11) implies in particular that a therapy cannot have superior short-time effects while being inferior in terms of chances of survival after a certain time point. In this case it would be hard to choose among therapies since the one that supports short-time survival could be inferior in terms of long time survival. Property (3.11), which excludes such effects, makes the model a *proportional continuation ratio model*.

One consequence of the property is that survival functions do not cross. If one compares two therapies represented by $x = 1$ and $x = 0$ with γ positive, one has $\lambda(t|x = 1) > \lambda(t|x = 0)$ for all t. Since the survival function is given by $S(t|\boldsymbol{x}) = \prod_{i=1}^{t}(1 - \lambda(i|\boldsymbol{x}))$ one obtains

$$S(t|x = 1) < S(t|x = 0)$$

for all t, which means the probability of survival for therapy $x = 1$ is smaller than for therapy $x = 0$ for all time points. Consequently, the survival functions do never cross.

Example 3.1 Copenhagen Stroke Study
For illustration we investigate survival in the Copenhagen Stroke Study with just one predictor in the model. Figure 3.2 presents the resulting estimates of the continuation ratio model for patients with diabetes and without diabetes. The upper panel of Fig. 3.2 shows the estimated hazard functions for the two populations whereas the lower panel shows the corresponding survival functions. Observed survival times (originally measured in days) were grouped into 12-month intervals. The coefficient γ for the diabetes group (represented by $x = 1$) was estimated as $\hat{\gamma} = 0.401$. From Eq. (3.11) it follows that the continuation ratio of the diabetes group increases by the factor $\exp(0.401) \approx 1.49$ for all time points (if compared to the non-diabetes group represented by $x = 0$). This implies that the risk of dying after hospital admission measured by the continuation ratio is approximately 1.5 times larger in the diabetes group than in the non-diabetes group. Details on how to estimate the parameters of the continuation ratio model will be presented in Sect. 3.4.

In addition to the continuation ratio estimates, the Kaplan–Meier estimates for the two groups are included in the lower panel of Fig. 3.2. It is seen that the continuation ratio model for discrete-time survival data yields a good approximation of the Kaplan–Meier estimates. Specifically, the model estimates are close to the life table estimates presented in Fig. 2.5, which were calculated *separately* for each of the two groups. □

Modeling of Hazards

Before considering alternative models let us make some remarks on the basic approach. Especially in discrete survival analysis the parameterization of the hazard function is the most widespread method: One models the effect of a set of covariates on the hazard. Subsequently one can consider the effect of the covariates on

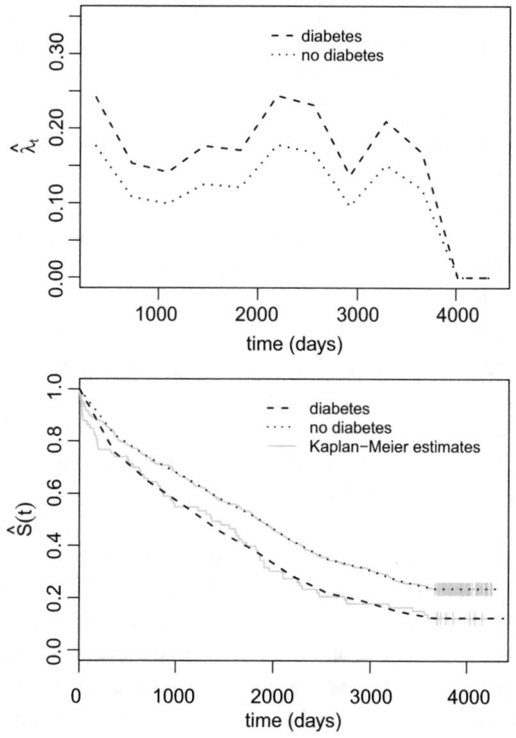

Fig. 3.2 Hazard rates (*upper panel*) and survival functions (*lower panel*) for the Copenhagen Stroke Study. Estimates were obtained by fitting a continuation ratio model with binary covariate diabetes/no diabetes

the distribution of the survival time or, equivalently, on the survival function. This approach differs from the common regression model, where one typically investigates the effect of covariates on the mean of the dependent variable. The advantages of modeling the hazard function have already been mentioned; in particular this approach allows to include time-varying covariates. Also, in modeling the transition process from one state to another it focusses on a feature that is of high interest in duration analysis.

Nevertheless, some care is needed when interpreting the form of the hazard function. If no covariates are involved (as in life tables) one observes the transition to other states in the population. In parametric regression models one conditions on the covariates, and the transition rate captured in the hazard function is conditional on covariates. This means that one observes transition rates in populations that are defined by the covariates. In particular when covariates are categorical, for example, defining gender, the underlying populations are clearly defined. But since usually not all relevant covariates are available, there might be considerable heterogeneity in the population that is not accounted for. Therefore one should not necessarily assume that each subject in a subpopulation defined by covariates has the same hazard function. For example, different individual hazard functions can yield the same population level hazard function. Also, constant hazards on the individual level will produce decreasing hazard functions on the population level, a phenomenon that is considered in Chap. 9. In *frailty models*, which are discussed in Chap. 9, one tries to explicitly account for the heterogeneity within the populations and to investigate the effects on the individual level. Since inference on the true hazard function on the individual level is hard to obtain, there is a tendency in biostatistics to focus on the effects of covariates on the survival function but not to (over)interpret the functional form of the hazard function. Nevertheless, in some areas the focus is on the individual hazards. When modeling the duration of unemployment, for example, it makes a difference whether a decreasing hazard observed in the population is caused by decreasing individual hazards, signaling declining chances in the labor market, or time-constant but population-varying individual hazards that yield decreasing hazard function in the populations because individuals with small hazards will stay unemployed for a longer time. In the latter case the individual hazards do not decrease but the population hazard does. In this spirit Van den Berg (2001) states that "the hazard function of the duration distribution is the focal point and basic building block of econometric duration models. Properties of the duration distribution are generally discussed in terms of properties of the hazard function. The individual hazard function and the way it depends on its determinants are the parameters of interest."

3.2.2 Alternative Models

In the logistic discrete hazard model the transition to the next category is modeled by a logistic distribution function. Alternative functions are in common use for binary models and yield alternative models. A special distribution function is the *minimum extreme value* or *Gompertz* distribution $h(\eta) = 1 - \exp(-\exp(\eta))$, which yields the model

$$\lambda(t|\boldsymbol{x}) = 1 - \exp(-\exp(\gamma_{0t} + \boldsymbol{x}^T\boldsymbol{\gamma}))$$

or equivalently

$$\log(-\log(P(T > t\,|\,T \geq t))) = \gamma_{0t} + \boldsymbol{x}^T\boldsymbol{\gamma}.$$

It is called the *grouped proportional hazards model* because it can be seen as a discretized version of Cox's proportional hazard model, which is the most widely used model for continuous time (see Sect. 3.3.2). In contrast to the logistic model, the response function $h(\eta) = 1 - \exp(-\exp(\eta))$ is not symmetric. Because of the form of the link function it is also often referred to as the *complementary log-log* ("clog-log") model.

Interestingly the model can also be written in the form

$$P(T \leq t\,|\,\boldsymbol{x}) = 1 - \exp(-\exp(\tilde{\gamma}_{0t} + \boldsymbol{x}^T\boldsymbol{\gamma})), \tag{3.12}$$

where $\tilde{\gamma}_{0t} = \log(\sum_{i=1}^{t} \exp(\gamma_{0i}))$ are transformations of the baseline parameters. Note that the $\tilde{\gamma}_{0t}$ are ordered, i.e., $\tilde{\gamma}_{0t} \leq \cdots \leq \tilde{\gamma}_{0k}$. The formulation in (3.12) links the model to the class of cumulative models, which are frequently used in the modeling of ordered response variables; cumulative models are extensively considered in Tutz (2012) and Agresti (2013).

A model that is closely linked to the grouped proportional hazards model uses the transformation function $h(\eta) = \exp(-\exp(-\eta))$. It is complementary to the Gompertz distribution, because if a random variable X follows a Gompertz distribution, the random variable $-X$ follows a Gumbel distribution, and vice versa. In general, if X has distribution function $F(\cdot)$, the random variable $-X$ has distribution function $F(x) = 1 - F(-x)$, which is exactly the transformation used to transform the Gompertz distribution into the Gumbel distribution.

An overview over the various models is given in the box on page 43 (Fig. 3.3). Note that the box also includes the exponential model, which has the disadvantage

Discrete Hazard Models

Logistic Model (logit link)

$$\lambda(t|\boldsymbol{x}) = \frac{\exp(\gamma_{0t}+\boldsymbol{x}^T\boldsymbol{\gamma})}{1+\exp(\gamma_{0t}+\boldsymbol{x}^T\boldsymbol{\gamma})},\ \log\left(\frac{P(T=t|\boldsymbol{x})}{P(T>t|\boldsymbol{x})}\right) = \gamma_{0t} + \boldsymbol{x}^T\boldsymbol{\gamma}$$

Probit Model (probit link)

$$\lambda(t|\boldsymbol{x}) = \Phi(\gamma_{0t} + \boldsymbol{x}^T\boldsymbol{\gamma}),\ \Phi^{-1}(\lambda(t|\boldsymbol{x})) = \gamma_{0t} + \boldsymbol{x}^T\boldsymbol{\gamma}$$

Gompertz or Grouped Proportional Hazards Model (clog-log link)

$$\lambda(t|\boldsymbol{x}) = 1 - \exp(-\exp(\gamma_{0t} + \boldsymbol{x}^T\boldsymbol{\gamma})),\ \log(-\log(P(T > t|T \geq t, \boldsymbol{x})) = \gamma_{0t} + \boldsymbol{x}^T\boldsymbol{\gamma}$$

Gumbel model (log-log link)

$$\lambda(t|\boldsymbol{x}) = \exp(-\exp(-(\gamma_{0t} + \boldsymbol{x}^T\boldsymbol{\gamma}))),\ -\log(-\log(\lambda(t|\boldsymbol{x}))) = \gamma_{0t} + \boldsymbol{x}^T\boldsymbol{\gamma}$$

Exponential Model (log link)

$$\lambda(t|\boldsymbol{x}) = \exp(\gamma_{0t} + \boldsymbol{x}^T\boldsymbol{\gamma}),\ \log(\lambda(t|\boldsymbol{x})) = \gamma_{0t} + \boldsymbol{x}^T\boldsymbol{\gamma}$$

Fig. 3.3 Overview of discrete hazard models

that the parameter space needs to be restricted because the hazard rate is restricted (i.e., $\lambda(t|\boldsymbol{x}) \in [0, 1]$). For an application of the exponential model see Weinberg and Gladen (1986). The box also includes the probit model, which uses the cumulative standard normal distribution $\Phi(\cdot)$, which apart from scaling is very similar to the logistic distribution function. In particular in economic applications the probit model is preferred over the logistic model when binary responses are modeled.

The use of common binary regression models for the modeling of the transition to period $t+1$ (given period t was reached) has the big advantage that software for binary models can be used to fit the corresponding discrete hazard models. However, alternative names are often used for the models. As already mentioned, the binary model behind the grouped proportional hazards model is often called "complementary log-log model" because of the used link function; the model behind the Gumbel model is known as "log-log model."

All models use a cumulative distribution function as response function $h(\cdot)$, for example, the logistic or the Gompertz distribution. The use of distribution functions has the nice side effect that the estimated hazard rates are between zero and one. However, if one wants to compare estimated coefficients for alternative models one should keep in mind that the distribution functions correspond to underlying random variables with different variances. For example, the logistic distribution function $h(\eta) = \exp(\eta)/(1 + \exp(\eta))$ corresponds to a random variable with variance $\pi^2/3$, whereas the Gompertz distribution refers to a random variable with variance $\pi^2/6$ (with $\pi = 3.14159\ldots$). Therefore comparisons of estimates obtained from different link functions should be based on standardized coefficients. Standardization to response functions that refer to random variables with variance 1 is obtained by computing γ_i/σ_h, where σ_h^2 denotes the variance of the distribution function $h(\cdot)$ (see, for example, Tutz 2012, Sect. 5.1). In Example 3.2 various models with different link functions are fitted and compared.

Example 3.2 Copenhagen Stroke Study

We consider survival in the Copenhagen Stroke Study to illustrate the fitting of various discrete hazard models. We start with one predictor and then include all of the available predictors. Figure 3.4 presents the estimated survival functions of patients that suffered a previous stroke and of patients without previous stroke. Five different survival models (logistic, probit, Gompertz, Gumbel, and exponential) were fitted with observations grouped into 12-month intervals. It is seen from Fig. 3.4 that the estimated survival functions obtained for the five models are very similar. The model-free Kaplan Meier estimates, which are also shown, indicate that the structure of the patient group without previous stroke is captured relatively well by the models, whereas survival in the previous-stroke group is overestimated in the interval [1000, 2100] days (corresponding to an interval of approximately 3–6 years after admission to hospital). It is seen that the risk of dying is considerably larger in the previous-stroke group than in the group of patients with a first-time stroke.

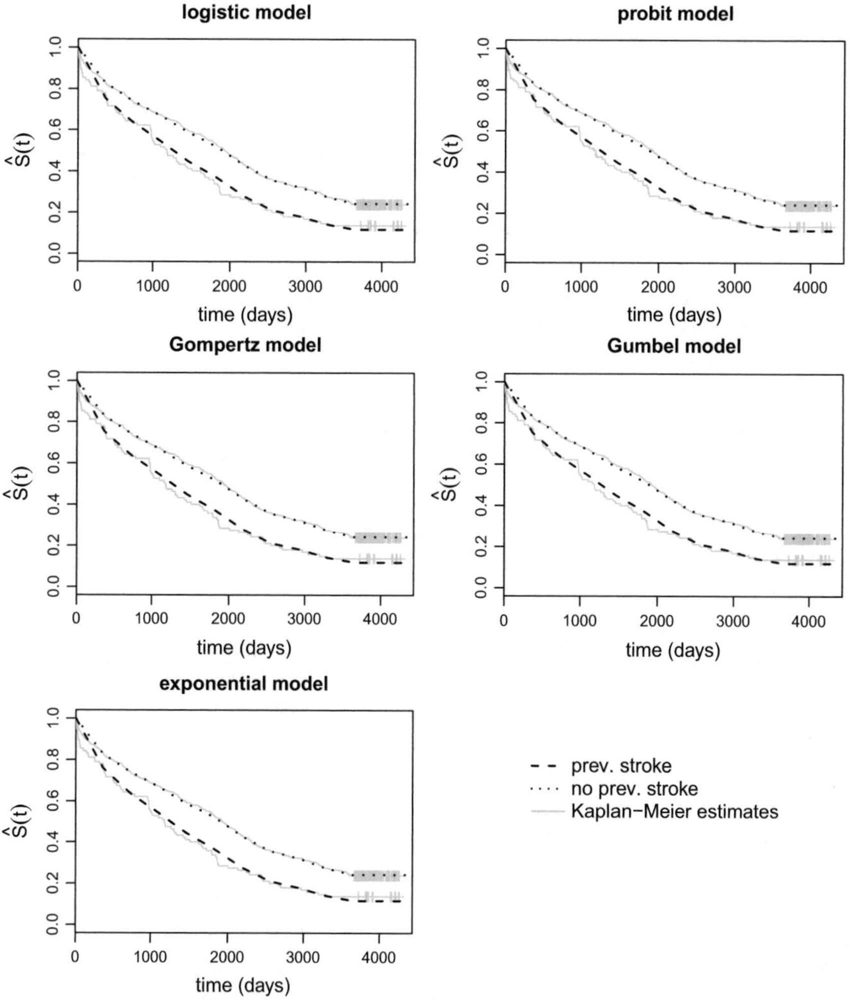

Fig. 3.4 Copenhagen Stroke Study. The figures show the estimated survival functions of patients that suffered a previous stroke and of patients without previous stroke. Different link functions were used to fit discrete hazard models

Table 3.1 shows the coefficient estimates that were obtained from the Copenhagen Stroke Study when all covariates were included in the hazard models. Positive coefficient estimates imply that the corresponding covariates have a positive effect on hazards (and hence a negative effect on survival). For example, patients with diabetes and a previous stroke have a higher estimated risk of dying than patients without diabetes or previous stroke. As expected, because of the negative coefficient signs, patients with a large Scandinavian stroke score tend to have a decreased risk of dying early. In addition to the coefficient estimates, Table 3.1 shows the estimated standard deviations and the p-values obtained from statistical hypotheses tests. Generally, p-values are a measure of the statistical significance of a covariate; they indicate whether the effect of a covariate on survival is systematically different from zero or not. In Table 3.1, for example, p-values for

Table 3.1 Copenhagen Stroke Study. The table presents the parameter estimates that were obtained from fitting discrete hazard models with different link functions (coef = parameter estimate, se = estimated standard deviation, $p = p$-value obtained from t-test)

	Logistic			Probit			Gompertz		
	Coef	se	p	Coef	se	p	Coef	se	p
Age	0.058	0.007	0.000	0.031	0.004	0.000	0.053	0.006	0.000
Sex (male)	0.458	0.128	0.000	0.255	0.070	0.000	0.412	0.115	0.000
Hypertension (yes)	0.233	0.123	0.058	0.132	0.068	0.050	0.206	0.110	0.061
Ischemic heart disease (yes)	0.128	0.143	0.372	0.079	0.079	0.316	0.094	0.128	0.461
Previous stroke (yes)	0.213	0.148	0.150	0.125	0.083	0.130	0.179	0.131	0.172
Other disabling disease (yes)	0.148	0.153	0.333	0.086	0.086	0.318	0.119	0.136	0.379
Alcohol intake (yes)	−0.107	0.133	0.420	−0.058	0.072	0.423	−0.090	0.121	0.458
Diabetes (yes)	0.325	0.165	0.049	0.188	0.092	0.040	0.280	0.146	0.055
Smoking status (yes)	0.345	0.127	0.006	0.204	0.069	0.003	0.301	0.114	0.008
Atrial fibrillation (yes)	0.407	0.172	0.018	0.233	0.099	0.019	0.367	0.148	0.013
Hemorrhage (yes)	0.009	0.274	0.973	0.025	0.150	0.868	−0.018	0.246	0.941
Scandinavian stroke score	−0.025	0.004	0.000	−0.014	0.003	0.000	−0.022	0.004	0.000
Cholesterol	0.010	0.045	0.821	0.004	0.025	0.882	0.009	0.041	0.833

	Gumbel			Exponential		
	Coef	se	p	Coef	se	p
Age	0.025	0.003	0.000	0.048	0.006	0.000
Sex (male)	0.215	0.057	0.000	0.372	0.101	0.000
Hypertension (yes)	0.114	0.056	0.041	0.184	0.097	0.057
Ischemic heart disease (yes)	0.077	0.066	0.242	0.067	0.112	0.549
Previous stroke (yes)	0.113	0.070	0.107	0.148	0.113	0.189
Other disabling disease (yes)	0.077	0.073	0.291	0.088	0.117	0.451
Alcohol intake (yes)	−0.047	0.059	0.423	−0.069	0.107	0.520
Diabetes (yes)	0.169	0.078	0.030	0.234	0.125	0.061
Smoking status (yes)	0.184	0.057	0.001	0.262	0.101	0.009
Atrial fibrillation (yes)	0.201	0.088	0.022	0.336	0.122	0.006
Hemorrhage (yes)	0.045	0.125	0.715	−0.042	0.219	0.846
Scandinavian stroke score	−0.012	0.002	0.000	−0.019	0.003	0.000
Cholesterol	0.001	0.020	0.954	0.007	0.036	0.851

the covariates age, sex, smoking status, atrial fibrillation, and Scandinavian stroke score were smaller than 0.05 in all five models. This result indicates that the corresponding covariates had a significant effect on survival (at significance level 0.05). When comparing the different models, most of the p-values were similar in size. Nevertheless, there were also differences. For example, in the logistic, probit, and Gumbel models diabetes had a significant negative effect on survival (if one considers the often-used significance level 0.05) while p-values were slightly larger than 0.05 in the Gompertz and exponential models. Also, the p-values of hypertension on survival showed some variation around 0.05. In some cases even the signs of the coefficient estimates changed. For example, estimates seem to indicate for hemorrhage patients an increased risk of dying in the logistic, probit, and Gumbel models and a decreased risk in the Gompertz and exponential models. But standard deviations and p-values are so large that the effects could have also been due to chance. Details on statistical hypotheses tests will be presented in Chap. 4.

Table 3.2 presents the *standardized* coefficient estimates of the four models, which were calculated by dividing the coefficient estimates by the standard deviations of the respective response function. More specifically, the standard deviations are given by $\pi/\sqrt{3}$ for the logistic model, $\pi/\sqrt{6}$ for the Gompertz and Gumbel models, and 1 for the probit and exponential models. As mentioned earlier, the standardized estimates are measured on the same scale and are more suitable for the comparison of coefficients than the raw estimates. Similar to the results presented in Fig. 3.4, the estimates obtained from the five modeling approaches (logistic, probit, Gompertz, Gumbel, and exponential) are similar with respect to the standardized coefficient estimates. Note that, in addition to comparing standardized coefficient estimates, it is also necessary to evaluate which of the five modeling approaches fitted the data best. Strategies for model comparison are presented in Chap. 4. □

Table 3.2 Copenhagen Stroke Study. The table presents the standardized coefficient estimates that were obtained from fitting discrete hazard models with different link functions

	Logistic	Probit	Gompertz	Gumbel	Exponential
Age	0.032	0.031	0.041	0.020	0.048
Sex (male)	0.253	0.255	0.321	0.167	0.372
Hypertension (yes)	0.128	0.132	0.161	0.089	0.184
Ischemic heart disease (yes)	0.070	0.079	0.074	0.060	0.067
Previous stroke (yes)	0.117	0.125	0.139	0.088	0.148
Other disabling disease (yes)	0.082	0.086	0.093	0.060	0.088
Alcohol intake (yes)	−0.059	−0.058	−0.070	−0.037	−0.069
Diabetes (yes)	0.179	0.188	0.218	0.132	0.234
Smoking status (yes)	0.190	0.204	0.234	0.144	0.262
Atrial fibrillation (yes)	0.224	0.232	0.286	0.156	0.336
Hemorrhage (yes)	0.005	0.025	−0.014	0.035	−0.042
Scandinavian stroke score	−0.014	−0.014	−0.017	−0.010	−0.019
Cholesterol	0.006	0.004	0.007	0.001	0.007

Concerning the choice among the models, two aspects are of major importance: The first one is goodness-of-fit (i.e., how well the model fits the underlying data), and the second one is ease of interpretation (i.e., how easily the model parameters can be interpreted). The difference between models can be small if the grouping intervals are very short. For example, Thompson (1977) showed that estimates are typically very similar for the grouped proportional hazards model and the logistic model in this case. Although differences between the standard links considered here can be small, in some applications quite different link functions can be more appropriate. In Chap. 4 more general families of response functions are considered. Some of the families contain the logistic and the clog-log model as special cases. By fitting a whole family one tries to find the most appropriate link function, which can be the logistic link function but can also be far away from it. Example 4.7 demonstrates that in some applications the underlying random variable can be strongly skewed. Even more flexible models are obtained by allowing for nonparametrically estimated response functions. These more general approaches focussing on the choice of the link are deferred to Chap. 4.

Proportionality

It should be noted that all models considered in this chapter postulate some proportionality property that is important w.r.t. the interpretation of parameters. Because $h(\cdot)$ is a monotonic function in the model equation $\lambda(t|\boldsymbol{x}) = h(\gamma_{0t} + \boldsymbol{x}^T\boldsymbol{\gamma})$, one can always compare two populations characterized by the values of the predictors $\boldsymbol{x}$ and $\tilde{\boldsymbol{x}}$ by

$$h^{-1}(\lambda(t|\boldsymbol{x})) - h^{-1}(\lambda(t|\tilde{\boldsymbol{x}})) = (\boldsymbol{x} - \tilde{\boldsymbol{x}})^T\boldsymbol{\gamma}, \tag{3.13}$$

which does not depend on t. Therefore, if a population has a larger hazard rate than the other, this ordering is the same over time. Which specific property holds for which model can be derived from computing the left-hand side of (3.13). As shown before, for the logistic model one obtains the log continuation ratios, which are postulated to not depend on time. For the grouped proportional hazards model it can be shown that the ratio of the logarithms of the survival functions is given by

$$\frac{\log(S(t|\boldsymbol{x}))}{\log(S(t|\tilde{\boldsymbol{x}}))} = \exp((\boldsymbol{x} - \tilde{\boldsymbol{x}})^T\boldsymbol{\gamma})$$

and therefore depends on $\boldsymbol{x}$ and $\tilde{\boldsymbol{x}}$ but not on time. It means that the logarithms of the discrete survival functions for two populations are proportional over time. For the Gumbel model the corresponding quantity is the logarithm of $\log(\lambda(t|\boldsymbol{x}))/\log(\lambda(t|\tilde{\boldsymbol{x}}))$, which seems less easy to interpret.

3.3 Discrete and Continuous Hazards

Models for continuous survival time use the same concepts as discrete survival models. But the definition of the hazard function and the link between the hazard function and the survival function is different. In the following we will shortly sketch the concepts for continuous time and the link between continuous time survival and discrete time survival. In particular the discretized version of the widely used Cox model is considered.

3.3.1 Concepts for Continuous Time

Let T_c denote a continuous survival time, which has density function $f(\cdot)$. The survival function, which represents the probability of survival until time t, is now given without ambiguity by

$$S_c(t) = P(T_c > t) = 1 - F_c(t),$$

where $F_c(t) = P(T_c \le t) = \int_0^t f(u)du$ denotes the distribution function of T_c. The hazard function for continuous time is defined as a limit by

$$\lambda_c(t) = \lim_{\Delta t \to 0} \frac{P(t \le T_c < t + \Delta t \,|\, T_c \ge t)}{\Delta t}. \tag{3.14}$$

In contrast to the discrete-time hazard function defined in (3.1), it is not a conditional probability and can take any positive value. An additional concept that is useful in continuous survival analysis is the cumulative hazard function

$$\Lambda_c(t) = \int_0^t \lambda_c(u)du. \tag{3.15}$$

Generally, the stochastic properties of a survival time are fixed if one of the following quantities is specified: distribution function, density, hazard function, or cumulative hazard function. It is straightforward to derive the connection between these quantities:

$$\lambda_c(t) = \frac{f(t)}{S_c(t)},$$

$$S_c(t) = \exp\left(-\int_0^t \lambda_c(u)du\right) = \exp(-\Lambda_c(t)),$$

$$f(t) = \lambda_c(t)\exp\left(-\int_0^t \lambda_c(u)du\right) = \lambda_c(t)\exp(-\Lambda_c(t))$$

(see, for example, Lawless 1982). The simplest model for continuous time assumes that the hazard is constant over time, $\lambda_c(t) = \lambda_c$ for $t \in [0, \infty)$. In this case the survival function is the exponential function $S_c(t) = \exp(-\lambda_c t)$. The corresponding cumulative distribution function is $F_c(t) = 1 - \exp(-\lambda_c t)$ and the density is $f(t) = \lambda_c \exp(-\lambda_c t)$. The distribution function and the density are familiar from introductory courses to statistics as describing a random variable that is exponentially distributed with parameter λ_c. Therefore the assumption of an exponential distribution is equivalent to postulating that the underlying hazard function is constant over time. The exponential distribution is also known as a distribution without memory, having the property $P(T_c > t + \Delta \,|\, T_c > t) = P(T_c > \Delta)$. This means the probability of a duration time longer than $t + \Delta$ given $T_c > t$ is the same as the probability of a duration time longer than Δ right from the beginning. In other words, when starting at $T_c > t$ the conditional distribution is the same as when starting at zero. This is another way of expressing that the hazard does not depend on time. More flexible models such as, for example, the Weibull distribution, are considered extensively in the literature on continuous time survival (Lawless 1982; Klein and Moeschberger 2003). A very flexible regression model that comprises all these models is the Cox model considered in the next section.

3.3.2 The Proportional Hazards Model

The most widely used model in continuous survival modeling is *Cox's proportional hazard model* (Cox 1972), which specifies

$$\lambda_c(t|\boldsymbol{x}) = \lambda_0(t)\exp(\boldsymbol{x}^T\boldsymbol{\gamma}). \tag{3.16}$$

The model is composed of two parts, namely the unknown baseline hazard $\lambda_0(t)$ and the effects of the covariates on λ_c given by $\exp(\boldsymbol{x}^T\boldsymbol{\gamma})$. Thus the variation of the hazard over time is separated from the effects of the covariates. The important consequence is that effects are constant over time. This becomes clear when considering two populations defined by the values of the predictor $\boldsymbol{x}$ and $\tilde{\boldsymbol{x}}$: One obtains that the ratio of the continuous hazards

$$\frac{\lambda_c(t|\boldsymbol{x})}{\lambda_c(t|\tilde{\boldsymbol{x}})} = \exp((\boldsymbol{x}-\tilde{\boldsymbol{x}})^T\boldsymbol{\gamma}) \tag{3.17}$$

does not depend on time. This property makes the model a *proportional hazards model*. The model is usually referred to as "Cox model" or simply as "proportional hazards model." The fact that hazards are proportional helps in the interpretation of the parameters. For example, in a treatment study where the hazard refers to survival, let $\boldsymbol{x} = 1$ indicate treatment 1 and $\tilde{\boldsymbol{x}} = 0$ indicate treatment 2. Then for positive γ the hazard for treatment 1 is $\exp(\gamma)$ times the hazard for treatment 2 at all times, which makes treatment 2 the better choice. It is crucial that the ratio of the hazards does not depend on time because then one of the treatments is to be preferred regardless of the survival time.

A different view on the proportional hazards property is obtained by considering the corresponding survival functions. It is easily derived that the survival function $S_c(t|\boldsymbol{x}) = P(T_c > t\,|\,\boldsymbol{x})$ of the Cox model has the form

$$S_c(t|\boldsymbol{x}) = \exp\left(-\int_0^t \lambda_0(u)du\right)^{\exp(\boldsymbol{x}^T\boldsymbol{\gamma})} = S_0(t)^{\exp(\boldsymbol{x}^T\boldsymbol{\gamma})}, \tag{3.18}$$

where $S_0(t) = \exp(-\int_0^t \lambda_0(u)du)$ is the baseline survival function. Therefore, the survival function given $\boldsymbol{x}$ is given as the baseline survival function to the power of $\exp(\boldsymbol{x}^T\boldsymbol{\gamma})$. The proportional hazards assumption has the consequence that the survival functions for distinct values of explanatory variables $\boldsymbol{x}$ and $\tilde{\boldsymbol{x}}$ do never cross. Thus, $S_c(t|\boldsymbol{x}) > S_c(t|\tilde{\boldsymbol{x}})$ (or $S_c(t|\boldsymbol{x}) < S_c(t|\tilde{\boldsymbol{x}})$) holds for all values of t, indicating that one of the values, $\boldsymbol{x}$ or $\tilde{\boldsymbol{x}}$, yields higher chances of survival at all times.

The Discretized Proportional Hazards Model

Let now time be coarsened by use of the intervals $[0, a_1), [a_1, a_2), \ldots\ldots, [a_{q-1}, a_q)$, $[a_q, \infty)$, and assume that the proportional hazards model holds. If discrete time is observed, that is, if one observes $T = t$ if failure occurs within the interval $[a_{t-1}, a_t)$, the *discrete* hazard $\lambda(t|\boldsymbol{x}) = P(T = t \mid T \geq t, \boldsymbol{x})$ takes the form

$$\lambda(t|\boldsymbol{x}) = 1 - \exp(-\exp(\gamma_{0t} + \boldsymbol{x}^T\boldsymbol{\gamma})), \tag{3.19}$$

where the parameters

$$\gamma_{0t} = \log(\exp(\theta_t) - \exp(\theta_{t-1})) \quad \text{with} \quad \theta_t = \log \int_0^{a_t} \lambda_0(u)du$$

are derived from the baseline hazard function $\lambda_0(u)$ (Exercise 3.1). Model (3.19) is equivalent to the Gompertz model or clog-log model for discrete hazards. It is essential that the effect of covariates contained in the parameter $\boldsymbol{\gamma}$ is the same as in the original Cox model for continuous time. Therefore, if the data generating model is the Cox model but data come in a coarsened form by grouping into intervals one can use the clog-log model for inference on the effect of covariates specified by the Cox model. Of course if continuous lifetimes are available the grouped version of the models uses less information than the original Cox model specified in (3.16). We defer the investigation of the resulting information loss to Sect. 3.6 after estimation concepts for discrete hazards have been considered.

When considering proportionality one should be careful if one refers to proportions in continuous time or discrete time. In fact, the proportionality in (3.17) holds for continuous time. However, proportionality takes a different form for the corresponding time-discrete version. With the clog-log model, proportionality does not refer to the discrete hazards but to discrete survival functions, that is, one obtains

$$\log(S(t|\boldsymbol{x}))/\log(S(t|\tilde{\boldsymbol{x}}))$$

(compare (3.13)). Nevertheless we will call the clog-log model also "grouped proportional hazards model." The latter name refers to the connection to the proportional hazards model for continuous time and is in common use.

3.4 Estimation

Let the basic discrete survival model $\lambda(t|\boldsymbol{x}_i) = h(\gamma_{0t} + \boldsymbol{x}_i^T\boldsymbol{\gamma})$ be given in the form

$$\lambda(t|\boldsymbol{x}_i) = h(\boldsymbol{x}_{it}^T\boldsymbol{\beta}), \tag{3.20}$$

where the vector of explanatory variables is $\boldsymbol{x}_{it}^T = (0, \ldots, 0, 1, 0, \ldots, 0, \boldsymbol{x}_i^T)$ with 1 being the t-th digit and all parameters collected in $\boldsymbol{\beta}^T = (\gamma_{01}, \ldots, \gamma_{0q}, \boldsymbol{\gamma}^T)$. Thus, to obtain a simple closed form, in $\boldsymbol{x}_{it}$ the time dependence is included although the explanatory variables $\boldsymbol{x}_i$ themselves do not depend on time.

Estimation

In the following we assume that observations are subject to *censoring*, that means that only a portion of the observed times can be considered as exact survival times. For the rest of the observations one only knows that the survival time exceeds a certain time point. We assume random censoring, that is, each individual i has a survival time T_i and a censoring time C_i, where T_i and C_i are independent random variables. In this framework the observed time is given by $t_i := \min(T_i, C_i)$ as the minimum of the survival time T_i and the censoring time C_i. It is often useful to introduce an indicator variable for censoring given by

$$\delta_i = \begin{cases} 1 \text{ if } T_i \leq C_i, \\ 0 \text{ if } T_i > C_i, \end{cases}$$

where it is implicitly assumed that censoring occurs at the end of the interval. Let the total data with potential censoring be given by $(t_i, \delta_i, \boldsymbol{x}_i), i = 1, \ldots, n$, where n is the sample size. It is useful to first consider non-censored and censored observed data separately. Since time and censoring are independent by assumption, the probability of observing the exact survival time $(t_i, \delta_i = 1)$ is given by

$$P(T_i = t_i, \delta_i = 1) = P(T_i = t_i)\, P(C_i \geq t_i), \tag{3.21}$$

and the probability of observing censoring at time t_i is given by

$$P(C_i = t_i, \delta_i = 0) = P(T_i > t_i)\, P(C_i = t_i). \tag{3.22}$$

A failure in interval $[a_{t_i-1}, a_{t_i})$ implies $C_i \geq t_i$, and censoring in interval $[a_{t_i-1}, a_{t_i})$ (i.e., $C_i = t_i$) implies survival beyond a_{t_i}. The contribution of the ith observation to the likelihood function is therefore given by

$$L_i = P(T_i = t_i)^{\delta_i} P(T_i > t_i)^{1-\delta_i} P(C_i \geq t_i)^{\delta_i} P(C_i = t_i)^{1-\delta_i}.$$

If one assumes that the censoringcontributions involving C_i do not depend on the parameters that determine the survival time ("noninformative censoring" in the sense of Kalbfleisch and Prentice 2002), one can separate the factor $c_i := P(C_i \geq t_i)^{\delta_i} P(C_i = t_i)^{1-\delta_i}$ to obtain the simpler form

$$L_i = c_i\, P(T_i = t_i)^{\delta_i} P(T_i > t_i)^{1-\delta_i}. \tag{3.23}$$

By using the discrete hazard function and including the covariates, one obtains with the help of (3.2) and (3.4)

$$L_i = c_i\, \lambda(t_i|\boldsymbol{x}_i)^{\delta_i}(1-\lambda(t_i|\boldsymbol{x}_i))^{1-\delta_i} \prod_{j=1}^{t_i-1}(1-\lambda(j|\boldsymbol{x}_i)). \tag{3.24}$$

This likelihood seems to be very specific for a discrete survival model with censoring. But closer inspection shows that it is in fact equivalent to the likelihood of a sequence of binary responses. By defining for a non-censored observation ($\delta_i = 1$) the sequence $(y_{i1}, \dots, y_{it_i}) = (0, \dots, 0, 1)$ and for a censored observation ($\delta_i = 0$) the sequence $(y_{i1}, \dots, y_{it_i}) = (0, \dots, 0)$, the likelihood (omitting c_i) can be written as

$$L_i = \prod_{s=1}^{t_i} \lambda(s|\boldsymbol{x}_i)^{y_{is}}(1-\lambda(s|\boldsymbol{x}_i))^{1-y_{is}}.$$

Thus L_i is equivalent to the likelihood of a binary response model with values $y_{is} \in \{0, 1\}$. Generally, for each i one has t_i such observations. Note, however, that the binary observations are not just artificially constructed values. In fact, the values y_{is} code the binary decisions for the transition to the next period. Specifically, y_{is} codes the transition from interval $[a_{s-1}, a_s)$ to $[a_s, a_{s+1})$ in the form

$$y_{is} = \begin{cases} 1, & \text{if individual fails in } [a_{s-1}, a_s), \\ 0, & \text{if individual survives } [a_{s-1}, a_s), \end{cases}$$

$s = 1, \dots, t_i$. For exact survival times one has the observation vector $(0, \dots, 0, 1)$ of length t_i, that is, survival for the first t_i intervals and failure in the t_i-th interval. For censored observations, it is known that the first t_i intervals have been survived.

As a consequence, the total log-likelihood of the discrete survival model is given by

$$l \propto \sum_{i=1}^{n}\sum_{s=1}^{t_i} y_{is} \log \lambda(s|\boldsymbol{x}_i) + (1-y_{is}) \log(1-\lambda(s|\boldsymbol{x}_i)). \tag{3.25}$$

Note that the log-likelihood is equivalent to the log-likelihood of the binary observations $y_{11}, \dots, y_{1,t_1}, y_{21}, \dots, y_{n,t_n}$ from the binary response model $P(y_{ij} = 1|x_i) = h(\boldsymbol{x}_{ij}^T\boldsymbol{\beta})$. In total one has $t_1 + \cdots + t_n$ binary observations. Therefore, the number of binary observations depends on the observed censoring and lifetimes. Thus, even if the number of observations n is considered fixed, the number of binary observations is not. It is a random variable that depends on the underlying survival and censoring process.

Nevertheless, the representation as a log-likelihood of a binary regression models allows to use software that is designed for these models. The only task is to generate the binary observations before fitting the binary model for transitions. For illustration let us consider the discrete hazard model with linear predictor $\eta_{ir} = \boldsymbol{\gamma}_{or} + \boldsymbol{x}_i^T \boldsymbol{\gamma}$. In closed form the linear predictor is given by $\boldsymbol{x}_{ir}^T \boldsymbol{\beta}$ with parameter vector $\boldsymbol{\beta}^T = (\gamma_{01}, \dots \gamma_{0q}, \boldsymbol{\gamma}^T)$. For the linear predictors of the binary model one has to adapt the covariate vector to the observations under consideration. For the generation of the design matrix one has to distinguish between censored and non-censored observations. If $T = t_i$ and $\delta_i = 1$, the t_i binary observations and design variables are given by the *augmented* data matrix.

Binary observations	Design variables					
0	1	0	0	...	0	$\boldsymbol{x}_i^T$
0	0	1	0	...	0	$\boldsymbol{x}_i^T$
0	0	0	1	...	0	$\boldsymbol{x}_i^T$
$\vdots$						
1	0	0	0	...	1	$\boldsymbol{x}_i^T$

Similarly, if $T = t_i$ and $\delta_i = 0$, the t_i binary observations and design variables are given by the augmented data matrix

Binary observations	Design variables					
0	1	0	0	...	0	$\boldsymbol{x}_i^T$
0	0	1	0	...	0	$\boldsymbol{x}_i^T$
0	0	0	1	...	0	$\boldsymbol{x}_i^T$
$\vdots$						
0	0	0	0	...	1	$\boldsymbol{x}_i^T$

Instead of constructing the design matrix one can also construct the observations with running time t, which has to be considered as a factor when using appropriate software. Then for $T = t_i$, $\delta_i = 1$ one uses the coding

Binary observations	Design variables	
0	1	$\boldsymbol{x}_i^T$
0	2	$\boldsymbol{x}_i^T$
0	3	$\boldsymbol{x}_i^T$
$\vdots$		
1	t_i	$\boldsymbol{x}_i^T$

Similarly, for $T = t_i$, $\delta_i = 0$ one uses the coding

Binary observations	Design variables	
0	1	$\boldsymbol{x}_i^T$
0	2	$\boldsymbol{x}_i^T$
0	3	$\boldsymbol{x}_i^T$
$\vdots$		
0	t_i	$\boldsymbol{x}_i^T$

Modeling the Censoring Time

In the previous section the contribution of censoring to the likelihood has been essentially ignored. However, the censoring process can also be analyzed by specifying a discrete hazard model. To this purpose let $\lambda_{\text{cens}}(t|\boldsymbol{x}_i) = P(C = t \mid C \geq t, \boldsymbol{x}_i)$ denote the hazard function for the censoring time. With censoring at the end of the interval the contribution of the ith observation to the likelihood, as considered before, is

$$L_i = c_i\, \lambda(t_i|\boldsymbol{x}_i)^{\delta_i}(1 - \lambda(t_i|\boldsymbol{x}_i))^{1-\delta_i} \prod_{j=1}^{t_i-1}(1 - \lambda(j|\boldsymbol{x}_i)),$$

where $c_i = P(C_i \geq t_i)^{\delta_i} P(C_i = t_i)^{1-\delta_i}$ contains the contribution of the censored observations. It is straightforward to derive

$$c_i = \lambda_{\text{cens}}(t_i|\boldsymbol{x}_i)^{1-\delta_i} \prod_{s=1}^{t_i-1}(1 - \lambda_{\text{cens}}(s|\boldsymbol{x}_i)).$$

If $\delta_i = 0$ one obtains

$$c_i = \prod_{s=1}^{t_i} \lambda_{\text{cens}}(s|\boldsymbol{x}_i)^{y_{is}^{(c)}} (1 - \lambda_{\text{cens}}(s|\boldsymbol{x}_i))^{1-y_{is}^{(c)}},$$

where $(y_{i1}^{(c)}, \dots, y_{i,t_i-1}^{(c)}, y_{it_i}^{(c)}) = (0, \dots, 0, 1)$. The $y_{is}^{(c)}$'s again code the transition to the next period. If the observation is not censored, implying $\delta_i = 1$ and $(y_{i1}^{(c)}, \dots, y_{i,t_i-1}^{(c)}) = (0, \dots, 0)$, one obtains

$$c_i = \prod_{s=1}^{t_i-1} (1 - \lambda_{\text{cens}}(s|\boldsymbol{x}_i))^{1-y_{is}^{(c)}},$$

which means that censoring has not occurred up to and including period $t_i - 1$.

In closed form the contribution of the ith observation to the likelihood function is given by

$$c_i = \prod_{s=1}^{t_i-\delta_i} \lambda_{\text{cens}}(s|\boldsymbol{x}_i)^{y_{is}^{(c)}} (1 - \lambda_{\text{cens}}(s|\boldsymbol{x}_i))^{1-y_{is}^{(c)}}.$$

Concerning the design matrix, one obtains for the censoring process with running time t and $\delta_i = 0$ the t_i observations

Binary observations	Design variables	
0	1	$\boldsymbol{x}_i^T$
0	2	$\boldsymbol{x}_i^T$
0	3	$\boldsymbol{x}_i^T$
$\vdots$		
1	t_i	$\boldsymbol{x}_i^T$

For the censoring process with running time t and $\delta_i = 1$ one obtains the $t_i - 1$ observations.

Binary observations	Design variables	
0	1	$\boldsymbol{x}_i^T$
0	2	$\boldsymbol{x}_i^T$
0	3	$\boldsymbol{x}_i^T$
$\vdots$		
0	$t_i - 1$	$\boldsymbol{x}_i^T$

Simultaneous maximum likelihood estimation for the failure time and censoring processes uses the log-likelihood $l = l_T + l_C$, where

$$l_T = \sum_{i=1}^{n} \sum_{s=1}^{t_i} (y_{is} \log \lambda(s|\boldsymbol{x}_i) + (1 - y_{is}) \log(1 - \lambda(s|\boldsymbol{x}_i)))$$

is the log-likelihood that depends on the discrete hazard of failure (i.e., on $\lambda(s|\boldsymbol{x}_i)$), and

$$l_C = \sum_{i=1}^{n} \sum_{s=1}^{t_i-\delta_i} y_{is}^{(c)} \log(\lambda_{\text{cens}}(s|\boldsymbol{x}_i)) + (1 - y_{is}^{(c)}) \log((1 - \lambda_{\text{cens}}(s|\boldsymbol{x}_i)))$$

is the log-likelihood that depends on the discrete hazard of censoring (i.e., on $\lambda_{\text{cens}}(s|\boldsymbol{x}_i)$). If failure and censoring do not share parameters, l_T and l_C can be maximized separately.

Censoring at the Beginning of the Interval

The derivation of the log-likelihood in the previous sections was based on the assumption that censoring occurs at the end of the interval. Definitions and derivations change if one assumes censoring at the beginning of the interval. In this case one has

$$\delta_i = \begin{cases} 1 \text{ if } T_i < C_i, \\ 0 \text{ if } T_i \geq C_i, \end{cases}$$

and

$$P(T_i = t_i, \delta_i = 1) = P(T_i = t_i)P(C_i > t_i),$$
$$P(C_i = t_i, \delta_i = 0) = P(T_i \geq t_i)P(C_i = t_i).$$

The contribution of the ith observation to the likelihood is now given by

$$L_i = P(T_i = t_i)^{\delta_i} P(T_i \geq t_i)^{1-\delta_i} P(C_i > t_i)^{\delta_i} P(C_i = t_i)^{1-\delta_i}.$$

Without censoring this yields

$$L_i = c_i\, \lambda(t_i|\boldsymbol{x}_i)^{\delta_i} \prod_{j=1}^{t_i-1} (1 - \lambda(j|\boldsymbol{x}_i)). \tag{3.26}$$

By defining the sequence $(y_{i1}, \ldots, y_{it_i}) = (0, \ldots, 0, 1)$ for a non-censored observation ($\delta_i = 1$), the likelihood (omitting c_i) can be written as

$$L_i = \prod_{s=1}^{t_i} \lambda(s|\boldsymbol{x}_i)^{y_{is}} (1 - \lambda(s|\boldsymbol{x}_i))^{1-y_{is}}.$$

For a censored observation one defines the sequence $(y_{i1}, \ldots, y_{i,t_i-1}) = (0, \ldots, 0)$, yielding

$$L_i = \prod_{s=1}^{t_i-1} \lambda(s|\boldsymbol{x}_i)^{y_{is}}(1-\lambda(s|\boldsymbol{x}_i))^{1-y_{is}}.$$

In closed form the contribution of the ith observation to the likelihood is given by

$$L_i = \prod_{s=1}^{t_i-(1-\delta_i)} \lambda(s|\boldsymbol{x}_i)^{y_{is}}(1-\lambda(s|\boldsymbol{x}_i))^{1-y_{is}},$$

and the total log-likelihood for the model is given by

$$l \propto \sum_{i=1}^{n} \sum_{s=1}^{t_i-(1-\delta_i)} (y_{is} \log \lambda(s|\boldsymbol{x}_i) + (1-y_{is}) \log(1-\lambda(s|\boldsymbol{x}_i)))\,.$$

The log-likelihood is again equivalent to the log-likelihood of the binary response model $P(y_{ij}=1\,|\,\boldsymbol{x}_i) = h(\boldsymbol{x}_i^T\boldsymbol{\beta})$ with binary observations $y_{11}, \ldots, y_{1,t_1-(1-\delta_1)}$, $y_{21}, \ldots, y_{n,t_n-(1-\delta_n)}$. In total one has $\sum_i (t_i - 1 + \delta_i)$ binary observations, where the sum varies with the number of censored observations and also depends on the observed lifetimes.

3.4.1 Standard Errors

Let us consider the case where censoring occurs at the end of the interval. Then the log-likelihood (3.25) can be used to derive approximate standard errors for the coefficient estimates of a discrete hazard model. It is straightforward to derive the *information matrix*, which is given by

$$\boldsymbol{F}(\boldsymbol{\beta}) := \mathrm{E}\left(-\frac{\partial^2 l(\boldsymbol{\beta})}{\partial\boldsymbol{\beta}\partial\boldsymbol{\beta}^T}\right) = \sum_{i=1}^{n}\sum_{s=1}^{t_i} \boldsymbol{x}_{it}\boldsymbol{x}_{it}^T \left(\frac{\partial h(\eta_{it})}{\partial \eta}\right)^2 / \sigma_{it}^2,$$

where $\eta_{it} = \boldsymbol{x}_{it}^T\boldsymbol{\beta}$ (with $\boldsymbol{x}_{it}$ from model (3.20)) and $\sigma_{it}^2 = h(\eta_{it})(1-h(\eta_{it}))$. By standard arguments, asymptotic standard errors of the maximum likelihood estimator $\hat{\boldsymbol{\beta}}$ are obtained from the approximation

$$\hat{\boldsymbol{\beta}} \overset{a}{\sim} \mathrm{N}\left(\boldsymbol{\beta}, F(\hat{\boldsymbol{\beta}})^{-1}\right). \tag{3.27}$$

For example, the asymptotic standard errors presented in Table 3.1 have been computed by using the above approximation. Note that the approximation in (3.27) also allows to construct *Wald confidence intervals* at the level $1-\alpha$ for $\hat{\boldsymbol{\beta}}$, which are given by

$$\hat{\beta}_k \pm z_{1-\alpha/2}\sqrt{F(\hat{\boldsymbol{\beta}})_{kk}^{-1}}\,, \tag{3.28}$$

where $\hat{\beta}_k$ is the k-th element of $\hat{\boldsymbol{\beta}}$, $F(\hat{\boldsymbol{\beta}})_{kk}^{-1}$ is the k-th diagonal element of $F(\hat{\boldsymbol{\beta}})^{-1}$, and $z_{1-\alpha/2}$ is the $1-\alpha/2$ quantile of the standard normal distribution.

3.5 Time-Varying Covariates

In the previous sections it has been assumed that predictors are fixed values that were observed at the beginning of the duration under investigation. Although we sometimes wrote the model as $\lambda(t|x_i) = h(\boldsymbol{x}_{it}^T\boldsymbol{\beta})$, this was just a convenient form to denote the variation of the intercept over time. In fact, the actual model was always $\lambda(t|\boldsymbol{x}_i) = h(\gamma_{0t} + \boldsymbol{x}_i^T\boldsymbol{\gamma})$ with fixed predictor value $\boldsymbol{x}_i$.

In practice, however, it is not uncommon that potential explanatory variables vary over time. For example, general measures of economic activity like business cycles may have an impact on the duration of unemployment of individuals. The corresponding measurements will vary over an individual's duration of unemployment.

In the following we will show how time-dependent covariate information may be incorporated into discrete-time hazard models. To this purpose, let $\boldsymbol{x}_{i1},\ldots,\boldsymbol{x}_{it}$ denote the sequence of observations of covariates for the ith unit (or individual) until time t, where $\boldsymbol{x}_{it}$ is a vector observed at discrete time t (or, if "discrete time" refers to intervals, at the beginning of the interval $[a_{t-1}, a_t)$). When modeling the hazard one might want to include part of the history up to time point t, $\{\boldsymbol{x}_{is}\}_{s\le t}$. Let this more general hazard be given by

$$\lambda(t|\{\boldsymbol{x}_{is}\}_{s\le t}) = P(T = t\,|\,T \ge t, \{\boldsymbol{x}_{is}\}_{s\le t}) = h(\eta_{it}),$$

where $h(\cdot)$ is the chosen response function and η_{it} contains the explanatory variables. The choice of η_{it} determines the complexity of the model. The simplest model uses only the current value of the time-varying covariates in a linear form,

$$\eta_{it} = \gamma_{0t} + \boldsymbol{x}_{it}^T\boldsymbol{\gamma}\,.$$

With time lags one may specify

$$\eta_{it} = \gamma_{0t} + \boldsymbol{x}_{it}^T\boldsymbol{\gamma} + \boldsymbol{x}_{i,t-1}^T\boldsymbol{\gamma}_1 + \boldsymbol{x}_{i,t-2}^T\boldsymbol{\gamma}_2 + \ldots$$

To obtain the probability of a transition, the sequence $\boldsymbol{x}_{i1},\dots,\boldsymbol{x}_{it}$ is considered as a stochastic process. More specifically, with indicator variables $y_{i1},\dots,y_{it}$ that represent the survival time such that $(y_{i1},\dots,y_{it_i}) = (0,\dots,0,1)$ if $T = t_i$, one obtains the stochastic process $\{y_{is},\boldsymbol{x}_{is}\}_s$. If, for simplicity, the covariate process is discrete, the probabilities can again be written as a product

$$P(\{y_{is},\boldsymbol{x}_{is}\}_{s\le t}) = P(y_{it},\boldsymbol{x}_{it}|\{y_{is},\boldsymbol{x}_{is}\}_{s<t})\cdot P(y_{i,t-1},\boldsymbol{x}_{i,t-1}|\{y_{is},\boldsymbol{x}_{is}\}_{s<t-1})\cdot\ldots\cdot P(y_{i1},\boldsymbol{x}_{i1}).$$

Since for any t

$$P(y_{it},\boldsymbol{x}_{it}|\{y_{is},\boldsymbol{x}_{is}\}_{s<t}) = P(y_{it}\,|\boldsymbol{x}_{it},\{y_{is},\boldsymbol{x}_{is}\}_{s<t})\;P(\boldsymbol{x}_{it}|\{y_{is},\boldsymbol{x}_{is}\}_{s<t})\,,$$

one obtains for $(y_{i1},\dots,y_{it}) = (0,\dots,0,1)$

$$P(y_{it},\boldsymbol{x}_{it}|\{y_{is},\boldsymbol{x}_{is}\}_{s<t}) = \lambda(t|\{\boldsymbol{x}_{is}\}_{s\le t})\;P(\boldsymbol{x}_{it}|\{y_{is},\boldsymbol{x}_{is}\}_{s<t}),$$

and for $(y_{i1},\dots,y_{it}) = (0,\dots,0)$

$$P(\{y_{is},\boldsymbol{x}_{is}\}_{s\le t}) = (1-\lambda(t|\{\boldsymbol{x}_{is}\}_{s\le t})\;P(\boldsymbol{x}_{it}|\{y_{is},\boldsymbol{x}_{is}\}_{s<t}).$$

Therefore, if $P(\boldsymbol{x}_{it}|\{y_{is},\boldsymbol{x}_{is}\}_{s<t})$ is not informative for the parameters in the hazard rate, one obtains for an observation $T_i = t_i$, which corresponds to $(y_{i1},\dots,y_{it_i}) = (0,\dots,0,1)$,

$$P(\{y_{is},\boldsymbol{x}_{is}\}_{s\le t_i}) = P(T_i = t_i,\{\boldsymbol{x}_{is}\}_{s\le t_i}) = c_i\;\lambda(t_i|\{\boldsymbol{x}_{is}\}_{s\le t})\prod_{l=1}^{t_i-1}(1-\lambda(l|\{\boldsymbol{x}_{is}\}_{s\le l})), \tag{3.29}$$

where c_i is determined by the non-informative probabilities $P(\boldsymbol{x}_{it}|\{y_{is},\boldsymbol{x}_{is}\}_{s<t})$.

In this representation the crucial assumption is that $P(\boldsymbol{x}_{it}|\{y_{is},\boldsymbol{x}_{is}\}_{s<t})$ is not informative. In particular, when the covariate process depends on survival, that is, on $\{y_{is}\}_{s<t}$ this assumption is questionable. But if, for example, the aim is to model the duration of unemployment, then covariate processes such as countrywide economic activity are hardly determined by the duration of unemployment of single persons. One can also postulate $P(\boldsymbol{x}_{it}|\{y_{is},\boldsymbol{x}_{is}\}_{s<t}) = P(\boldsymbol{x}_{it}|\{\boldsymbol{x}_{is}\}_{s<t})$, which corresponds to the concept of an external covariate process (Kalbfleisch and Prentice 2002). A much more general framework for the use of time-varying covariates is provided by counting processes and martingales, see, for example, Fleming and Harrington (2011).

The advantage of representation (3.29) is that under similar assumptions on the censoring process one can rely on the likelihood (3.25). For illustration we consider the case where the hazard depends on the current $\boldsymbol{x}_{it}$ only. If all assumptions hold, one obtains for the log-likelihood of the corresponding model $\lambda(t|\{\boldsymbol{x}_{is}\}_{s\leq t}) = h(\gamma_{0t} + \boldsymbol{x}_{it}^T\boldsymbol{\gamma})$

$$l \propto \sum_{i=1}^{n}\sum_{s=1}^{t_i} y_{is}\log\lambda(s|\boldsymbol{x}_{it}) + (1-y_{is})\log(1-\lambda(s|\boldsymbol{x}_{it})).$$

When using software for the corresponding binary response model that describes the transitions, one has to construct again the corresponding design matrices and distinguish between censored and non-censored observations.

If $T = t_i$, $\delta_i = 1$ the t_i binary observations and design variables are given by

Binary observations	Design variables					
0	1	0	0	...	0	$\boldsymbol{x}_{i1}^T$
0	0	1	0	...	0	$\boldsymbol{x}_{i2}^T$
0	0	0	1	...	0	
⋮						
1	0	0	0	...	1	$\boldsymbol{x}_{it_i}^T$

Similarly, if $T = t_i$, $\delta_i = 0$ the t_i binary observations and design variables are given by

Binary observations	Design variables					
0	1	0	0	...	0	$\boldsymbol{x}_{i1}^T$
0	0	1	0	...	0	$\boldsymbol{x}_{i2}^T$
0	0	0	1	...	0	
⋮						
0	0	0	0	...	0	$\boldsymbol{x}_{it_i}^T$

The crucial modification compared to the design matrices in Sect. 3.4 is that the covariate values vary over time.

Example 3.3 German Socio-Economic Panel (SOEP)
The Socio-Economic Panel is an ongoing longitudinal survey of about 12,000 private households in Germany. Data collection started in 1984 and is focussed on topics such as employment, income, quality of life, and health. In this example the event of interest is drop-out of the SOEP. Since data are collected annually, the time until drop-out is measured in years (median duration = 3 years). Approximately 37 % of the households are censored, meaning that they continue to participate in the study. The data are available after registration at http://www.diw.de/de/soep; for a complete description of the household data we refer to https://data.soep.de/datasets/11 and https://data.soep.de/datasets/14. For survival modeling we applied various pre-processing steps to the SOEP data. In particular, we considered categories such as "could be any value" and "does not apply" as missing values. Also, the categories "answer improbable" and "no answer" were set to missing.

To illustrate discrete survival modeling with time-varying covariates, we fitted a continuation ratio model using the time to drop out of the SOEP (measured in years) as outcome variable. The following covariates were considered: adjusted monthly household net income (in EUR, abbreviated by *HGAHINC*), household typology (summarized to the seven categories "1-person household," "single parent, 1 child," "single parent, more than 1 child," "couple, 1 child," "couple without children," "couple, more than 1 child," "3- and more-generation HH," *HGTYP2HH*), month of the interview (*HGHMONTH*), and interview method (ten categories, see Table 3.5, *HGHMODE*). All four covariates were time-varying, e.g., their values or categories could be subject to changes over time.

Figure 3.5 displays the baseline hazard coefficients with 95 % Wald confidence intervals. It is seen that all intervals have similar lengths. In the starting year the baseline hazard is quite low. As expected, a trend is observable in the estimates: The longer a household participates in the survey, the higher is the hazard that the household will drop out.

Tables 3.3, 3.4, 3.5, and 3.6 contain the coefficient estimates, standard errors and p-values for the covariates of the continuation ratio model. Regarding interpretation, estimates can be transformed to the odds ratio scale by taking $\exp(\hat{\gamma})$. For example, in case of a categorical covariate the odds ratio of a specific category increases by the factor $\exp(\hat{\gamma})$ compared to the reference category. For instance, in Table 3.6 (referring to the "month of the interview"), it is seen that the odds of dropping out of the SOEP increase by $\exp(\hat{\gamma}_{HGHMONTH\,Sep}) = 2.754$ if the interview is done in September instead of February (provided that the values of all other covariates are constant). □

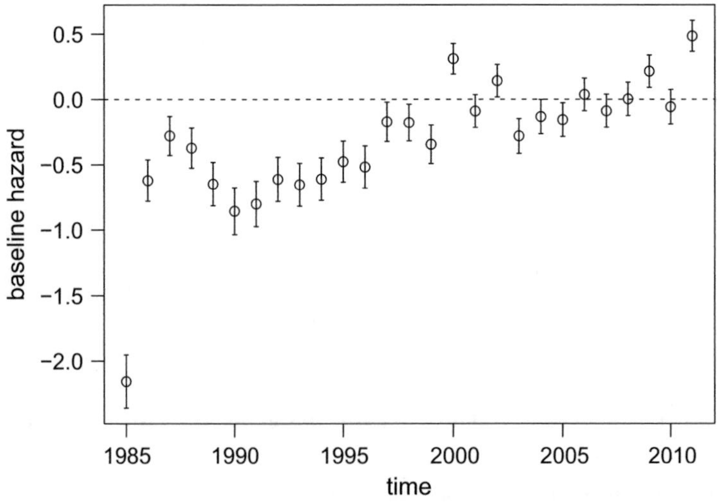

Fig. 3.5 Coefficient estimates for the baseline hazard rate in Example 3.3 (SOEP data); confidence intervals are 95 % Wald intervals

Table 3.3 Estimated effect of the continuous covariate in Example 3.3 (SOEP data)

Covariate	$\hat{\gamma}$	sd($\hat{\gamma}$)	p
HGAHINC	−0.000059	0.00000654	<0.0001

Table 3.4 Estimated effects of the categorical covariate "household typology" (*HGTYP2HH*) in Example 3.3 (SOEP data)

Category	$\hat{\gamma}$	sd($\hat{\gamma}$)	p
1-Person HH (ref. category)	0.0000	–	–
Single parent, 1 child	−0.3301	0.04788	< 0.001
Single parent, more than 1 child	−0.1223	0.05883	0.038
Couple two children	−0.2098	0.02327	< 0.001
Couple, 1 child	−0.2640	0.02954	< 0.001
Couple, more than 1 child	−0.2430	0.02814	< 0.001
3- and more-generation HH	−0.2836	0.08896	0.001

Table 3.5 Estimated effects of the categorical covariate "interview method" (*HGHMODE*) in Example 3.3 (SOEP data)

Category	$\hat{\gamma}$	sd($\hat{\gamma}$)	p
With interviewer assistance (ref. category)	0.0000	–	–
Oral interview	−0.3157	0.0887	0.0004
Written ques. interviewer	−0.2670	0.9009	0.0030
Written ques. no interviewer	−0.6012	0.1142	< 0.0001
Oral and written	−0.3103	0.1059	0.0034
With interpreter	−0.1371	0.1436	0.3398
Exc interpreter	−0.1459	0.0992	0.1415
CAPI - Wave O onwards	−0.2532	0.0897	0.0047
Written, by mail	0.2630	0.0905	0.0036
Phone interview	0.5464	0.2276	0.0163

Table 3.6 Estimated effects of the time-dependent categorical covariate "month of interview" (*HGHMONTH*) in Example 3.3 (SOEP data). The reference category with $\hat{\gamma} = 0$ is February. There were no interviews in January, March, and May

Category	$\hat{\gamma}$	sd($\hat{\gamma}$)	p
April	0.345	0.0225	<0.001
June	0.668	0.0315	<0.001
July	0.786	0.0357	<0.001
Aug	0.938	0.0333	<0.001
Sep	1.013	0.0548	<0.001
Oct	1.306	0.0742	<0.001
Nov	1.160	0.1596	<0.001
Dec	1.309	0.1682	<0.001

3.6 Continuous Versus Discrete Proportional Hazards

As outlined in Sect. 3.3.2 the Cox (or proportional hazards) model for continuous time, given by $\lambda_c(t|\boldsymbol{x}) = \lambda_0(t)\exp(\boldsymbol{x}^T\boldsymbol{\gamma})$, yields for data that are grouped in fixed intervals the discrete hazard model $\lambda(t|\boldsymbol{x}) = 1 - \exp(-\exp(\gamma_{0t} + \boldsymbol{x}^T\boldsymbol{\gamma}))$, which is called the grouped proportional hazards model.

If the Cox model holds and continuous lifetimes are observed, estimation is typically based on the maximization of the *partial likelihood*

$$PL(\boldsymbol{\gamma}) := \prod_{i=1}^{k} \frac{\exp(\boldsymbol{x}_{(i)}^T\boldsymbol{\gamma})}{\sum_{j\in\mathcal{R}(t_{(i)})}\exp(\boldsymbol{x}_j^T\boldsymbol{\gamma})}\,, \tag{3.30}$$

where $t_{(1)} < \cdots < t_{(k)}$ refer to the ordered observed event times in the data (assuming that there are k events) and $\boldsymbol{x}_{(1)}, \ldots, \boldsymbol{x}_{(k)}$ refer to the corresponding vectors of explanatory variables. Since T is continuous, all event times are assumed to be distinct. The terms $\mathcal{R}(t_{(i)})$, $i = 1, \ldots, k$, are the so-called risk sets, i.e., the groups of observations that are still alive at time point $t_{(i)}$. By definition of the Cox model in continuous time, the term $\exp(\boldsymbol{x}_{(i)}^T\boldsymbol{\gamma})$ is a time-constant inflation factor of the conditional hazard of observation i. Therefore, the partial likelihood can be interpreted as the product of k risk probability factors, where each factor quantifies the conditional risk of observing an event in observation i at time point $t_{(i)}$.

It follows from (3.30) that the estimation of a Cox model in continuous time is based on a finite set of discrete-time points $t_{(i)}$ and is therefore similar to the estimation of a discrete survival model with intervals $[0, t_{(1)}), [t_{(1)}, t_{(2)}), \ldots [t_{(k)}, \infty)$. The main conceptual difference between the estimation of discrete survival models and the estimation of a continuous Cox model is that the interval borders $t_{(i)}$ are *random* (and therefore data-dependent) whereas in the case of discrete survival data they are *fixed*. Also, unlike in discrete survival modeling, each of the intervals $[t_{(i)}, t_{(i+1)})$ contains exactly one observation.

Because of rounded database entries, in practice often ties occur even when the survival times have not been grouped. If the Cox model is applied to such data, the partial log-likelihood in (3.30) has to be modified, as some of the event times $t_{(i)}$ are not unique but refer to *several* observations. One way to adjust (3.30) in the presence of ties is to construct the so-called *exact partial likelihood* (Cox 1972). Assuming that the data contain k_i events in observations $j_1, \ldots, j_{k_i}$ at time point $t_{(i)}$, the factors in (3.30) are replaced by the conditional risks of realizing these events *given* that there are k_i events at $t_{(k)}$ (Box-Steffensmeier and Jones 2004). The tie-handling method based on the exact partial likelihood is sometimes referred to as the *discrete method* (for example, within the software system SAS). Other methods for tie handling, which are not considered here, are the Breslow and Efron approximations, and the *exact marginal likelihood* technique (Kalbfleisch and Prentice 2002).

Applying the exact partial likelihood correction technique reveals another interesting relationship between the continuous Cox model and discrete survival modeling. It can be shown that the optimization of the exact partial likelihood is exactly the same as fitting a so-called *conditional logistic regression model* to the data. The latter model is based on the same assumptions as the continuation ratio model in Sect. 3.2.1 but does not involve estimation of the baseline parameters γ_{0t} (Chamberlain 1980). As a consequence, fitting a Cox model with the exact partial likelihood to survival data (even if there are may ties and strong grouping effects) will often yield results that are similar to those obtained from a continuation ratio model. Finally, it is important to note that if a Cox model in continuous time holds, estimates obtained for grouped observations when using the original Cox model differ from those obtained from the grouped proportional hazards model (with clog-log link). This situation is illustrated in Fig. 3.6, which was produced using simulated data ($n = 100$) that were generated from an exponential survival model. The exponential survival model is a special case of the continuous proportional hazards model with time-constant hazard function $\lambda(t) = \exp(\gamma_0 + \boldsymbol{x}^\top \boldsymbol{\gamma})$. For the simulation study we considered five independent normally distributed covariates $\boldsymbol{x} = (x_1, \ldots, x_5)^\top$ with mean $\mu = (4.5, 4.5, 4.5, 4.5, 4.5)^\top$ and unit covariance matrix. The coefficient vector was set to $\boldsymbol{\gamma} = -(0.1, 0.2, 0.3, 0.4, 0.5)^\top$, yielding survival times with median $\approx$530 and 75 % quantile $\approx$1550. Censoring times were generated independently from an exponential distribution with mean 2500. Survival times that were larger than 1500 were also considered censored, yielding an overall censoring rate of $\approx$35 %

In Fig. 3.6, estimates that use the originally continuous survival data, but also estimates that use grouped data with different interval lengths are considered. Specifically, the continuous Cox model based on the exact partial likelihood, the discrete continuation ratio logit model, and the discrete grouped proportional hazards model were fitted. The upper panel of Fig. 3.6 shows boxplots for the estimates of γ_2, which corresponds to the parameter for covariate x_2, for varying interval lengths (based on $B = 100$ simulation runs). The first number on the abscissa refers to the interval length while the second number refers to the resulting number of intervals. For example, 30 (50) means that the interval length was 30 yielding 50 intervals. White box plots refer to the estimates for the discrete clog-log model, and gray box plots refer to the estimates for the continuous Cox model based on the exact partial likelihood. It is seen that estimates based on the grouped proportional hazards model show larger variability than estimates based on the continuous Cox model if many intervals (and hence almost the exact times) are used. However, for strong grouping the variability is smaller for the grouped proportional hazards model.

The lower panel of Fig. 3.6 depicts the corresponding values of the root mean squared error

$$\mathrm{RMSE}_2 = \sqrt{\frac{1}{B}\sum_{j=1}^{B}(\gamma_2 - \hat{\gamma}_2)^2} \tag{3.31}$$

of the estimator $\hat{\gamma}_2$. As expected, estimates obtained from the Cox model in continuous time (based on the exact partial likelihood) are highly similar to those

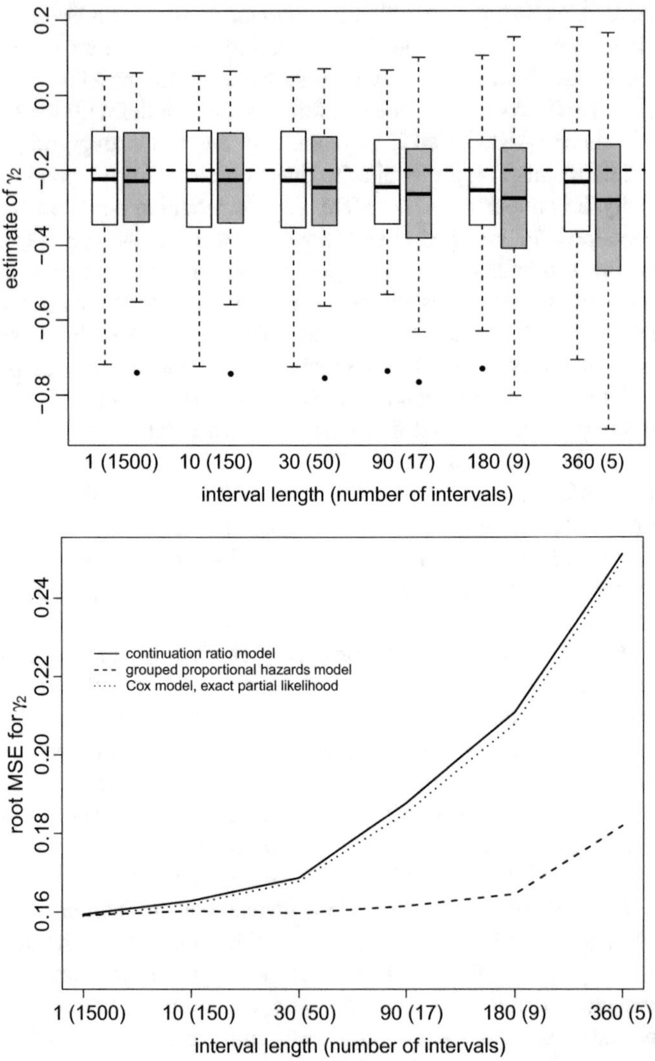

Fig. 3.6 Results from a simulation study with five normally distributed covariates. Survival times and covariate data ($n = 100$) were generated from a survival model with exponentially distributed outcome and five covariates. The number of simulation runs was $B = 100$. The *upper panel* shows box plots of the estimates of the regression coefficient γ_2 referring to the second covariate. White box plots refer to the discrete clog-log model, and gray box plots refer to the continuous Cox model based on the exact partial likelihood. The *numbers in brackets* refer to the number of time intervals; the *dashed line* refers to the true value of γ_2. The *lower panel* shows the respective RMSE estimates for various grouping scenarios

obtained from the continuation ratio model with logistic link function. However, there are notable differences between the root mean squared error values of the proportional hazards models in continuous and discrete time. Since by definition the grouped proportional hazards model is correctly specified even if the interval lengths (and hence the number of ties) are large, RMSE values of this model are smaller than those of the Cox model in continuous time. It is also seen that larger interval lengths result in larger RMSE values and thus in a worse performance of the estimators. This result is to be expected, as stronger grouping usually entails a loss of information. Nevertheless it is remarkable that the performance of the grouped proportional hazards model is quite stable. Its performance in terms of MSE deteriorates only when the number of intervals is quite small; for example, at the right end the data have been grouped into only five intervals. Very similar results were obtained for the estimates of the other coefficients, see, for example, Fig. 3.7.

3.7 Subject-Specific Interval Censoring

In grouped survival it is typically assumed that time is measured on a coarse scale determined by the intervals $[0, a_1), [a_1, a_2), \ldots \ldots, [a_{q-1}, a_q), [a_q, \infty)$. What one in fact observes are *interval censored data*. A more specific pattern of interval censoring occurs if the intervals are specific to the individuals under investigation. For example, in a clinical trial or a longitudinal study with a periodic follow-up an individual who is monitored weekly for a change may miss visits for a few weeks. Then, if a change is observed it is only known that it happened within the interval between two appointments. The observed interval refers to a specific individual, yielding *individual-specific interval censoring*.

Following Finkelstein (1986) the data for individual-specific censoring can be represented by $([l_i, r_i), \boldsymbol{x}_i)$, $i = 1, \ldots, n$, where $[l_i, r_i)$ is the interval during which the response occurred. If the survival time is right censored one has $r_i = \infty$. Under the assumption that the censoring mechanism is independent of both the response time distribution and the covariates, and that each subject will eventually fail unless it is censored before failure, the likelihood contribution of the ith individual is proportional to

$$L_i = P(T_c \in [l_i, r_i)|\boldsymbol{x}_i) = S_c(l_i|\boldsymbol{x}_i) - S_c(r_i|\boldsymbol{x}_i),$$

where $S_c(t|\boldsymbol{x}) = P(T > t\,|\,\boldsymbol{x})$ is the continuous time survival function. For right censored data with $r_i = \infty$ the contribution is reduced to $S_c(l_i|\boldsymbol{x}_i)$. For the case of fixed intervals $[0, a_1), [a_1, a_2), \ldots \ldots, [a_{q-1}, a_q)$ and individuals that do not miss visits one obtains the same log-likelihood contribution as in discrete survival (Eq. (3.23)) but with censoring at the end of the interval.

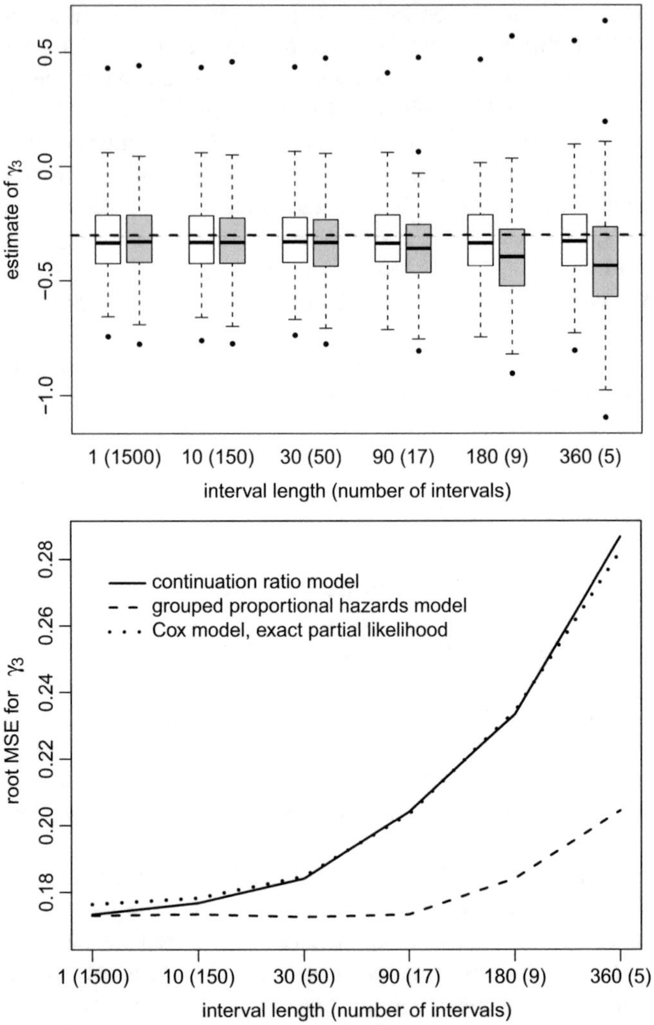

Fig. 3.7 Results from a simulation study with five normally distributed covariates. Survival times and covariate data ($n = 100$) were generated from a survival model with exponentially distributed outcome and five covariates. The number of simulation runs was $B = 100$. The *upper panel* shows boxplots of the estimates of the regression coefficient γ_3 referring to the third covariate. White boxplots refer to the discrete clog-log model, and gray boxplots refer to the continuous Cox model based on the exact partial likelihood. The *numbers in brackets* refer to the number of time intervals; the dashed line refers to the true value of γ_3. The *lower panel* shows the respective RMSE estimates for various grouping scenarios

Finkelstein (1986) considered in particular the proportional hazards model in continuous time with survival function $S_c(t|\boldsymbol{x}) = S_0(t)^{\exp(\boldsymbol{x}^T\boldsymbol{\gamma})}$, where $S_0(t)$ is the baseline survival function. Then the likelihood contribution of the ith individual is

$$L_i = S_0(l_i)^{\exp(\boldsymbol{x}^T\boldsymbol{\gamma})} - S_0(r_i)^{\exp(\boldsymbol{x}^T\boldsymbol{\gamma})}.$$

The total log-likelihood can be written in a more convenient form. From the sets $(l_i, r_i), i = 1, \ldots n$, one determines the set of times $0 = a_0 < a_1 < \cdots < a_{q+1} = \infty$, such that each l_i and r_i is contained in the set. Then, the contribution of the i-th observation to the likelihood can be expressed as $\sum_{j=1}^{q+1} \alpha_{ij}\{S_c(a_{i-1}|\boldsymbol{x}_i) - S_c(a_i|\boldsymbol{x}_i)\}$, where $\alpha_{ij} = 1$ if $[a_{i-1}, a_j)$ is a subset of $[l_i, r_i)$, and 0 otherwise. If one assumes a proportional hazards model in continuous time, one obtains for the total log-likelihood

$$\begin{aligned} l &= \sum_{i=1}^{n}\sum_{j=1}^{q+1} \alpha_{ij}\left\{S_c(a_{j-1}|\boldsymbol{x}_i) - S_c(a_j|\boldsymbol{x}_i)\right\} \\ &= \sum_{i=1}^{n}\sum_{j=1}^{q+1} \alpha_{ij}\left\{S_0(a_{j-1})^{\exp(\boldsymbol{x}^T\boldsymbol{\gamma})} - S_0(a_j)^{\exp(\boldsymbol{x}^T\boldsymbol{\gamma})}\right\} \\ &= \sum_{i=1}^{n}\sum_{j=1}^{q+1} \alpha_{ij}\left\{\exp(-\exp(\tau_{j-1} + \boldsymbol{x}^T\boldsymbol{\gamma}) - \exp(-\exp(\tau_j + \boldsymbol{x}^T\boldsymbol{\gamma})\right\}, \end{aligned}$$

where $\tau_j = \log(-\log(S_0(a_j)))$ represents a parameterization of the baseline survival function. Finkelstein (1986) derived the first and second derivatives for the log-likelihood function to obtain maximum likelihood estimates for the survival function and the parameter $\boldsymbol{\gamma}$.

It should be noted that for the intervals that were built from all interval boundaries for estimation one can also use the representation of the proportional hazards as model with clog-log link as considered in (3.19). The main difference is that in (3.19) the parameters $\gamma_{0j} = \log(\int_{a_{j-1}}^{a_j} \lambda_0(u)du) = \log(\log S_0(a_{j-1}) - \log S_0(a_j))$ are used to parameterize the baseline hazard while here the parameters τ_j are used. When using the likelihood for grouped data as given in Sect. 3.4, one just has to include the weights α_{ij}, which encode the intervals in which censoring occurred.

More on the modeling of individual-specific interval-censored data is found, for example, in Rabinowitz et al. (1995), Lindsey and Ryan (1998), Cai and Betensky (2003), Sun (2006), and Chen et al. (2012).

3.8 Literature and Further Reading

Discrete Hazard Models. Thompson (1977) and Prentice and Gloeckler (1978) were among the first to consider discrete survival data in biometrics. While Thompson (1977) focussed on the logistic model, Prentice and Gloeckler (1978) considered the grouped Cox model and derived a score test for hypothesis testing. Early references for the representation of hazard models as binary Bernoulli trials are Brown (1975) and Laird and Olivier (1981). An overview of discrete survival models was given by Fahrmeir (1998).

Extensions. Mantel and Hankey (1978) replaced the parameters of the baseline hazard by a polynomial. Similarly, Efron (1988) proposed regression splines to model the large number of baseline hazard parameters. He also discussed extensively the use of the binary response model representation of the discrete hazard model.

Regression Models for Interval-Censored Data. The proportional hazards model for interval-censored data was proposed by Finkelstein (1986). Extensions to additive models with smooth effects were considered in Cai and Betensky (2003). Estimation techniques for accelerated failure time models were proposed by Rabinowitz et al. (1995) and Betensky et al. (2001); additive hazards models were studied by Zeng et al. (2006) and Wang et al. (2010).

Bayesian Approaches. Fahrmeir and Knorr-Held (1997) proposed a flexible Bayesian nonparametric analysis for dynamic models with time-varying effects. Fahrmeir and Kneib (2011) considered simulation-based full Bayesian Markov chain Monte Carlo (MCMC) inference for longitudinal and event history data.

3.9 Software

Discrete hazard models can be fitted in R by using the *dataLong* function that is part of the R package *discSurv* and by applying the *glm* function for generalized linear models. In the first step, *dataLong* is used to convert a set of discrete survival data to its corresponding binary representation (as demonstrated in Sect. 3.4). Next, binomial regression models can be fitted by using *glm* with appropriate link function. When specifying *family = binomial()*, a logistic discrete hazard model is fitted. Gompertz and exponential models can be fitted by specifying *family = binomial(link = "cloglog")* and *family = binomial(link = "log")*, respectively. Gumbel models can be fitted by specifying *family = binomial(gumbel())*, with the *gumbel()* link function being available as part of the *discSurv* package.

3.10 Exercises

3.1 Assume that the proportional hazards model holds for continuous time T_c, i.e.,

$$\lambda_c(t|\boldsymbol{x}) = \lambda_0(t)\exp(\boldsymbol{x}^T\boldsymbol{\gamma}).$$

Let now time be coarsened by use of the intervals $[0, a_1), [a_1, a_2), \ldots\ldots, [a_{q-1}, a_q)$, $[a_q, \infty)$ and let T denote discrete time with $T = t$ if failure occurs within the interval $[a_{t-1}, a_t)$. Show that the discrete hazard $\lambda(t|\boldsymbol{x}) = P(T = t \mid T \geq t, \boldsymbol{x})$ is given by

$$\lambda(t|\boldsymbol{x}) = 1 - \exp(-\exp(\gamma_{0t} + \boldsymbol{x}^T\boldsymbol{\gamma}))$$

and write the parameters γ_{0t} as functions of quantities of the proportional hazards model. (Basic concepts of continuous survival are given in Sect. 3.3.1.)

3.2 Consider the congressional careers data described in Example 1.4 with response "losing the general election."

1. Convert the data to a set of augmented data with binary response.
2. Fit a proportional continuation ratio model with logistic link function and with covariates *age*, *priorm*, *prespart*, *leader*, *scandal*, and *redist* to the data.
3. Illustrate the baseline hazard rates graphically over time.
4. Interpret the covariate effects. Which effects are significant at level $\alpha = 0.05$ (according to the respective t-tests)?
5. Fit the same model using probit and complementary log-log link functions. Compare the models with respect to their fitted hazard rates and coefficient estimates.

3.3 Consider a data set collected for the Second National Survey on Fertility of Italian women. This data set and its covariates are described in detail in Chap. 4 (Example 4.1). In the following, the time to first childbirth (measured in years) will be the outcome of interest.

1. Convert the data to a set of augmented data. Use 16 intervals for categorizing the continous event times: $[0, 1], (1, 2], \ldots, (14, 15], (15, 30]$.
2. Fit a proportional continuation ratio model to the data and illustrate the baseline hazard rates graphically over time.
3. Interpret the covariate effects obtained from the proportional continuation ratio model. Which effects are significant at level $\alpha = 0.05$?

3.4 Derive the total log-likelihood of a discrete-time survival model with interval-censored observations, assuming that the censoring process does not depend on the parameters of the survival time.

3.5 Recall the definition of the hazard function λ with discrete time T (Eq. (3.1)). Discuss the relationship between this function and the hazard function for continuous time, which is given by

$$\lambda_c(t|\boldsymbol{x}) = \lim_{\Delta t \to 0} \frac{P(t \leq T_c < t + \Delta t \,|\, T_c \geq t, \boldsymbol{x})}{\Delta t}$$

with $\Delta t > 0$.

3.6 Show that the identities for λ_c, S_c, and f stated in Sect. 3.3.1 hold for continuous survival time. Derive the corresponding relations for discrete time.

3.7 Consider the *Weibull model* in continuous time, which is defined as

$$\log(T_c) = \boldsymbol{x}^T \boldsymbol{\xi} + \sigma \cdot \epsilon,$$

where $\boldsymbol{\xi}$ is a vector of coefficients, σ is a positive constant, and ϵ is a noise variable such that the density of T_c becomes equal to the Weibull density

$$f(t) = \varphi\alpha(\varphi t)^{\alpha-1} \exp\left(-(\varphi t)^{\alpha}\right)$$

with $\alpha := 1/\sigma$ and $\boldsymbol{x}^T \boldsymbol{\xi} = -\log(\varphi)$, $\varphi > 0$. Show that this model satisfies the proportional hazards assumption, i.e., verify that its hazard rate can be written as

$$\lambda_c(t|\boldsymbol{x}) = \lambda_0(t) \exp(\boldsymbol{x}^T \boldsymbol{\gamma}),$$

where the baseline hazard $\lambda_0(t)$ does not depend on $\boldsymbol{x}^T \boldsymbol{\gamma}$.

Chapter 4
Evaluation and Model Choice

In Chap. 3 basic hazard models for discrete survival have been introduced and estimation methods have been discussed. In the present chapter we consider diagnostic tools for these models. In particular we discuss test statistics that evaluate the significance of predictors, consider goodness-of-fit tests and residuals as well as measures for the predictive performance and more flexible links. A summary of the concepts presented in this chapter is given in Fig. 4.1.

4.1 Relevance of Predictors: Tests

The discrete survival model considered in the previous chapter has the form

$$\lambda(t|\boldsymbol{x}_i) = h(\gamma_{0t} + \boldsymbol{x}_i^T \boldsymbol{\gamma}), \tag{4.1}$$

where $\boldsymbol{\gamma}$ represents the weights on the explanatory variables. When modeling survival one is in particularly interested in the impact of explanatory variables. For example, in treatment studies one wants to know if there are treatment effects on survival or not. Of course, one also wants to know if the other variables in the model that account for the heterogeneity in the population are relevant. One strategy to evaluate the relevance of variable j within the model uses tests of the null hypothesis

$$H_0 : \gamma_j = 0 \text{ against } H_1 : \gamma_j \neq 0.$$

But this simple pair of hypotheses works only if a variable is represented by only one parameter. If, for example, one has a factorial explanatory variable or if quadratic terms of a continuous variable are included, one has to test simultaneously if all the corresponding parameters are zero. A more general pair of hypotheses that covers

G. Tutz, M. Schmid, *Modeling Discrete Time-to-Event Data*,
Springer Series in Statistics, DOI 10.1007/978-3-319-28158-2_4

Concepts for the evaluation of ...

... relevant predictor variables:

- conduct statistical hypothesis tests, e.g., likelihood ratio, Wald or score tests
- plot residuals, e.g., martingale residuals

... goodness-of-fit:

- compute goodness-of-fit tests
- plot residuals, e.g., deviance residuals or adjusted deviance residuals

... prediction accuracy:

- calculate R^2 coefficients from the test data
- draw prediction error curves and calculate the integrated prediction error $\widehat{PE}_{\text{int}}$
- calculate the Brier score
- draw time-dependent AUC curves and calculate the concordance index C^*

... link / response functions:

- embed the response function in a family of response functions (such as the generalized logistic family)
- estimate the response function nonparametrically

Fig. 4.1 Summary of basic concepts for the evaluation of discrete hazard models

these cases are the linear hypotheses of the form

$$H_0 : \boldsymbol{C\beta} = \boldsymbol{\xi} \text{ against } H_1 : \boldsymbol{C\beta} \neq \boldsymbol{\xi},$$

where $\boldsymbol{C}$ is a fixed matrix of full rank $s \leq p$ and $\boldsymbol{\xi}$ is a fixed vector. The vector $\boldsymbol{\beta}$ in the linear hypothesis $\boldsymbol{C\beta} = \boldsymbol{\xi}$ collects all the parameters of the model, that is, $\boldsymbol{\beta}^T = (\gamma_{01}, \ldots, \gamma_{0q}, \boldsymbol{\gamma}^T)$. For example, if the model contains one factorial explanatory variable with three categories (represented by the coefficients $\boldsymbol{\gamma}^\top = (\gamma_1, \gamma_2)$) and if the aim is to test this covariate against zero, $\boldsymbol{C}$ becomes

$$\begin{bmatrix} 0 \ldots 0\ 1\ 0 \\ 0 \ldots 0\ 0\ 1 \end{bmatrix}$$

with $\boldsymbol{\beta}^T = (\gamma_{01}, \ldots, \gamma_{0q}, \gamma_1, \gamma_2)$ and $\boldsymbol{\xi} = (0, 0)^\top$.

Tests can be derived from the binomial representation of the log-likelihood in (3.25). This approach allows for using tools from binary regression. For example, a common test statistic for linear hypotheses is the likelihood ratio test. It is based on the comparison between two models, the model without constraints and the model fitted under the linear constraints. Let $\hat{\boldsymbol{\beta}}$ denote the ML estimate for the full model (4.1) and $\tilde{\boldsymbol{\beta}}$ denote the estimate under the constraint $\boldsymbol{C}\boldsymbol{\beta} = \boldsymbol{\xi}$. Then the *likelihood ratio statistic* is given by

$$\mathrm{LR} = -2\{l(\tilde{\boldsymbol{\beta}}) - l(\hat{\boldsymbol{\beta}})\},$$

which quantifies the change of the log-likelihood l (given in (3.25)) when evaluated at $\hat{\boldsymbol{\beta}}$ and $\tilde{\boldsymbol{\beta}}$. Under regularity conditions LR follows asymptotically a χ^2-distribution with $s = rk(\boldsymbol{C})$ degrees of freedom, where $rk(\boldsymbol{C})$ denotes the rank of the matrix $\boldsymbol{C}$. That means one fits the model twice, once without constraints and once with the constraints. Then one computes the differences in the log-likelihoods.

Alternative test statistics that can be derived as approximations of LR are the Wald statistic and the score statistic. The *Wald statistic* has the form

$$w = (\boldsymbol{C}\hat{\boldsymbol{\beta}} - \boldsymbol{\xi})^T[\boldsymbol{C}\boldsymbol{F}^{-1}(\hat{\boldsymbol{\beta}})\boldsymbol{C}^T]^{-1}(\boldsymbol{C}\hat{\boldsymbol{\beta}} - \boldsymbol{\xi}),$$

where $\boldsymbol{F}(\boldsymbol{\beta}) = \mathrm{E}(-\partial^2 l(\boldsymbol{\beta})/\partial\boldsymbol{\beta}\partial\boldsymbol{\beta}^T)$ denotes the Fisher information matrix. An advantage of the Wald statistic is that only the full model has to be fitted to obtain $\hat{\boldsymbol{\beta}}$, but no fit under constraints is needed. Note that for scalar $\boldsymbol{\xi}$ the Wald test is equivalent to the t test that is implemented in the R function *glm* (and that was already mentioned in Chap. 3). The third statistic is the *score statistic*

$$u = s^T(\tilde{\boldsymbol{\beta}})\boldsymbol{F}^{-1}(\tilde{\boldsymbol{\beta}})s(\tilde{\boldsymbol{\beta}}),$$

where $s(\boldsymbol{\beta}) = \partial l(\boldsymbol{\beta})/\partial\boldsymbol{\beta} = (\partial l(\boldsymbol{\beta})/\partial\beta_1, \ldots, \partial l(\boldsymbol{\beta})/\partial\beta_p)^T$ is the score function evaluated at the fit of the constrained model.

Asymptotically all three test statistics, the likelihood ratio statistic, the Wald statistic, and the score statistic, have the same distribution

$$\mathrm{LR}, w, u \overset{(a)}{\sim} \chi^2(\mathrm{rank}\,\boldsymbol{C}),$$

see, for example, Fahrmeir and Tutz (2001).

Example 4.1 Time Between Cohabitation and First Childbirth

For illustration we analyze a data set that was collected for the Second National Survey on Fertility. This survey is a retrospective study on Italian women born between 1946 and 1975. An aim of the study was to investigate the effects of socio-economic and demographic factors on fertility patterns in Italy. Using a subsample of $n = 3164$ women (originally analyzed by Muggeo et al. 2009), we consider the time between the beginning of cohabitation and first childbirth (measured in years, median: 1.25 years, censoring rate: 14 %) as the primary outcome. Because multiple events (here, childbirths) were recorded for some of the women, another outcome variable is the time between first and second childbirth ($n = 2720$, median: 3.33 years, censoring rate: 35 %). Explanatory variables include age at the beginning of cohabitation, geographic area, and the number of siblings in the families of origin of the women (see Table 4.1).

Table 4.1 Explanatory variables for the time between cohabitation and first childbirth (Second National Survey on Fertility in Italy)

Variable	Categories/unit	Sample proportion/median (range)
Age at the beginning of cohabitation	Years	22.7 (12.20–49.10)
Cohort of birth	1946–1950	20 %
	1951–1955	21 %
	1956–1960	20 %
	1961–1965	21 %
	1966–1975	18 %
Educational attainment	First stage basic	21 %
	Second stage basic	33 %
	Upper secondary	37 %
	Degree	9 %
Geographic area	North	45 %
	Center	22 %
	South	33 %
Occupational status	Worker	48 %
	Non-worker	52 %
Siblings in the family of origin of the woman	0	7 %
	1	29 %
	2	24 %
	≥ 3	40 %

In the following we will analyze the results of various statistical hypothesis tests that were obtained from modeling the time to first childbirth (grouped in years). Predictor variables included all six covariates presented in Table 4.1. Observations with missing values in any of the predictor variables were excluded from the analysis (resulting in a reduced sample size of $n = 3147$). Also, event times that were larger than 10 years were considered censored (resulting in a censoring rate equal to 14.8 %).

Table 4.2 shows the results that were obtained from fitting a discrete-time hazard model with logistic link to the data. The parameter estimates $\hat{\gamma}$ in Table 4.2 confirm several often observed results: For example, women with a high educational attainment tend to give birth to their first children later than women with low educational attainment. Also, women belonging to later cohorts (1960+) tend to give birth to their first children later than earlier cohorts born before 1961. Table 4.3 shows the corresponding p-values obtained from likelihood ratio, Wald, and score tests. Each test was applied to each of the covariates separately in order to investigate statistical significance ("marginal"/"type II" tests). Obviously, all covariates are significant at level $\alpha = 0.05$, with only small differences between the covariate-specific test statistics. □

Table 4.2 Years between cohabitation to first childbirth. The table shows the parameter estimates and estimated standard deviations that were obtained from fitting a logistic discrete-time hazard model to the data (ageCo = age at cohabitation, edu = educational attainment, area = geographic area, cohort = cohort of birth, occ = occupational status, sibl = number of siblings)

Covariate	Parameter estimate	Est. std. error
ageCo	−0.0499	0.0069
edu First stage basic (Ref. category)		
edu Second stage basic	0.0249	0.0745
edu Upper secondary	−0.2106	0.0786
edu degree	−0.2693	0.1090
cohort 1946–1950 (Ref. category)		
cohort 1951–1955	−0.0253	0.0764
cohort 1956–1960	−0.2346	0.0781
cohort 1961–1965	−0.2920	0.0790
cohort 1966–1975	−0.7555	0.0907
area North (Ref. category)		
area Center	0.2844	0.0624
area South	0.6695	0.0617
occ worker (Ref. category)		
occ non-worker	0.2296	0.0528
sibl	0.0549	0.0267

Table 4.3 Years between cohabitation to first childbirth. The table shows the test statistics and *p*-values of likelihood ratio, Wald, and score tests that were obtained from fitting a logistic discrete-time hazard model to the data (ageCo = age at cohabitation, edu = educational attainment, area = geographic area, cohort = cohort of birth, occ = occupational status, sibl = number of siblings)

	LR test		Wald test		Score test	
Covariate	Statistic	*p* value	Statistic	*p*-value	Statistic	*p* value
ageCo	53.395	<0.00001	51.774	<0.00001	53.395	<0.00001
edu	18.721	0.00031	18.768	0.00031	18.721	0.00030
cohort	92.095	<0.00001	88.456	<0.00001	92.095	<0.00001
area	117.863	<0.00001	117.898	<0.00001	117.863	<0.00001
occ	18.862	0.00001	18.905	0.00001	18.862	0.00001
sibl	4.220	0.03993	4.217	0.04002	4.220	0.03997

4.2 Residuals and Goodness-of-Fit

In the preceding section, maximum likelihood estimation of discrete hazard models was based on the binary representation of transitions between categories. However, when the issue is to analyze residuals and goodness-of-fit, one should bear in mind that the original data consist of n independent observations $(t_i, \delta_i, \boldsymbol{x}_i)$. Therefore the deviances and residuals obtained from fitting a binary model are not appropriate here. In the following we will present strategies on how to construct valid residuals and goodness-of-fit statistics for discrete survival data.

4.2.1 No Censoring

In a model without censoring, the discrete time $T_i \in \{1, \ldots, q\}$ follows a multinomial distribution. In general, a vector $\boldsymbol{Y}^T = (Y_1, \ldots, Y_k)$ is multinomially distributed, $\boldsymbol{Y} \sim M(n, (\pi_1, \ldots, \pi_k))$, if the probability mass function is given by

$$f(y_1, \ldots, y_k) = \begin{cases} \frac{n!}{y_1! \ldots y_k!} \pi_1^{y_1} \ldots \pi_k^{y_k} & y_i \in \{0, \ldots, n\}, \\ & \sum_i y_i = n, \\ 0 & \text{otherwise}, \end{cases}$$

where $\boldsymbol{\pi}^T = (\pi_1, \ldots, \pi_k)$ is a probability vector, that is, $\pi_i \in [0, 1]$, $\sum_i \pi_i = 1$.

In discrete survival one considers the multinomially distributed vector $(T_{i1}, \ldots, T_{ik}) \sim M(n_i, (\pi_1, \ldots, \pi_k))$, where T_{is} counts the number of responses in period s given that n_i observations are available at the same measurement value $\boldsymbol{x}_i$. If $n_i = 1$ just one of the variables $T_{i1}, \ldots, T_{ik}$ takes value 1.

Let us first consider the case without censoring and data collected at N measurement values $\boldsymbol{x}_i$, $i = 1, \ldots, N$, with n_i observations at $\boldsymbol{x}_i$. In other words, the covariate values (and thus the observations) can be grouped into N groups. Tests are the same as in categorical data analysis (see Tutz 2012 or Agresti 2013). With $\hat{\boldsymbol{\beta}}$ denoting the maximum likelihood estimate, one obtains the fitted hazard $\hat{\lambda}(t|\boldsymbol{x}_i) = h(\gamma_{0t} + \boldsymbol{x}_i^T \hat{\boldsymbol{\gamma}})$ and the fitted probabilities

$$\hat{\pi}_{it} = \hat{P}(T = t|\boldsymbol{x}_i) = \hat{\lambda}(t|\boldsymbol{x}_i) \prod_{s=1}^{t-1} (1 - \hat{\lambda}(s|\boldsymbol{x}_i)).$$

Moreover, let p_{it} denote the proportion of observations in period t in subpopulation i. An appropriate goodness-of-fit measure is the *Pearson statistic*

$$\chi_P^2 = \sum_{i=1}^{N} \sum_{t=1}^{k} n_i \frac{(p_{it} - \hat{\pi}_{it})^2}{\hat{\pi}_{it}},$$

where the inner sum represents the squared *Pearson residual*

$$r_{P,i}^2 = \sum_{t=1}^{k} n_i \frac{(p_{it} - \hat{\pi}_{it})^2}{\hat{\pi}_{it}}.$$

The smaller the Pearson statistic (i.e., the smaller the sum of Pearson residuals), the better the model fit. An alternative goodness-of-fit statistic is the *deviance*

$$D = 2\sum_{i=1}^{N} n_i \sum_{t=1}^{k} p_{it} \log\left(\frac{p_{it}}{\hat{\pi}_{it}}\right),$$

with the corresponding quadratic *deviance residuals* given by

$$r_{D,i}^2 = 2n_i \sum_{t=1}^{k} p_{it} \log\left(\frac{p_{it}}{\hat{\pi}_{it}}\right).$$

Similar to the Pearson statistic, the deviance becomes small in situations where the model fits the data well. Under the assumptions of the fixed cells asymptotic ($n_i/N \to \gamma_i \in (0,1)$) and regularity conditions, χ_P^2 and D are asymptotically χ^2-distributed with $N(k-1)-p$ degrees of freedom, where p is the number of estimated parameters. When using a significance level α the model is considered inappropriate if both or one of the test statistics are larger than the $1-\alpha$-quantile of the corresponding distribution, $\chi_{1-\alpha}^2(N(k-1)-p)$. It should be noted that these tests serve as goodness-of-fit tests only if n_i is not too small. For $n_i = 1$, with only one observation being available at fixed value $\boldsymbol{x}_i$, they are useless since no asymptotic distribution is available.

Nevertheless, residuals can also be used as diagnostic tools in the case $n_i = 1$. In this case the squared deviance residual for observation i is

$$r_{D,i}^2 = 2\log\left(\frac{1}{\hat{\pi}_{it_i}}\right) = -2\log(\hat{\lambda}_{it_i}) - \sum_{s=1}^{t_i-1} 2\log(1-\hat{\lambda}_{is}),$$

where $\hat{\lambda}_{is} = \hat{\lambda}(s|\boldsymbol{x}_i)$. It can be re-written in a form that is familiar from binary response models,

$$r_{D,i}^2 = -2\sum_{s=1}^{t_i} \{y_{is}\log(\hat{\lambda}_{is}) + (1-y_{is})\log(1-\hat{\lambda}_{is})\}, \quad (4.2)$$

where $(y_{i1},\ldots,y_{it_i}) = (0,\ldots,0,1)$ denotes the transitions over periods. Thus, the deviance residual can be written as the residual for the binary response vector that codes the non-transitions. How observations and fit are compared becomes even more obvious in the representation

$$r_{D,i}^2 = 2\sum_{s=1}^{t_i} \left\{y_{is}\log\left(\frac{y_{is}}{\hat{\lambda}_{is}}\right) + (1-y_{is})\log\left(\frac{1-y_{is}}{1-\hat{\lambda}_{is}}\right)\right\}, \quad (4.3)$$

which shows that at each time point the discrepancy between data and fit is measured by $\log(y_{is}/\hat{\lambda}_{is})$ if $y_{is} = 1$ and by $\log(1 - y_{is})/(1 - \hat{\lambda}_{is})$ if $y_{is} = 0$. For the Pearson statistic no such representation seems available.

A transformation of the deviance residuals that typically is closer to a normal distribution (in case of a well fitting model) is the *adjusted deviance residual*

$$d_i = \sum_{s=1}^{t_i} \left\{ \text{sign}(y_{is} - \hat{\lambda}_{is}) \sqrt{y_{is} \log\left(\frac{y_{is}}{\hat{\lambda}_{is}}\right) + (1 - y_{is}) \log\left(\frac{1 - y_{is}}{1 - \hat{\lambda}_{is}}\right)} \right\}$$
$$+ \sum_{s=1}^{t_i} \left\{ (1 - 2\hat{\lambda}_{is}) / \sqrt{\hat{\lambda}_{is}(1 - \hat{\lambda}_{is}) \cdot 36} \right\} . \quad (4.4)$$

Note that we assume $0 \cdot \log(0) \equiv 0$ in (4.4). When considering this type of residual, model fit can be assessed by inspecting normal quantile–quantile plots.

4.2.2 *Deviance in the Case of Censoring*

In the presence of censoring, analysis of the fitted model is more complicated. In this case one models the observed time periods $\min(T_i, C_i)$. In particular, with $q = k - 1$ one can only observe the combined events

$$(t, \delta = 1) : \{T = t, C \geq t\}, t = 1, \dots, q,$$
$$(t, \delta = 0) : \{T > t, C = t\}, t = 1, \dots, q.$$

Therefore one has to distinguish between $2q$ categories. Under the random censoring assumption the corresponding probabilities are

$$\pi_t^{(\delta)} = \begin{cases} P(T = t)P(C \geq t) \text{ if } \delta = 1, \\ P(T > t)P(C = t) \text{ if } \delta = 0, \end{cases}$$

which in closed form can be written as

$$\pi_t^{(\delta)} = P(T = t)^{\delta} P(T > t)^{1-\delta} P(C \geq t)^{\delta} P(C = t)^{1-\delta}.$$

Let the probabilities for observation i be collected in $\boldsymbol{\pi}_i^T = ((\boldsymbol{\pi}_i^{(1)})^T, (\boldsymbol{\pi}_i^{(0)})^T)$, where $\boldsymbol{\pi}_i^{(1)} := (\pi_{i1}^{(1)}, \dots, \pi_{iq}^{(1)})^T$, and $\boldsymbol{\pi}_i^{(0)} := (\pi_{i1}^{(1)}, \dots, \pi_{iq}^{(0)})^T$. Then the corresponding deviance for grouped observations has the form

$$D = 2\sum_{i=1}^{N} n_i \left\{ \sum_{r=1}^{q} p_{ir}^{(1)} \log\left(\frac{p_{ir}^{(1)}}{\hat{\pi}_{ir}^{(1)}}\right) + \sum_{r=1}^{q} p_{ir}^{(0)} \log\left(\frac{p_{ir}^{(0)}}{\hat{\pi}_{ir}^{(0)}}\right) \right\}$$

with the terms on the right-hand side given by

$$\log\left(\frac{p_{ir}^{(1)}}{\hat{\pi}_{ir}^{(1)}}\right) = \log\left(\frac{P(T_i = r)}{\hat{P}(T_i = r)}\right) + \log\left(\frac{P(C_i \geq r)}{\hat{P}(C_i \geq r)}\right),$$

$$\log\left(\frac{p_{ir}^{(0)}}{\hat{\pi}_{ir}^{(0)}}\right) = \log\left(\frac{P(T_i > r)}{\hat{P}(T_i > r)}\right) + \log\left(\frac{P(C_i = r)}{\hat{P}(C_i = r)}\right).$$

In order to use the deviance as a goodness-of-fit statistic one has to specify two models, one for the survival time and one for the censoring process. Goodness-of-fit then refers to both models. This is somewhat unsatisfying since one would prefer to evaluate the fit of the survival model separately.

Although the likelihood based on the binary variables that code transitions does not yield a goodness-of-fit statistic, it can be used to define residuals also in the case of censored observations. For single observations (i.e., $n_i = 1$) the contribution of the ith observation to the corresponding "deviance" $D = -2l$ (with l denoting the log-likelihood (3.25)) is

$$\begin{aligned} r_{D,i}^2 &= -2\left\{\delta_i \log(\hat{P}(T_i = t_i)) + (1-\delta_i)\log(\hat{P}(T_i > t_i))\right\} \\ &= -2\sum_{s=1}^{t_i} y_{is}\log(\hat{\lambda}_{is}) + (1-y_{is})\log(1-\hat{\lambda}_{is}), \end{aligned} \quad (4.5)$$

which is the same as (4.2). We consider it as "squared deviance residuals" also in the case of censored observations.

4.2.3 Martingale Residuals

An alternative type of residual that takes censoring into account and is particularly suited for assessing the functional forms of predictor effects is the *martingale residual* defined by

$$m_i = \delta_i - \sum_{s=1}^{t_i} \hat{\lambda}_{is}, \quad i = 1, \ldots, n, \quad (4.6)$$

where $\hat{\lambda}_{is} = \hat{\lambda}(s|\boldsymbol{x}_i)$. Here, $\Lambda(t_i) = \sum_{s=1}^{t_i} \hat{\lambda}_{is}$ measures the cumulative risk of observation i up to time t_i. This definition is equivalent to the cumulative hazard function in survival analysis for continuous time (see Sect. 3.3.1 or Klein and Moeschberger 2003). The idea of the martingale residual is to compare for each individual the *observed* number of events up to t_i (measured by δ_i) with the *expected* number of events up to t_i (measured by $\Lambda(t_i)$). If one uses the binary variables representation with $(y_{i1}, \ldots, y_{it_i}) = (0, \ldots, 0, \delta_i)$ the residuals can be defined as

$$m_i = \sum_{s=1}^{t_i} (y_{is} - \hat{\lambda}_{is}), \quad i = 1, \ldots, n.$$

Thus the martingale residuals use the differences between the transition indicators and the estimated probabilities of failure, in contrast to the deviance residuals, which use the log-transformed proportion of observation and fit (Eq. (4.3)). It can be shown that for the logistic model the martingale residuals sum up to zero (Exercise 4.1).

For a well fitting model that includes all relevant predictors, the martingale residuals should be "random" and uncorrelated with the covariate values. Following this idea, martingale residuals can be used to assess the importance and the functional forms of the covariates in a discrete-time survival model. For each covariate this is done by plotting the residuals vs. the covariate values of interest. Adding a smooth estimate to the plot (e.g., obtained via a P-spline estimator) provides further information on the functional form of the respective covariate effect (see Example 4.2).

Example 4.2 Promotions in Rank for Biochemists

For illustration we consider a data set from the book by Allison (1995). It contains information on the careers of 301 biochemists who were employed as assistant professors at graduate departments in the USA. The event of interest is the promotion of a biochemist to the rank of associate professor during his/her career. The data are available under the link http://support.sas.com/publishing/bbu/zip/61339.zip. Observed event times were measured in years and ranged from 1 year to 10 years; 28 % of the event times were censored. The variables that will be used to model the time to promotion are presented in Table 4.4.

In the following we will analyze the martingale and deviance residuals obtained from a discrete-time hazard model with logit link. Two models are considered: The first model is the full model with the six covariates "Ph.D. from medical school?", "prestige of the Ph.D. institution," "prestige of the first employing institution," "selectivity of the undergraduate institution," "cumulative number of articles," and "cumulative number of citations." This model is compared to a "reduced" model, which is the same as the full model but without the covariate "cumulative number of articles." Note that the covariates "cumulative number of articles" and "cumulative number of citations" are time-dependent. We start with the reduced model: In Fig. 4.2 the martingale residuals of the reduced model are plotted vs. the number of articles in year 1. In addition, the plot contains a trend line that was estimated via a P-spline with cross-validated smoothing parameter. The functional form of the trend line suggests that the number of articles in year 1 is an influential covariate and should be included in the model, as there is a positive linear effect of this variable on the martingale residuals. Similarly, the normal quantile–quantile plot of the adjusted deviance residuals of the reduced model (Fig. 4.3) indicates deviations from normality, suggesting that the model fit is suboptimal.

Table 4.4 Variables that are used to model the time to promotion in rank for biochemists (Allison 1995). Note: None of the biochemists had more than two employers during the observation period

Variable	Categories/unit	Sample proportion/median (range)
Selectivity of undergraduate institution	Score	5 (1–7)
Ph.D. from medical school?	Yes/no	63 %/37 %
Prestige of the Ph.D. institution	Score	3.36 (0.92–4.62)
Number of articles published in year 1		3 (0–22), $n = 301$
Number of articles published in year 2		4 (0–27), $n = 299$
Number of articles published in year 3		5 (0–36), $n = 292$
Number of articles published in year 4		7 (0–44), $n = 263$
Number of articles published in year 5		7 (0–35), $n = 211$
Number of articles published in year 6		8 (0–36), $n = 149$
Number of articles published in year 7		8 (0–32), $n = 96$
Number of articles published in year 8		8 (0–44), $n = 59$
Number of articles published in year 9		6 (2–49), $n = 42$
Number of articles published in year 10		6 (2–35), $n = 29$
Number of citations in year 1		20 (0–420), $n = 301$
Number of citations in year 2		25 (0–421), $n = 299$
Number of citations in year 3		32.5 (0–566), $n = 292$
Number of citations in year 4		41 (0–566), $n = 263$
Number of citations in year 5		45 (0–579), $n = 211$
Number of citations in year 6		53 (0–430), $n = 149$
Number of citations in year 7		53 (0–496), $n = 96$
Number of citations in year 8		39 (0–724), $n = 59$
Number of citations in year 9		29.5 (1–864), $n = 42$
Number of citations in year 10		30 (1–566), $n = 29$
Prestige of first employing institution	Score	2.56 (0.65–4.64)
Prestige of second employing institution (= prestige of 1st institution if biochemist did not change employer)	Score	2.52 (0.65–4.64)
Year of employer change (if biochemist changed employer)		4.5 (2–10), $n = 74$

Figure 4.4 shows the martingale residuals obtained from the full model (including the cumulative number of articles as time-dependent covariate). Now the P-spline estimate is close to zero, indicating only very little correlation between the number of articles in year 1 and the residuals. Also, the adjusted deviance residuals of the full model (Fig. 4.5) are slightly closer to normality than the respective residuals of the reduced model in Fig. 4.3. These findings indicate that the model fit improves by adding the cumulative number of articles to the model. Still, Fig. 4.5 shows that there remain deviations of the residuals from normality, which might have been caused by other missing covariates or by an insufficient small-sample approximation of the normal distribution.

□

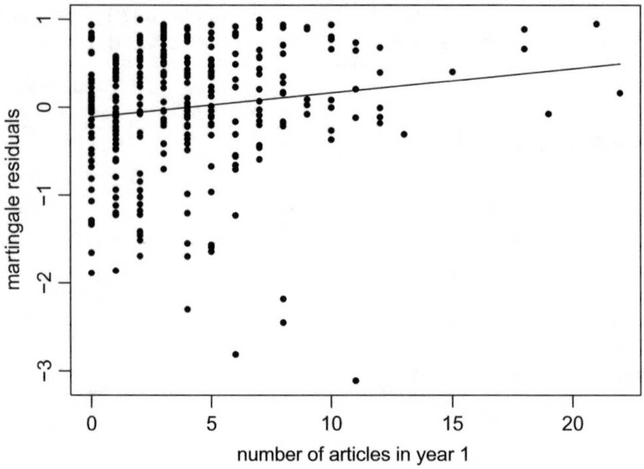

Fig. 4.2 Promotions in rank for biochemists. The plot shows the martingale residuals obtained from the reduced model with covariates "Ph.D. from medical school?", "prestige of the Ph.D. institution," "prestige of the first employing institution," "selectivity of the undergraduate institution," and "cumulative number of citations." The residuals are plotted vs. the values of the variable "number of articles in year 1." The trend line was obtained via a P-spline with cross-validated smoothing parameter. Obviously, there is a positive effect of the variable on the residuals, indicating that the number of published articles should be added to the model equation

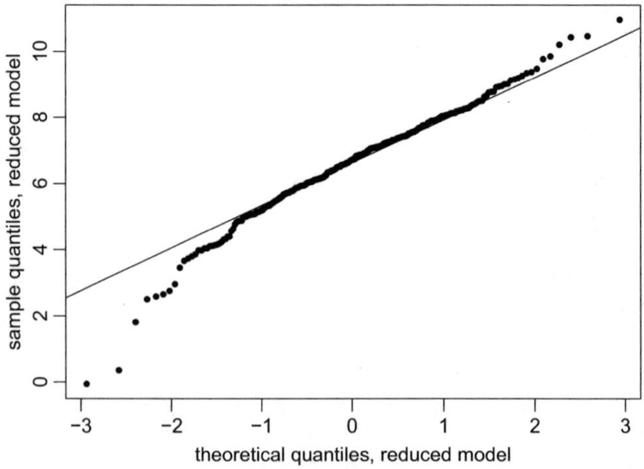

Fig. 4.3 Promotions in rank for biochemists. The figure contains a normal quantile–quantile plot of the adjusted deviance residuals obtained from the reduced model with covariates "Ph.D. from medical school?", "prestige of the Ph.D. institution," "prestige of the first employing institution," "selectivity of the undergraduate institution," and "cumulative number of citations." The plot indicates deviations from normality.

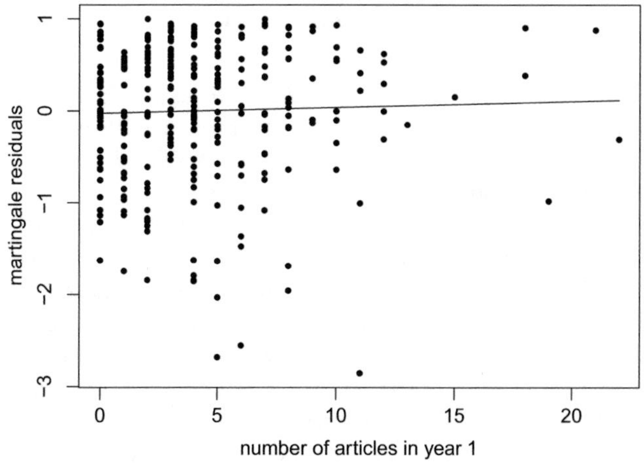

Fig. 4.4 Promotions in rank for biochemists. The plot shows the martingale residuals obtained from the full model with covariates "Ph.D. from medical school?", "prestige of the Ph.D. institution," "prestige of the first employing institution," "selectivity of the undergraduate institution," "cumulative number of citations," and "cumulative number of articles." The residuals are plotted vs. the values of the variable "number of articles in year 1." The trend line (obtained via fitting a P-spline with cross-validated smoothing parameter) suggests that there is only little correlation between the number of articles in year 1 and the residuals

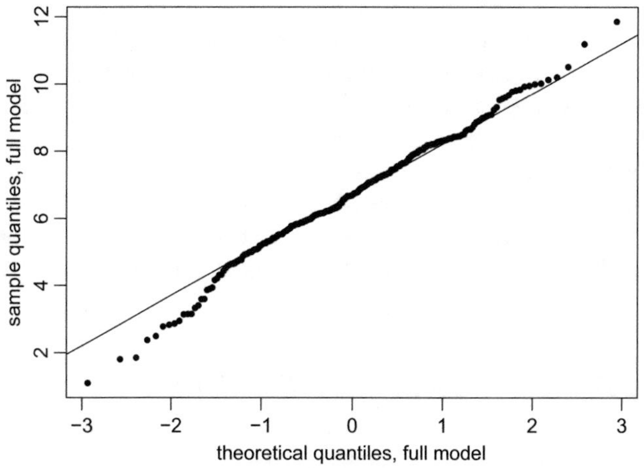

Fig. 4.5 Promotions in rank for biochemists. The figure contains a normal quantile–quantile plot of the adjusted deviance residuals obtained from the full model with covariates "Ph.D. from medical school?", "prestige of the Ph.D. institution," "prestige of the first employing institution," "selectivity of the undergraduate institution," "cumulative number of citations," and "cumulative number of articles." The figure indicates a slightly improved model fit compared to the reduced model (Fig. 4.3)

4.3 Measuring Predictive Performance

In the previous section we considered methods for assessing the goodness-of-fit of parametric regression models. These methods provide information on whether a survival model is well *calibrated*, i.e., on how well the fitted survival probabilities agree with their corresponding observed proportions.

In addition to assessing goodness-of-fit, it is often of interest to measure the performance of survival models with respect to *predicting* survival of future observations. This issue is important in many applications, because a high goodness-of-fit in the observed data does not necessarily imply that the model will perform equally well on future data. Also, statistical hypothesis tests often provide only little information about whether a covariate (or the whole model) is important for the prediction of future survival. For example, if sample sizes are large, covariate effects might be significant even if their effect on survival (measured, e.g., by the magnitude of the parameters $\boldsymbol{\gamma}$) is small.

In the following we will consider three approaches that are designed to measure the prediction accuracy of survival models. For all approaches we assume that the survival model was fitted on a learning data set $(t_i, \delta_i, \boldsymbol{x}_i)$, $i = 1, \ldots, n$ (as in Chap. 3) and that prediction accuracy is evaluated on an additional independent test data set $(t_j^{\mathcal{T}}, \delta_j^{\mathcal{T}}, \boldsymbol{x}_j^{\mathcal{T}})$, $j = 1, \ldots, n^{\mathcal{T}}$, that follows the same distribution as the learning data. The superscript $\mathcal{T}$ indicates that the respective observations are from the test data.

Note that using independent sets of learning and test data is important for measuring predictive performance, as this strategy helps to avoid overoptimistic predictions that would be obtained if the same data were used for both model fitting and the evaluation of prediction accuracy. In situations where an independent test data set is not available, cross-validation techniques may be applied. In this case the idea is to split the data multiple times into subsets of learning and test data. Cross-validated predictions are then obtained by (1) fitting the model to all learning data subsets, (2) evaluating the model fits on the respective test data subsets, and (3) averaging the resulting estimates of prediction accuracy. For an overview of cross-validation methods see, for example, Molinaro et al. (2005) and Kim (2009).

4.3.1 Predictive Deviance and R^2 Coefficients

The predictive deviance evaluated on the test data is given by

$$D = -2\sum_{j=1}^{n^{\mathcal{T}}}\{\delta_j^{\mathcal{T}}\log(\hat{P}(T_j^{\mathcal{T}} = t_j^{\mathcal{T}})) + (1-\delta_j^{\mathcal{T}})\log(\hat{P}(T_j^{\mathcal{T}} > t_j^{\mathcal{T}}))\}$$

$$= -2\sum_{j=1}^{n^{\mathcal{T}}}\sum_{s=1}^{t_j^{\mathcal{T}}}\{y_{js}^{\mathcal{T}}\log(\hat{\lambda}_{js}) + (1-y_{js}^{\mathcal{T}})\log(1-\hat{\lambda}_{js})\}, \qquad (4.7)$$

where $\hat{\lambda}_{js} = \hat{P}(T_j^{\mathcal{T}} = s \mid T_j^{\mathcal{T}} \geq s, \boldsymbol{x}_j^{\mathcal{T}})$ and where $T_j^{\mathcal{T}}$ are the (unobserved) true survival times in the test data. As before, $(y_{j1}^{\mathcal{T}}, \ldots, y_{jt_j^{\mathcal{T}}}^{\mathcal{T}}) = (0, \ldots, 0, 1)$ if $\delta_j^{\mathcal{T}} = 1$ and $(y_{j1}^{\mathcal{T}}, \ldots, y_{jt_j^{\mathcal{T}}}^{\mathcal{T}}) = (0, \ldots, 0, 0)$ if $\delta_j^{\mathcal{T}} = 0$ denote the transitions over periods.

The predictive deviance is equivalent to the negative log-likelihood (3.25) of a binomial regression model evaluated on the test data. Consequently, prediction accuracy is large if (4.7) is small and vice versa.

Note that the predictive deviance is an unbounded measure. To facilitate interpretation, it is sometimes convenient to consider R^2-type coefficients given by

$$R^2 = \frac{1 - \exp\left((\sum_{j=1}^{n^{\mathcal{T}}} t_j^{\mathcal{T}})^{-1}(D - D_0)\right)}{1 - \exp(-(\sum_{j=1}^{n^{\mathcal{T}}} t_j^{\mathcal{T}})^{-1} D_0)}, \qquad (4.8)$$

where D_0 is the predictive deviance obtained from a *null model* without covariate information. It can be shown that (4.8) is equal to 1 if prediction accuracy is perfect and equal to zero if predictions are based on the null model (Nagelkerke 1991). However, R^2 coefficients have several problems when used in practical applications. In particular, R^2 coefficients are often much smaller than 1 even in case of very well-predicting models, which makes interpretation difficult. Also, in contrast to the predictive deviance, it is unclear whether R^2 coefficients are "proper" in the sense that they become maximal if computed from the true underlying model (cf. Gneiting and Raftery 2007).

Example 4.3 Promotions in Rank for Biochemists

In Chap. 3 we introduced five different types of link functions for discrete-time hazard models (logistic, probit, Gompertz, Gumbel, and exponential). Because the models result in different interpretations regarding the magnitude of coefficients and the significance of predictor effects, it is of interest to investigate which model is most suitable to predict future or unseen survival times.

Here we use the predictive deviance to investigate which link function results in the best prediction accuracy for the biochemists data. For statistical analysis we used the six covariates "Ph.D. from medical school?", "prestige of the Ph.D. institution," "prestige of the first employing institution," "selectivity of the undergraduate institution," "cumulative number of articles," and "cumulative number of citations." To compare the models with respect to their predictive performance, we calculated the predictive deviance in combination with resampling. This was done as follows: First, we used 50 random splits of the data and generated 50 learning data sets (of size $2/3 \cdot n \approx 200$ each) and 50 test data sets (of size $1/3 \cdot n \approx 101$ each). The discrete-time hazard models were fitted to each of the 50 training data sets, and the respective predictive deviances were computed from the 50 test data sets.

The resulting 50 values of the predictive deviance are visualized in Fig. 4.6 for the logistic, probit, Gompertz, and Gumbel models. It is seen that the logistic model resulted in the best performance among the models. The Gumbel model showed the worst performance; the probit and Gompertz models also performed slightly worse than the logistic model. Note that the exponential model was excluded from this study because of its numerical instability (which is due to the restrictions that have to be imposed on the parameter space, cf. Sect. 3.2.2). □

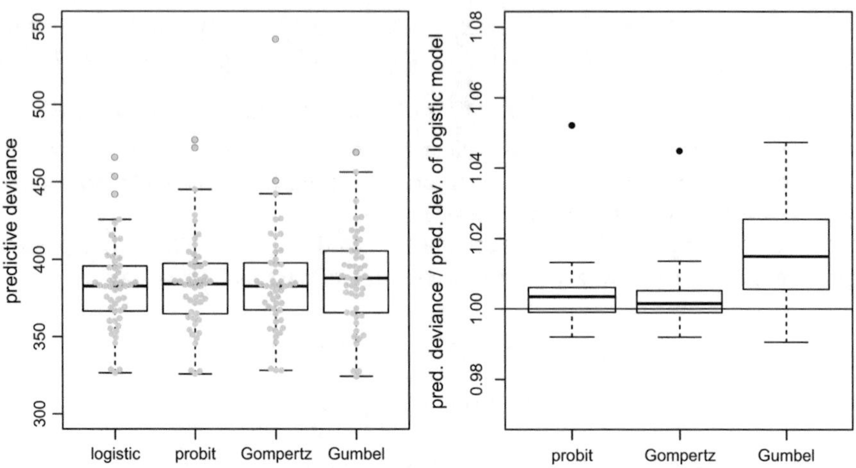

Fig. 4.6 The *left panel* shows the predictive deviances for the biochemists data, as obtained from 50 test samples of size $n^{\mathcal{T}} = 101$. The *right panel* shows the predictive deviances of the probit, Gompertz, and Gumbel models divided by the respective predictive deviances obtained from the logistic model. Therefore, the *right panel* provides information on the percentage decrease in prediction accuracy that resulted from using the probit, Gompertz, and Gumbel link functions instead of the logistic link function. Note that two outlying values in the Gompertz and Gumbel models were omitted from the panels

4.3.2 Prediction Error Curves

Prediction error curves (*PE curves*) are a time-dependent measure of prediction error that is based on the squared distance between the *predicted* survival functions $\hat{S}_j(t) = \prod_{s=1}^{t}(1 - \hat{\lambda}_{js})$, $j = 1, \ldots, n^{\mathcal{T}}$, and the corresponding *observed* survival functions $\tilde{S}_j(t) = I(t < t_j^{\mathcal{T}})$, where $I(\cdot)$ denotes the indicator function. By definition, $I(t < t_j^{\mathcal{T}}) = 1$ if $t < t_j^{\mathcal{T}}$ and 0 otherwise. Therefore, the observed survival functions are equal to 1 as long as an observation is still alive and become 0 after the event of interest has occurred. For each time point t under consideration, PE curves measure the deviation of what we *observe* (i.e., $\tilde{S}_j(t)$) from what is *predicted* from a statistical model (i.e., $\hat{S}_j(t)$).

For fixed t, the PE curve (which includes *inverse probability of censoring weights* $w_j^{\mathcal{T}}(t)$) is given by

$$\widehat{\mathrm{PE}}(t) = \frac{1}{n^{\mathcal{T}}} \sum_{j=1}^{n^{\mathcal{T}}} \left[\frac{\delta_j^{\mathcal{T}}(1 - \tilde{S}_j(t))}{\hat{G}_j(t_j^{\mathcal{T}} - 1)} + \frac{\tilde{S}_j(t)}{\hat{G}_j(t)} \right] \left(\hat{S}_j(t) - \tilde{S}_j(t) \right)^2$$

$$= \frac{1}{n^{\mathcal{T}}} \sum_{j=1}^{n^{\mathcal{T}}} w_j^{\mathcal{T}}(t) \left(\hat{S}_j(t) - \tilde{S}_j(t) \right)^2 . \quad (4.9)$$

The weights $w_j^{\mathcal{T}}(t)$ contain the expression $\hat{G}_j(t) = \hat{P}(C_j > t \,|\, \boldsymbol{x}_j^{\mathcal{T}})$, which is the estimated survival function of the censoring process obtained from the learning data. Their role will be discussed later. The second factor in (4.9) represents the basic measure of discrepancy, namely the squared deviation between observed and predicted survival for fixed t. One problem with this squared distance is that it can only be computed from the test data

(a) if an event was observed at or before t (implying that one knows that $\tilde{S}_j(t) = 0$), or
(b) if the person is still alive at t (implying that one knows that the event occurred after t, that is, $\tilde{S}_j(t) = 1$).

Situations (a) and (b) are reflected by the two summands in the first factor of (4.9): The numerator $\delta_j^{\mathcal{T}}(1-\tilde{S}_j(t))$ of the first summand becomes equal to 1 in situation (a) and 0 otherwise, whereas the numerator $\tilde{S}_j(t)$ of the second summand becomes equal to 1 in situation (b) and zero otherwise, yielding the weights $w_j^{\mathcal{T}} = 1/\hat{G}_j(t_j^{\mathcal{T}} - 1)$ for (a) and $w_j^{\mathcal{T}} = 1/\hat{G}_j(t)$ for (b).

Problems arise for observations that were censored before t because the squared deviation in (4.9) cannot be computed in this case. Thus, these observations are not used in the computation of the PE curve at t. On the other hand, completely ignoring the observations that were censored before t would lead to a bias. This is the main reason why the inverse probability of censoring weights $w_j^{\mathcal{T}}, j = 1, \ldots, n^{\mathcal{T}}$, are included in (4.9). The idea of inverse probability of censoring weighting is as follows: Assume that we were in the (hypothetical) situation where all survival times had been fully observed (no censoring). In this situation, we could calculate $\widehat{\mathrm{PE}}(t)$ by computing the squared deviation $(\hat{S}_j(t) - \tilde{S}_j(t))^2$ for all t using the full data sample containing all observations. As explained above, however, this calculation is not possible in the presence of censoring, implying that—for a fixed time point t—we have to rely on the reduced sample of observations that were not censored before t. The idea is then to "reconstruct" the characteristics of the unknown full data sample by using the weights $w_j^{\mathcal{T}}$. These weights account for the inverse probability that an observation in the test data is censored after t. Assume, for example, that $\hat{G}_j$ is large (e.g., close to 1) for a fixed time point under consideration. Then it is highly likely that the censoring event will occur after this time point, implying that $w_j^{\mathcal{T}}$ is close to 1 as well. Hence the value of $w_j^{\mathcal{T}}$ reflects the fact that one is confident that what is contained in the observed data corresponds approximately to what would have been contained in the full data sample without censoring. On the other hand, if $\hat{G}_j$ is small, it is likely that the observations that have been fully observed up to the time point of interest constitute only a small fraction of those observations that would be available in the full data sample. Consequently, they are up-weighted to reconstruct the structure of the full data sample.

The inverse probability of censoring approach is similar to strategies for avoiding selection bias and for dealing with missing data in survey research. For example, in surveys underrepresented groups of observations are often up-weighted by their inverse probabilities of being included in the survey to obtain unbiased estimates. Similarly, groups with missing data are often up-weighted by their inverse probabilities of being completely observed. Mathematically, inverse probability of censoring weighting guarantees the consistency of the estimator $\widehat{PE}(t)$ for the mean of the random variable $(\hat{S}_j(t) - \tilde{S}_j(t))^2$; for details, see in particular van der Laan and Robins (2003) and also Gerds and Schumacher (2006).

Obtaining Estimates of the Censoring Process

In order to compute the inverse probability of censoring weights, the survival function of the censoring process, $G_j(t) = P(C_j > t \,|\, \boldsymbol{x}_j^T)$, has to be estimated. Estimates of $\hat{G}_j$ can be obtained from the learning data analogously to those of the survival function S_j, that is, by representing the censoring model as a binary regression model. But now censoring is the event of interest, and the observation of survival plays the role of the censoring process. Consider, for example, the situation where $\delta_i = 1$ and the observed survival time is t_i. It follows that the censoring event must take place after $t_i - 1$ and that the unobserved censoring time C_i has been larger than $t_i - 1$ (because $T_i \le C_i$ in this case). Consequently, the binary observations and design variables for the estimation of the censoring process are given by

Binary Observations	Design Variables	
0	1	$\boldsymbol{x}_i^T$
0	2	$\boldsymbol{x}_i^T$
0	3	$\boldsymbol{x}_i^T$
⋮		
0	$t_i - 1$	$\boldsymbol{x}_i^T$

where the running time t has to be considered as a factor when using appropriate software. Similarly, if the observed survival time is t_i and $\delta_i = 0$, the censoring event has taken place at t_i and the censoring time C_i is therefore equal to t_i. In this case, the binary observations and design variables for the estimation of the censoring process are given by

Binary Observations	Design Variables	
0	1	$\boldsymbol{x}_i^T$
0	2	$\boldsymbol{x}_i^T$
0	3	$\boldsymbol{x}_i^T$
⋮		
1	t_i	$\boldsymbol{x}_i^T$

Because the PE curve given in (4.9) is an average over the $n^{\mathcal{T}}$ observations in the test sample, its value is often insensitive to the set of design variables that are included in the censoring model. For this reason, a popular strategy is to simply fit a covariate-free censoring model for the estimation of the censoring process (i.e., to use columns 1 and 2 of the above design matrices but not the covariates). This essentially corresponds to a life table estimate for the censoring process.

Properties and Integrated Prediction Error Curve

By definition, the PE curve becomes small if the predicted survival functions agree closely with the observed survival functions. It can further be shown that the PE curve is a "proper scoring rule" for each t in the sense that it becomes minimal if $\hat{S}$ is equal to the true survival function $P(t_j^{\mathcal{T}} > t \,|\, \boldsymbol{x})$ (Gneiting and Raftery 2007). A time-independent coefficient of prediction error is given by the *integrated* PE curve, which is defined as

$$\widehat{\mathrm{PE}}_{\mathrm{int}} = \hat{\mathrm{E}}_T[\widehat{\mathrm{PE}}(T)] = \sum_t \widehat{\mathrm{PE}}(t) \cdot \hat{P}(T = t) \,. \tag{4.10}$$

Generally, a well-predicting survival model should result in PE values that are smaller than 0.25 for all t. This is because 0.25 corresponds to the value of the PE curve obtained from a non-informative model with $\hat{S}(t) = 0.5$ for all t.

Example 4.4 Time from Cohabitation to First Childbirth
According to the hypothesis tests in Example 4.1, the geographic area had a highly significant effect on the time to first childbirth (measured in years). We now analyze whether this covariate also improves prediction accuracy on external or future data. To this purpose, we generated 50 learning samples of size $2/3 \cdot n = 2098$ each that were drawn randomly from the data. For each of the 50 learning samples, the remaining observations ($n^{\mathcal{T}} = 1049$) were used as test samples for the evaluation of prediction accuracy. We considered two logistic discrete-time hazard models: The full model (including all covariates presented in Table 4.2) and the reduced model without the geographic area.

Figure 4.7 shows the average prediction error curves that were obtained from the test data. The survival function of the censoring process (and hence the inverse probability of censoring weights) were estimated from a logistic model without covariates. It is seen that the addition of the covariate "geographic area" to the model leads to an increase in prediction accuracy, as the average PE curve of the full model is below the average curve of the reduced model at almost all time points. Also, the reduced model performs better than a null model without covariate information. Similar results were obtained from the integrated prediction errors shown in Table 4.5. □

Brier Score

In discrete response models an often used measure to evaluate probabilistic forecasts is the *Brier score*. For one observation it has the form

$$b_i = \delta_i(1 - \hat{\pi}_{it_i})^2 + \sum_{s \neq t_i} \hat{\pi}_{is}^2 \,.$$

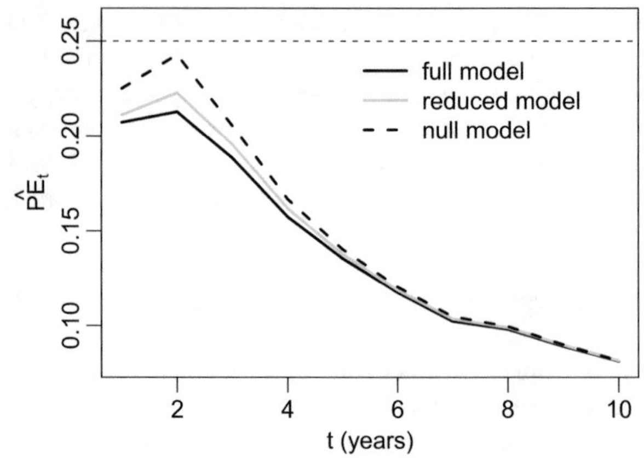

Fig. 4.7 Years from cohabitation to first childbirth. The plot shows the average prediction error curves obtained from the full and reduced models. Discrete-time hazard models with logit link were fitted to 50 learning samples of size $n = 2098$ each; predictions were obtained from the remaining sets of observations (of size $n^{\mathcal{T}} = 1049$ each)

Table 4.5 Years from cohabitation to first childbirth. Average integrated PE curves, as predicted from 50 learning and 50 test samples

$\widehat{PE}_{int}$	Mean	sd
Full model	0.18939	0.00372
Reduced model	0.19509	0.00372
Null model	0.20772	0.00302

Generally, the Brier score is small if prediction accuracy is high and vice versa. In contrast to the prediction error curves defined in the previous subsection (which are also based on quadratic deviations and are sometimes referred to as "Brier score" in the literature on continuous survival times, see Gerds and Schumacher 2006), the above definition does not involve the survival function but the estimated probabilities $\hat{\pi}_{it} = \hat{P}(T = t \,|\, \boldsymbol{x}_i)$.

4.3.3 Discrimination Measures

An alternative approach to evaluate prediction accuracy is to compute discrimination measures for the predictor $\eta := \boldsymbol{x}^T\boldsymbol{\gamma}$. The idea of discrimination measures is to consider survival outcomes as time-dependent binary variables with levels "event at t" and "event after t." Consequently, prediction accuracy can be measured by using established concepts for the evaluation of binary classification rules. This is done as follows: For each fixed time point t, one considers observations having an event at t as "cases" and observations having an event after t as "controls."

Using this definition, η has a high prediction accuracy if it has a *high discriminative power*, that is, if it is able to discriminate between cases and controls in the test data. Discriminative power can be measured using *time-dependent sensitivities* and *specificities*, which are defined as

$$\text{sens}(c, t) := \text{P}(\eta > c \mid T = t) \tag{4.11}$$

and

$$\text{spec}(c, t) := \text{P}(\eta \leq c \mid T > t) , \tag{4.12}$$

respectively (Heagerty and Zheng 2005). Here, c is a threshold of the predictor η. A large sensitivity $\text{P}(\eta > c \mid T = t)$ means that η and therefore the hazard $\lambda(t|\boldsymbol{x}) = h(\eta)$ tends to be large. This corresponds to the detection of "cases" and can be seen as "hit rate" if cases are seen as signals in signal detection theory. In contrast, a large specificity $\text{P}(\eta \leq c \mid T > t)$ means that the hazards for $T > t$ are small, indicating that "controls" are correctly identified. In signal detection theory this corresponds to "correct rejection," because the signal represented by "cases" is not present. By definition, sensitivity and specificity rates vary over thresholds. In the extreme case $c \to -\infty$ sensitivity tends to one and specificity to zero, whereas for $c \to \infty$ sensitivity becomes zero and specificity becomes one.

Summarizing $\text{sens}(c, t)$ and $\text{spec}(c, t)$ for fixed t yields the *time-dependent ROC curve*, which is defined as

$$\text{ROC}(c, t) := \{1 - \text{spec}(c, t), \text{sens}(c, t)\}_{c \in \mathbb{R}} . \tag{4.13}$$

The ROC curve plots the hit rate (sensitivity) against the false positive rate (1-specificity) for varying thresholds. It typically has a concave shape connecting the points (0,0) and (1,1). If η has a high discriminative power the curve is strongly concave and has a large area below the curve (see Example 4.5).

Analogously to ROC analysis for binary outcomes (as outlined, for example, in Pepe 2003) it is possible to calculate the areas under the time-dependent ROC curves for each time point t. This results in the *time-dependent AUC curve*, denoted by AUC(t). The AUC curve should be larger than 0.5 for all time points, because 0.5 corresponds to the AUC value that is obtained by a null model without covariate information.

Similar to the integrated prediction error curve, the area under the time-dependent AUC curve can be used as a time-independent measure of discriminative power. Following the approach by Heagerty and Zheng (2005), we consider the index

$$C^* = \sum_t \text{AUC}(t) \cdot w(t) \tag{4.14}$$

with weights $w(t) = P(T = t)\, P(T > t) / \sum_t P(T = t)\, P(T > t)$. It can be shown that C^* equals the probability $P(\eta_{j1}^{\mathcal{T}} > \eta_{j2}^{\mathcal{T}} \mid T_{j1}^{\mathcal{T}} < T_{j2}^{\mathcal{T}})$, which is a global concordance index measuring the probability that observations with large values of η have shorter survival times than observations with small values of η. Here, $\eta_{j_1}^{\mathcal{T}}$, $\eta_{j_2}^{\mathcal{T}}$, $T_{j_1}^{\mathcal{T}}$, and $T_{j_2}^{\mathcal{T}}$ denote the predictors and survival times of two randomly chosen observations j_1 and j_2 in the test sample. Analogously to the time-dependent AUC curve, C^* should be larger than 0.5 if the predictor η performs better than chance.

Following Uno et al. (2007), we estimate sens(c, t) and spec(c, t) by

$$\widehat{\text{sens}}(c,t) = \frac{\sum_j \delta_j^{\mathcal{T}} \text{I}\left(\hat{\eta}_j^{\mathcal{T}} > c \cap t_j^{\mathcal{T}} = t\right) / \hat{G}_j(t_j^{\mathcal{T}} - 1)}{\sum_j \delta_j^{\mathcal{T}} \text{I}\left(t_j^{\mathcal{T}} = t\right) / \hat{G}_j(t_j^{\mathcal{T}} - 1)}, \tag{4.15}$$

$$\widehat{\text{spec}}(c,t) = \frac{\sum_j \text{I}\left(\hat{\eta}_j^{\mathcal{T}} \le c \cap t_j^{\mathcal{T}} > t\right)}{\sum_j \text{I}\left(t_j^{\mathcal{T}} > t\right)}, \tag{4.16}$$

respectively, where $\hat{\eta}_j$, $j = 1, \ldots, n^{\mathcal{T}}$, denote the estimates of $\boldsymbol{x}^T\boldsymbol{\gamma}$ in the test data. Similar to the estimator of the prediction error curve in (4.9), the weights $1/\hat{G}_j(t_j^{\mathcal{T}} - 1)$ ensure the consistency of (4.15). Estimates of AUC(t) can be obtained by using numerical integration of the estimated ROC curve $\left\{1 - \widehat{\text{spec}}(c,t), \widehat{\text{sens}}(c,t)\right\}_{c \in \mathbb{R}, t \ge 0}$. The concordance index C^* can be estimated by

$$\hat{C}^* = \sum_t \widehat{\text{AUC}}(t)\, \hat{P}(T = t)\, \hat{P}(T > t) \Big/ \sum_t \hat{P}(T = t)\, \hat{P}(T > t)\,, \tag{4.17}$$

where $\widehat{\text{AUC}}(t)$ denotes the estimated time-dependent AUC curve.

Example 4.5 Promotions in Rank for Biochemists
The residual analysis in Example 4.2 suggested that the addition of the covariate "cumulative number of articles" improved the fit of the logistic discrete-time hazard model. We now analyze whether considering this covariate also improves prediction accuracy on external or future data. To this purpose, we generated a learning sample of size $n = 200$ that was drawn randomly from the biochemists data. The remaining observations ($n^{\mathcal{T}} = 101$) were used as a test sample for the evaluation of prediction accuracy. Again we considered two models: The full model (including the six covariates already used in Example 4.2) and the reduced model without the covariate "cumulative number of articles."

Figure 4.8 shows the ROC curves that were obtained from the test data at time point $t = 5$. It is seen that the addition of the cumulative number of published articles leads to an increase of prediction accuracy at $t = 5$, as the ROC curve of the full model is above the curve of the reduced model at almost all thresholds. The diagonal line (with AUC = 0.5) corresponds to a survival model without covariates. Therefore any model predicting better than chance should result in an ROC curve that is above the diagonal line. Generally, the closer the ROC curve is to the upper and left borders of the unit square, the better the predictive performance of the corresponding model will be. From Fig. 4.8 it is seen that the reduced model (being close to the diagonal line) predicts only slightly better than chance. Of course, this does not mean that the other covariates do not have any predictive value in the population. In fact, the relatively small sample size might also have contributed to the low prediction accuracy of the reduced model.

The AUC values at $t = 5$ (computed from the test data) were 0.562 for the full model and 0.512 for the reduced model, again indicating that the former model outperforms the latter one and that

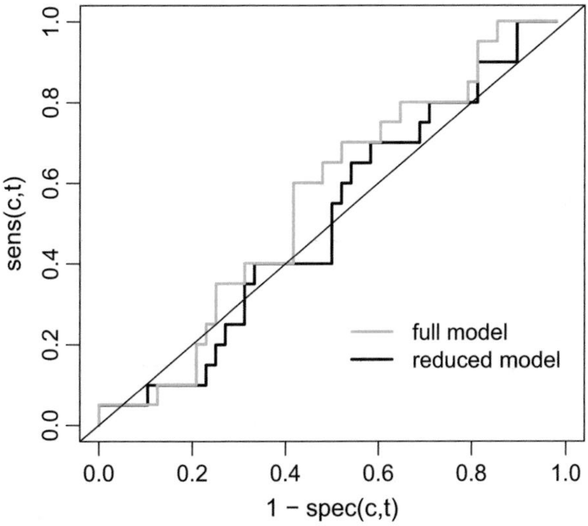

Fig. 4.8 Promotions in rank for biochemists. The plot shows the ROC curves (computed from the test data) that were obtained from the full and reduced models at $t = 5$. Discrete-time hazard models with logistic link were fitted to a learning sample of size $n = 200$; predictions were obtained from the remaining 101 observations in the data

the reduced model predicts only slightly better than chance at $t = 5$. The AUC curve for all time points is presented in Fig. 4.9. It shows that the reduced model performs worse than the full model at almost all time points, confirming the prognostic value of the cumulative number of articles.

In the final step we computed the summary index $\hat{C}^*$ for both models. We obtained $\hat{C}^* = 0.583$ for the full model and $\hat{C}^* = 0.561$ for the reduced model. This result is in line with the results obtained from the time-dependent AUC curves. □

In the literature on continuous survival times, the time-dependent sensitivity rate defined in (4.11) is usually known as *incident* sensitivity because cases are defined as observations with $T = t$. Another definition of time-dependent sensitivity, which is sometimes used in the literature, is the *cumulative* sensitivity

$$\text{sens}_{\text{cum}}(c, t) = \text{P}(\eta > c \,|\, T \leq t), \qquad (4.18)$$

which uses observations with $T \leq t$ as cases (Heagerty and Zheng 2005). Similar to the incident sensitivity, cumulative sensitivities can be used to define time-dependent ROC and AUC curves for assessing the prediction accuracy of a time-discrete survival model. In practice, however, the cumulative approach is less often used than the incident approach because there is no established summary index (such as the index C^* in (4.14)) based on cumulative sensitivities. In particular,

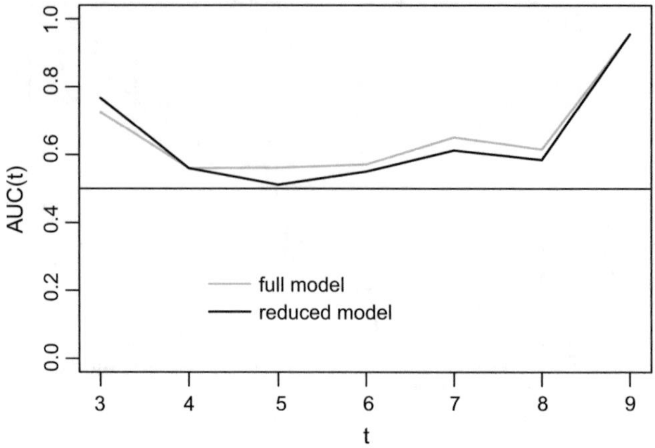

Fig. 4.9 Promotions in rank for biochemists. The plot shows the time-dependent AUC curves (computed from the test data) that were obtained from the full and reduced models. Discrete-time hazard models with logistic link function were fitted to a learning sample of size $n = 200$; predictions were obtained from the remaining 101 observations in the data

unlike $C^* = \mathrm{P}(\eta_{j1}^{\mathcal{T}} > \eta_{j2}^{\mathcal{T}} \mid T_{j1}^{\mathcal{T}} < T_{j2}^{\mathcal{T}})$, integrated versions of the AUC curve based on cumulative sensitivities do not seem to have an easy probabilistic interpretation.

4.4 Choice of Link Function and Flexible Links

In Chap. 3 discrete hazard models of the form

$$\lambda(t|\boldsymbol{x}) = h(\gamma_{0t} + \boldsymbol{x}^T \boldsymbol{\gamma})$$

with given response function $h(\cdot)$ have been considered and several choices of $h(\cdot)$ have been discussed. Although these response functions yield satisfactory results in many applications, it is sometimes possible to improve the model fit by considering more flexible choices of response functions. More flexible models can either be obtained if

(1) the response function is embedded into a *family* of response functions, or if
(2) the response function is estimated nonparametrically.

We first introduce families of response functions; afterwards nonparametric estimators of response functions are briefly described.

4.4.1 *Families of Response Functions*

Generalized Logistic Distribution Family

An interesting family that is a special case of the generalized logistic distribution uses the specification

$$\lambda(t|\mathbf{x}) = F_\xi(\gamma_{0t} + \mathbf{x}^T\boldsymbol{\gamma}),$$

where F_ξ is the distribution function

$$F_\xi(u) = 1 - (1 + \xi\exp(u))^{-1/\xi} \tag{4.19}$$

with $\xi > 0$. For $\xi = 1$ one obtains the logistic distribution function; for the limit $\xi \to 0$ one obtains the clog-log model $F_\xi(u) = 1 - \exp(-\exp(u))$ (Exercise 4.6). Thus the family comprises the two models that are most widely used in discrete survival modeling, namely the logistic and the grouped proportional hazards model. The function $F_\xi(u) = 1 - (1 + \xi\exp(u))^{-1/\xi}$ is also known as the distribution function of the *log-Burr distribution*. The corresponding density is given by $f_\xi(u) = (1 + \xi\exp(u))^{-1/\xi-1}\exp(u)$; it is left-skewed for $\xi < 1$ and right skewed for $\xi > 1$ (see Fig. 4.10). If $\xi = 1$ it is symmetric, which is a well-known property of the logistic distribution. The generalized logistic distribution has been considered by Prentice (1975) and Prentice (1976) in the modeling of binary data and by Hess (2009) in discrete survival modeling. Prentice showed that ξ can be consistently estimated along with the other parameters by maximum likelihood. A Wald test based on the estimate of ξ can be used to test the parameter within the family of distributions. If the logistic model holds ($\xi = 1$) the asymptotic distribution of the maximum likelihood estimator $\hat{\xi}$ is normal and can be approximated by $\mathrm{N}(1, 4(\pi^2 + 3)/(\tilde{n}(\pi^2 - 6)))$, where $\tilde{n}$ denotes the total number of binary observations in the uncensored case. In the limiting case $\xi \to 0$, the asymptotic distribution of $\hat{\xi}$ is equal to the distribution of a random variable defined as $\xi^{trunc} = \xi^*$ if $\xi^* \geq 0$ and $\xi^{trunc} = 0$ if $\xi^* < 0$, where $\xi^* \sim \mathrm{N}\left(0; \pi^2/(\tilde{n}(\pi^2 - 6))\right)$.

Example 4.6 Simulation Study on the Generalized Logistic Family
In the following the generalized logistic family is used to demonstrate that strongly biased effects can occur if the true model is far away from the typically used logistic and clog-log models. The illustration closely follows Hess et al. (2014), where the family was used to model the duration of trade relationships. First we consider a simulation study in which the true response function is given by the log-Burr distribution (4.19), with the parameter ξ given by $\xi = 5$. That means the true underlying model is definitely not a logistic model, but, as shown later, is not unrealistic in applications.

Let the model contain two explanatory variables, x_1, x_2 with parameters given by $\gamma_1 = \gamma_2 = 1$. The variables are generated as independent random draws from a normal distribution with zero mean and unit variance. The baseline hazard is given by $\gamma_{0t} = -\log(t)$. To illustrate the impact of response functions on estimation, four different hazard models are fitted: the models with $\xi = 0$ (clog-log) and $\xi = 1$ (logit), the true model with $\xi = 5$, and a probit model which is not nested in the class of the generalized logistic family. In all models the baseline hazard was modeled

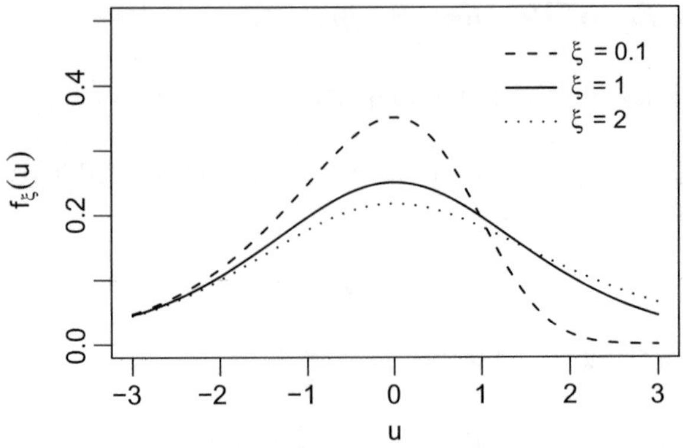

Fig. 4.10 Illustration of the generalized logistic distribution family. The figure depicts the density $f_\xi(u)$ for various values of the parameter ξ. For $\xi = 1$ the density is symmetric

Table 4.6 Estimated covariate effects for different response functions, as obtained from the simulation study described in Example 4.6 (genLog = generalized logistic)

	Estimated models			
	cloglog	logit	genLog ($\xi = 5$)	probit
$\hat{\gamma}_1$	0.713	0.815	0.953	0.843
$\hat{\gamma}_2$	0.590	0.738	0.967	0.788
$\hat{\gamma}_1/\hat{\gamma}_2$	1.209	1.104	0.986	1.070
Hazard ratio at $t = 1$	1.566	1.643	1.659	1.626
Hazard ratio at $t = 12$	1.625	1.784	2.177	1.968

by dummies for each discrete time point $t \in (1, \ldots, 12)$. To make parameters comparable, the parameters are transformed by using the conversion factors proposed by Amemiya (1981). The corresponding estimates are denoted by $\hat{\gamma}_1, \hat{\gamma}_2$. Table 4.6 shows an overview of the impact of response functions on the estimated covariate effects.

It is seen that the covariate effects show almost no bias if the correct response function is used, but are distinctly underestimated when the response function is misspecified. Table 4.6 also shows the ratios of the estimated covariate effects, and the results indicate that also the *relative* effects of explanatory variables are biased if the response function is misspecified. Moreover, estimated hazard ratios at the shortest ($t = 1$) and longest ($t = 12$) durations were considered. The hazard ratios were calculated for an increase in x_1 from zero to one, keeping $x_2 = 0$. For misspecified response functions the estimated hazard ratios are smaller than their counterparts obtained from the correct specification. Also the differences in the hazard ratios at $t = 1$ and $t = 12$ vary substantially across the fitted models. For the model with $\xi = 5$ and the probit model, the estimated hazard ratios increase by about 31 and 21 %, respectively, while they are rather constant for the clog-log model. The latter result was to be expected because the clog-log model is the grouped-duration analogue of Cox's proportional hazards model. The effect is also illustrated in Fig. 4.11, which shows the estimated hazard rates obtained from the clog-log model relative to the true hazard rates generated by the model with $\xi = 5$. It is seen that the hazard estimates obtained from the clog-log model are substantially biased. Small and large hazard rates are overestimated, whereas medium-sized hazard rates are underestimated. In summary, bias of various forms concerning parameter estimates, relative effects and hazard rates have to be expected if the true response function is strongly skewed but standard models are fitted. □

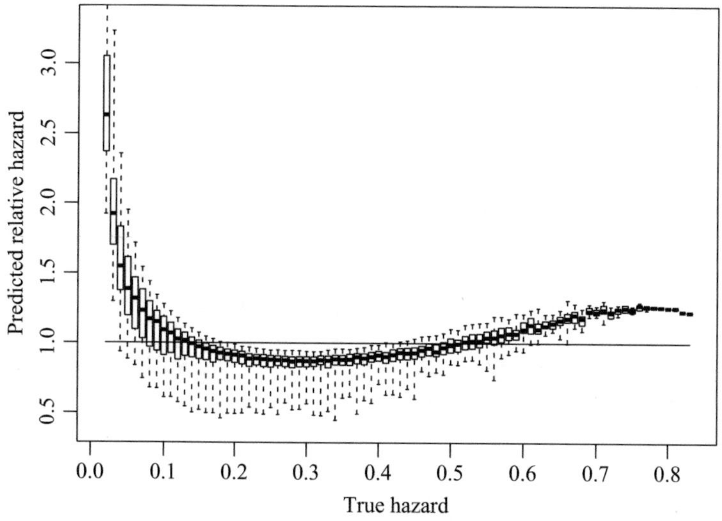

Fig. 4.11 Predicted hazards obtained from the simulation study described in Example 4.6. The true link function was a generalized logistic function with $\xi = 5$ while the estimated model was a clog-log model

Table 4.7 Coefficient estimates for the Duration of Trade Data

	cloglog ($\xi = 0$)	logit ($\xi = 1$)	Pareto ($\xi \approx 4.3$)	probit
Transportation costs	0.1482	0.1797	0.2297	0.1886
GDP	−0.0412	−0.0425	−0.0424	−0.0402
Tariff rate	−0.0395	−0.0413	−0.0434	−0.0409
Exchange rate	−0.1936	−0.2041	−0.1894	−0.1528
Coefficient of variation	−0.1336	−0.1434	−0.1513	−0.1418
Multiple spell dummy	0.5690	0.6741	0.8723	0.7202
Agricultural goods	0.1816	0.2455	0.3241	0.2546
Reference priced products	0.3066	0.3502	0.4090	0.3545
Homogeneous goods	0.4809	0.5758	0.7060	0.5947

Example 4.7 Duration of Trade Relationships
The data record annual US imports between 1972 and 1988 and include information on the value of imports, customs collected, and other relevant factors that might affect the duration of trade. They have been analyzed before by Besedes and Prusa (2006) and Hess and Persson (2012). The traded products are classified according to the 7-digit Tariff Schedule of the United States (TSUSA) which amounts to a total of some 20,000 products. A trade relationship is then defined as a certain product being imported from one specific exporter, and a trade spell is defined as a period of time with uninterrupted import of a given product from one specific country. These spells are calculated as the number of consecutive years with non-zero imports. When fitting the general model one obtains $\hat{\xi} = 4.4$. For comparison also the cloglog, logit, and probit models were fitted. The parameter estimates in Table 4.7, which are standardized using the conversion factors of Amemiya (1981), suggest that the estimated average effects of explanatory variables are affected by the response function chosen to specify the discrete hazard. For more details, see Hess et al. (2014). □

The Model Family of Aranda-Ordaz

Aranda-Ordaz (1983) proposed the model family

$$\lambda(t|\boldsymbol{x}) = F_\alpha(\gamma_{0t} + \boldsymbol{x}^T\boldsymbol{\gamma}),$$

where F_α is the distribution function

$$F_\alpha(u) = \begin{cases} 1 - \exp\left(-(1+\alpha u)^{1/\alpha}\right) & \text{for } u \in [-1/\alpha, \infty), \\ 0 & \text{otherwise,} \end{cases}$$

that depends on the parameter α. For $\alpha \to 0$ one obtains the grouped proportional hazards model. For $\alpha = 1$ one gets the model

$$-\log(1 - \lambda(t|\boldsymbol{x})) = \gamma_{0t} + \boldsymbol{x}^T\boldsymbol{\gamma},$$

where the constant 1 is absorbed into the parameters γ_{0t}. The model for $\alpha = 1$ is a discretized version of the additive continuous time model $\lambda_c(t|\boldsymbol{x}) = \lambda_0(t) + \boldsymbol{x}^T\boldsymbol{\gamma}$.

Therefore the family includes the grouped proportional hazards model and a discretized version of an additive model as special cases. A disadvantage of the family is that the range of predictors is restricted since the linear predictor has to fulfill $\gamma_{0t} + \boldsymbol{x}^T\boldsymbol{\gamma} > -1/\alpha$. An extension of the model that includes polynomial terms was proposed by Tibshirani and Ciampi (1983).

The Model Family of Pregibon

Pregibon (1980) considered a family of link function for binary responses. For discrete hazards, these link functions refer to the representation

$$g_{\alpha,\delta}(\lambda(t|\boldsymbol{x})) = \gamma_{0t} + \boldsymbol{x}^T\boldsymbol{\gamma},$$

with $g_{\alpha,\delta}(\cdot)$ given by

$$g_{\alpha,\delta}(\lambda) = \frac{\lambda^{\alpha-\delta} - 1}{\alpha - \delta} - \frac{(1-\lambda)^{\alpha-\delta} - 1}{\alpha + \delta}.$$

The family also contains the symmetric logit link as the limiting case $\alpha, \delta \to 0$, but is not symmetric for $\alpha, \delta > 0$. Pregibon (1980) also shows how to test the deviation of the link function from a hypothesized link function.

Several further families that include the link functions in common use have been proposed; see Morgan (1985), Stukel (1988), Czado (1992), Czado (1997), and Koenker and Yoon (2009).

4.4.2 *Nonparametric Estimation of Link Functions*

In binary regression several tools have been developed to estimate unknown link functions. Weisberg and Welsh (1994) proposed to estimate regression coefficients using the canonical link and then to estimate the link via kernel smoothers given the estimated parameters. In the next step, all the parameters are re-estimated, and alternating between estimation of link and parameters yields consistent estimates. The basic principle of alternating between these two estimates was also used by Yu and Ruppert (2002), but instead of kernel smoothers the unknown function is approximated by an expansion in basis functions. Alternatives have been considered by Ruckstuhl and Welsh (1999) and Muggeo and Ferrara (2008). Leitenstorfer and Tutz (2011) and Tutz and Petry (2012) used boosting techniques. The latter approach additionally includes variable selection.

4.5 Literature and Further Reading

Many of the concepts presented in this chapter were originally proposed to evaluate models for continuous event times. For example, *prediction error curves* for continuous survival models have been developed by Graf et al. (1999) and Gerds and Schumacher (2006). Similarly, *time-dependent discrimination measures* for continuous event times have been proposed by Heagerty et al. (2000) and Heagerty and Zheng (2005). Importantly, these authors established the connection between the integrated AUC curve and the concordance index C^*. The latter index was originally proposed by Harrell Jr et al. (1996) to evaluate predictions for binary responses; the censoring-adjusted versions of time-dependent discrimination measures and C^* were developed by Uno et al. (2007) and Uno et al. (2011). Comparisons of estimators for time-dependent discrimination measures have been presented in Schmid and Potapov (2012) and Schmid et al. (2015).

Martingale residuals for continuous event times have been described, e.g., in Klein and Moeschberger (2003), and *adjusted deviance residuals* for binary models have been treated in Tutz (2012).

The *Brier score* for probabilistic forecasts dates back to Brier (1950). A rigorous treatment of probabilistic forecasts and scoring rules has been presented by Gneiting and Raftery (2007).

R^2 *coefficients* have a long tradition in linear regression and have been generalized to other likelihood-based models by various authors (e.g., by Nagelkerke 1991).

4.6 Software

Statistical hypothesis tests for discrete-time hazard models can be conducted in R via the *Anova* function of the add-on package *car* (Fox and Weisberg 2015). This function includes various options for specifying test types and statistics, such as *test.statistic=c("LR")* for likelihood ratio tests and *test.statistic=c("Wald")* for Wald tests. Functions to evaluate R^2 coefficients are implemented in several R packages, for example, in the add-on packages *pscl* (Jackman 2015, function *pR2*), and *fmsb* (Nakazawa 2015, function *NagelkerkeR2*),. Prediction error curves and discrimination measures can be computed by using the functions *predErrDiscShort* (for prediction error curves), *tprUno* (for time-dependent sensitivities), *fprUno* (for time-dependent specificities), and *aucUno* (for time-dependent AUC curves), respectively, that are contained in the *discSurv* package. The *discSurv* package also contains R functions to compute martingale residuals, deviance residuals, and adjusted deviance residuals, which are implemented in *martingaleResid*, *devResid*, and *adjDevResid*, respectively.

4.7 Exercises

4.1 Let the logistic model be used to model the hazards. Show that the martingale residuals defined by $m_i = \delta_i - \sum_{s=1}^{t_i} \hat{\lambda}_{is}$, $i = 1, \ldots, n$ sum up to zero. Hint: Consider the log-likelihood for the binary representation of the transitions and use that the ML estimate is found if the derivative of the log-likelihood function (the score function) is zero.

4.2 Consider the pairfam data, which are described in detail in Chap. 9.

1. Estimate the hazard rate for the time to first childbirth by fitting a logistic discrete hazard model. Use the covariates "age of woman," "age of partner," "duration of relationship," and "status of the relationship."
2. Specify the expressions $\boldsymbol{C}$, $\boldsymbol{\beta}$, and $\boldsymbol{\xi}$ to test the null hypothesis that age of both partners does not have any effect on the time to first childbirth.
3. Calculate the likelihood ratio (LR) test statistic.
4. Calculate the p-value. Can H_0 be rejected?
5. Test the same hypothesis using a Wald test and compare the result to the result obtained from the LR test.
6. Conduct LR and Wald tests to investigate whether the relationship categories "living apart together" and "married" are significantly different from the category "living together."

4.3 Consider the TTP data from Exercise 2.4 and fit a grouped proportional hazards model (using the covariates presented in Table 2.4) to the data. Apply square root transformations to the continuous covariates before including them in the model.

1. Calculate the adjusted deviance residuals for the full model and for the intercept model without covariates.
2. Analyze the adjusted deviance residuals by inspecting normal quantile–quantile plots. How does the inclusion of the covariates affect the distribution of the adjusted deviance residuals?
3. Conduct a goodness-of-fit test on normality of the adjusted deviance residuals (for example, an Anderson–Darling or a Shapiro–Wilk test).

4.4 Consider the congressional careers data. The aim is to compare different modeling options for the response variable *time to loss of a general election* by carrying out tenfold cross-validation.

1. Subdivide the data randomly into tenfolds and create ten training samples for tenfold cross-validation.
2. Fit five logistic discrete hazard models to each of the ten training data sets. Specifically, use the following sets of predictor variables:

   (a) age, scandal, redist
   (b) age, prespart, opengub, redist, district
   (c) age, opengub, opensen, district
   (d) age, priorm, prespart, opengub, redist, district
   (e) age, priorm, prespart, opengub, opensen, redist

3. Compute predictions from the five models using the ten test samples.
4. Evaluate the predictive deviances of the five models.
5. Draw boxplots of the ten predictive deviances for each model and interpret the results. Which model has the best predictive performance?

4.5 Consider the US unemployment data of Example 1.1. The outcome variable of interest in Example 1.1 was the time to re-employment (regardless of whether re-employment was at a full-time job or at a part-time job).

1. Subdivide the observations into ten equally sized parts, to be used for tenfold cross-validation.
2. Convert all samples to sets of augmented data with binary outcome variables y_{is}.
3. Fit logistic discrete hazard models to the ten training samples. Use the covariates *age*, *filed unemployment claim*, *log weekly earnings in lost job*, and *tenure in lost job*.
4. For each of the ten test samples calculate the true positive rate (TPR), the false positive rates (FPR), and the area under the curve (AUC) at $t = 5$.
5. Compute the AUC values at each time point and draw the cross-validated time-dependent AUC curve. In addition, estimate the cross-validated concordance index. Evaluate the contributions of the four covariates to the prediction accuracy of the model.

4.6 Show that the generalized logistic distribution family defined in (4.19) converges to the clog-log model as $\xi \to 0$.

4.7 Consider a data set from Singer and Willett (2003) that was obtained from a sample of 180 middle-school boys. After each grade, the boys were asked whether they had sex for the first time (see Capaldi et al. 1996). As a consequence, all times to the event "first sex" were measured in years (median of observed event times = 11 years). Because boys were observed between the 7th and the 12th grade, the maximum observed event time was 12 years (median 11 years). The censoring rate was 30 %, implying that 30 % of the boys were still virgins after the 12th grade. The explanatory variable was a binary predictor that indicated wether a boy didn't live with his biological parents any more at the beginning of the 7th grade ("parental transition," observed for 60 % of the boys). The data are available at http://www.ats.ucla.edu/stat/examples/alda.

1. Convert the sample to a set of augmented data with binary outcome variable y_{is}.
2. Estimate the hazard rate for the time to first sex by fitting discrete hazard models. Use the logistic, probit, and cloglog link functions and compare the estimates.
3. Conduct LR and Wald tests to investigate whether the covariate "parental transition" has a significant effect on the time to first sex.
4. Fit a Cox proportional hazards model in continuous time to the non-augmented data. Compare the results to those obtained from the grouped proportional hazards model with cloglog link.

Chapter 5
Nonparametric Modeling and Smooth Effects

The basic discrete survival model considered in the previous chapters has the form $\lambda(t|\boldsymbol{x}_i) = h(\eta_{it})$ with the linear predictor given by

$$\eta_{it} = \gamma_0(t) + \boldsymbol{x}_i^T \boldsymbol{\gamma}, \tag{5.1}$$

where, for notational convenience, $\gamma_0(t)$ denotes the parameters that vary over time. The model is parametric, with the parameters given by $\gamma_0(1), \ldots, \gamma_0(q), \boldsymbol{\gamma}^T$. More specifically, the predictor η_{it} is *linear* in $\boldsymbol{\gamma}$, implying that each covariate contained in $\boldsymbol{x}_i$ has a linear effect on the transformed hazard $g(\lambda(t|\boldsymbol{x}_i))$. In practice, however, the linearity assumption is often too restrictive, for example, when there are quadratic or logarithmic predictor effects. In the following we will consider models that allow for a more flexible predictor which is not necessarily linear. We will first consider smooth nonlinear versions of the baseline hazard $\gamma_0(t)$. In the next step, *additive hazard models* that relax the linearity assumption for the covariate effects will be considered. Finally, we will introduce time-varying coefficients that allow parameter estimates to vary smoothly over time.

5.1 Smooth Baseline Hazard

The model with predictor (5.1) assumes that all parameters are fixed. The number of parameters in the model is determined by the number of intervals, because for each interval one has a separate intercept $\gamma_0(t)$. Thus, if the number of intervals is large, the number of parameters is large as well. In particular in this case one obtains more stable estimates if one assumes that the baseline hazard represented by the parameters $\gamma_0(1), \ldots, \gamma_0(q)$ is a smooth function in time. Then the smooth function can be specified by a simpler parameterization that contains fewer parameters.

G. Tutz, M. Schmid, *Modeling Discrete Time-to-Event Data*,
Springer Series in Statistics, DOI 10.1007/978-3-319-28158-2_5

A common way to fit a smooth function is to assume that the function can be approximated by a finite sum of basis functions. Let the parameters $\gamma_0(1), \ldots, \gamma_0(q)$ be approximated by

$$\gamma_0(t) = \sum_{s=1}^{m} \gamma_{0s}\phi_s(t) , \tag{5.2}$$

where $\phi_s(\cdot)$ are fixed basis functions. Common choices are *polynomial splines* in the form of the truncated power series basis and *B-splines*, which are considered later. The crucial point is that one considers the parameters $\gamma_0(t)$ as a function in t and approximates this function by a weighted sum of m basis functions. The number of basis functions, m, can usually be chosen much smaller than the number of intervals, q, without losing much in terms of accuracy of fit.

As a first example let us consider basis functions that are given in the form of polynomial splines. Polynomial regression splines are obtained by dividing the time domain into continuous intervals $[\tau_i, \tau_{i+1}]$ and representing the unknown function by a separate polynomial of degree d in each interval. In addition, the polynomials are supposed to join smoothly at the knots $\tau_1 < \ldots < \tau_{m_s}$, $m_s = m - 1$, which determine the boundaries of the intervals. In discrete hazard models the knots are chosen from the time domain $[0, q]$. A simple representation of polynomial splines of degree d is the *truncated power series basis*, which yields

$$\gamma_0(t) = \gamma_{00} + \gamma_{01}t + \ldots + \gamma_{0d}t^d + \sum_{i=1}^{m_s} \gamma_{k+i}(t - \tau_i)_+^d, \tag{5.3}$$

where $(t - \tau_i)_+^d$ are the truncated power functions defined by

$$(t - \tau)_+^d := \begin{cases} (t - \tau)^d & \text{if } t \geq \tau, \\ 0 & \text{if } t < \tau. \end{cases}$$

The representation (5.3) uses the $m = m_s + d + 1$ basis functions

$$\phi_1(t) = 1, \phi_2(x) = t, \ldots, \phi_{d+1}(t) = t^d,$$
$$\phi_{d+2}(t) = (t - \tau_1)_+^d, \ldots, \phi_{d+m_s+1}(t) = (t - \tau_{m_s})_+^d,$$

which form the truncated power series basis of *degree d* (or, alternatively, of *order* $d + 1$).

An alternative representation is by B-spline basis functions, which are defined recursively. Since the definition is not very instructive they are visualized in Fig. 5.1.

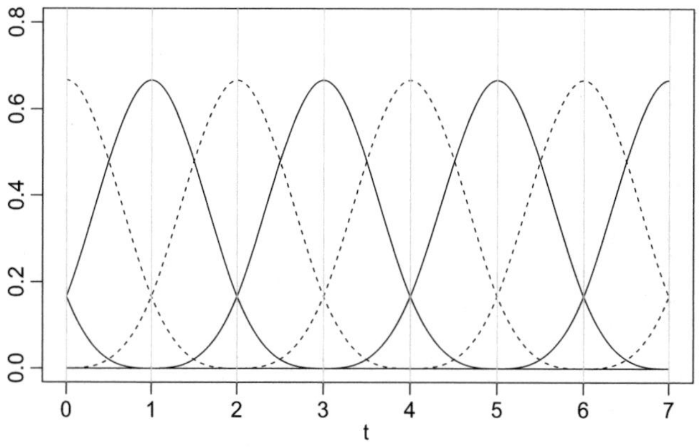

Fig. 5.1 Example of a set of B-spline basis functions of degree $d = 3$. The *gray lines* indicate the positions of the boundary knots (at $t = 0$ and $t = 7$) and the $m_s = 6$ interior knots. The *black lines* represent the $m_s + d + 1 = 10$ basis functions. Because $d = 3$, each basis function is larger than zero in $d + 1 = 4$ adjacing intervals. The $2 \cdot d = 6$ additional knots needed for the recursive construction of the B-spline basis are not shown here. They were at the positions $t = -3, -2, -1$ and $t = 8, 9, 10$

In this example, a set of B-spline basis functions was constructed by defining $m_s + 2$ equidistant knots that subdivide the time range into $m_s + 1$ intervals. The knot positions are indicated by the gray vertical lines, and the black lines in Fig. 5.1 represent the B-spline basis functions (obtained from using the recursive formula given in De Boor 1978). The middle m_s knots are referred to as "interior knots" whereas the outer two knots are called "boundary knots." Generally, defining m_s interior knots implies that there are $m = m_s + d + 1$ B-spline basis functions. For technical reasons, the recursive construction of the $m_s + d + 1$ basis functions requires the definition of d additional knots to the left and another d additional knots to the right of the boundary knots. In Fig. 5.1, these additional knots are not shown; they were defined by extending the equidistant grid to the left and to the right of the boundary knots. For details, see De Boor (1978). As seen from Fig. 5.1, B-spline basis functions are strictly local because they only differ from zero in $d + 1$ adjacing intervals. If compared to the truncated power series basis, the locality of B-spline basis functions is convenient because it leads to increased numerical stability.

Figure 5.2 shows how a spline function of degree $d = 3$ can be constructed from the set of B-spline basis functions presented in Fig. 5.1. This is essentially done by putting weights on the basis functions. One can imagine that quite different functional forms can be obtained by appropriately chosen weights.

Instead of using the truncated polynomials or the B-spline basis, which both yield polynomial splines, the basis functions can also be chosen as *radial basis functions*,

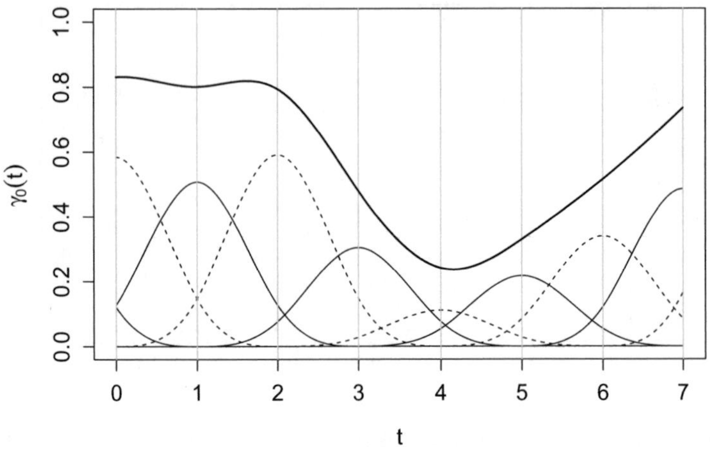

Fig. 5.2 This figure shows how a spline function of degree $d = 3$ (represented by the *thick black line*) can be constructed from the set of B-spline basis functions defined in Fig. 5.1. Each of the ten basis functions (represented by the *dashed and solid black lines* below the *thick black line*) was weighted by a coefficient γ_{0s}, $s = 1, \ldots, 10$. Summing up the weighted basis functions results in the smooth function represented by the *thick black line*

for example, by using the Gaussian density

$$\phi_s(t) = \exp\left(-\frac{(t-\tau_s)^2}{2\sigma^2}\right),$$

where τ_s is the center of the basis function and σ^2 is an additional parameter that determines the spread of the basis function. Radial basis functions have been used mainly in the machine learning community; for a more detailed description, we refer to Ripley (1996).

Generally, when time-varying parameters such as the baseline hazard $\gamma_0(t)$ are expanded in basis functions, two strategies are in common use:

- Choosing a small number of basis functions, say 4 or 5, such that numerically stable estimates of the coefficients exist.
- Choosing a relatively large number of basis functions and using a *penalty term* to obtain stable estimates. This approach has been propagated, in particular, by Eilers and Marx (1996). Generally, a large number of basis functions result in very flexible spline functions. On the other hand, estimates are usually wiggly and have many local optima. Therefore, in order to maintain the flexibility and to obtain sufficiently smooth spline estimates that are numerically stable, penalty terms are used. Illustrations and examples of penalty terms will be given in the next subsection.

5.1.1 Estimation

One advantage of the expansion in basis functions (5.2) is that the predictor is again linear, not in the covariates but in the coefficients γ_{0s}, which is the essential condition for using the GLM framework of Chap. 3. As has been shown in Sect. 3.4, the likelihood for an observation t_i is equivalent to the likelihood for the binary observations $(y_{i1}, \dots, y_{it_i}) = (0, \dots, 0, \delta_i)$, which code whether the failure has occurred over the first t_i intervals. The binary model for y_{it} has been specified in the form $\lambda(t|\boldsymbol{x}_i) = h(\gamma_0(t) + \boldsymbol{x}_i^T\boldsymbol{\gamma})$.

If $\gamma_0(t)$ is expanded in basis functions, one obtains the linear predictor

$$\eta_{it} = \gamma_0(t) + \boldsymbol{x}_i^T\boldsymbol{\gamma} = \sum_{s=1}^{m} \gamma_{0s}\phi_s(t) + \boldsymbol{x}_i^T\boldsymbol{\gamma}. \tag{5.4}$$

Since the values $\phi_s(t)$ are known, one has an "extended" linear predictor

$$\eta_{it} = (\phi_1(t), \dots, \phi_q(t), \boldsymbol{x}_i^T)\,\boldsymbol{\beta},$$

where all model coefficients are collected in the vector $\boldsymbol{\beta}$. Consequently, if one uses a small number of basis functions, fitting procedures for binary regression models can be used based on the likelihood representation (3.25).

If one uses a large number of basis functions to obtain increased flexibility, estimation is usually based on penalized log-likelihood approaches. In penalized likelihood estimation, the usual log-likelihood is replaced by

$$l_p(\boldsymbol{\beta}) = l(\boldsymbol{\beta}) - \frac{\lambda}{2}J(\boldsymbol{\beta}),$$

where $l(\boldsymbol{\beta})$ is the familiar log-likelihood function from Chap. 3, λ is a tuning parameter, and $J(\boldsymbol{\beta})$ is a penalty that puts restrictions on $\boldsymbol{\beta}$. Note that the tuning parameter λ should not be confused with the hazard function $\lambda(t|\boldsymbol{x})$. We will denote both terms by λ, as this is standard notation that is commonly used in the literature. Usually, these restrictions prevent the elements in $\boldsymbol{\beta}$ from having too large deviations from neighboring elements, thus controlling the roughness of the smooth function represented by the basis functions.

In the following we will assume throughout that basis functions are given by B-spline functions that are defined on an equidistant grid, as in Fig. 5.1. Then in discrete hazard models with smooth baseline hazard $\gamma_0(t)$ the parameter vector is $\boldsymbol{\beta}^T = (\gamma_{01}, \dots, \gamma_{0m}, \boldsymbol{\gamma}^T)$, and the penalty contains only the parameters corresponding to $\gamma_0(t)$. An often used penalty is the difference penalty

$$J_\delta = \sum_{j=\delta+1}^{m} (\Delta^\delta \gamma_{0j})^2, \tag{5.5}$$

where Δ is the difference operator on adjacent B-spline coefficients, that is, $\Delta\gamma_{0j} = \gamma_{0j} - \gamma_{0,j-1}$, $\Delta^2\gamma_{0j} = \Delta(\gamma_{0j} - \gamma_{0,j-1}) = \gamma_{0j} - 2\gamma_{0,j-1} + \gamma_{0,j+2}$, etc. This penalty has the effect that the parameters are estimated smoothly, with the degree of smoothness determined by the tuning parameter λ. If λ increases, smoothness is enforced. If one uses, for example, first differences $\gamma_{0j} - \gamma_{0,j-1}$ ($\delta = 1$), in the extreme case ($\lambda \to \infty$) the baseline hazard $\gamma_0(t)$ will become a constant. In general, if a penalty of order δ is used and the degree of the B-spline is higher than δ, for large values of λ the fit will approach a polynomial of degree $\delta - 1$. For this approach Eilers and Marx (1996) coined the term *P-splines* ("penalized splines").

With $\boldsymbol{\gamma}_0^T = (\gamma_{01}, \ldots, \gamma_{0q})$ the penalty (5.5) has the general form

$$J_\delta = \boldsymbol{\gamma}_0^T \boldsymbol{K}_0 \boldsymbol{\gamma}_0 = \boldsymbol{\beta}^T \boldsymbol{K} \boldsymbol{\beta}, \tag{5.6}$$

which is in wide use in penalty approaches. The matrices $\boldsymbol{K}_0$ and $\boldsymbol{K}$ are easily constructed for differences of fixed order (Exercise 5.2). It should be noted that using B-splines of degree 1 is equivalent to penalizing the size of the original parameters $\gamma_0(t)$ because then $\gamma_0(t) = \gamma_{0t}$. Maximization of the penalized log-likelihood can be obtained by modifying maximization methods used in GLMs (see, for example, Wood 2006). Alternative smoothing approaches that also use a quadratic form for a penalty are *smoothing splines*, which are based on non-equidistant knots but which are not considered in detail here (see, e.g., Hastie and Tibshirani 1990 for a description).

By using matrix notation, approximations to standard errors are obtained in a similar way as in generalized linear models. For example, approximate covariances are obtained by the sandwich matrix

$$\mathrm{cov}(\hat{\boldsymbol{\beta}}) \approx (\boldsymbol{F}(\hat{\boldsymbol{\beta}}) + 2\lambda\boldsymbol{K})^{-1}\boldsymbol{F}(\hat{\boldsymbol{\beta}})(\boldsymbol{F}(\hat{\boldsymbol{\beta}}) + 2\lambda\boldsymbol{K})^{-1},$$

where $\boldsymbol{F}(\boldsymbol{\beta})$ denotes the information matrix of the ML estimate (see Eilers and Marx 1996).

In R, smooth estimates of the baseline hazard can be obtained by using the *gam* function in the package *mgcv*. For estimation one uses the codings

Binary observations	Design variables	
0	1	$\boldsymbol{x}_i^T$
0	2	$\boldsymbol{x}_i^T$
0	3	$\boldsymbol{x}_i^T$
$\vdots$		
1	t_i	$\boldsymbol{x}_i^T$

for $T = t_i$, $\delta_i = 1$ and

Binary observations	Design variables	
0	1	$\boldsymbol{x}_i^T$
0	2	$\boldsymbol{x}_i^T$
0	3	$\boldsymbol{x}_i^T$
$\vdots$		
0	t_i	$\boldsymbol{x}_i^T$

for $T = t_i$, $\delta_i = 0$. These codings are essentially the same as those used in Sect. 3.4. However, the time column is no longer coded as factor variable but is treated as a numerical covariate.

If the intervals from which the discrete time has been generated have varying length and one wants to approximate the underlying continuous time, one might want to modify the expansion in basis functions. Let $\{m_1, \ldots, m_q\}$ denote the mean values of the intervals, that is, $m_i = (a_i - a_{i-1})/2$. Then the knots are chosen from $[a_0, a_q]$ and the expansion $\gamma_0(t) = \sum_{s=1}^{m} \gamma_{0s}\phi_s(t)$ is considered for values $t \in \{m_1, \ldots, m_q\}$. Also the penalty term should be modified because simple differences do not reflect the varying interval lengths. As in smoothing splines one can use the penalty term $\int (\gamma_0^{(2)}(t))^2 dt$, where $\gamma_0^{(2)}(t)$ denotes the second derivative. Generally, the second derivative is a measure of the wiggliness of a function and is related to the second-order difference penalty, see Eilers and Marx (1996). The penalty term can also be written as the quadratic form $\boldsymbol{\gamma}_0^T \boldsymbol{K}_0 \boldsymbol{\gamma}_0$, with the entries of the matrix $\boldsymbol{K}_0 = (k_{ij})$ given by $k_{ij} = \int \phi_i^{(2)}(t)\phi_j^{(2)}(t)dt$.

Example 5.1 Munich Founder Study

For illustration we use the Munich Founder study where the dependent variable is the failure time measured in months (Example 1.2). Figure 5.3 shows the estimates of a continuation ratio model for founders with working experience less than 10 years and 10 or more years. The black lines in the upper panel are the estimates of the survival functions ("time to failure") of the two groups that were obtained from a continuation ratio model with non-smooth intercepts γ_{0t}. In contrast, the black lines in the lower panel were obtained by smoothing these estimates, i.e., by fitting a continuation ratio model that treats time as a continuous variable. Smoothing was accomplished by using P-spline basis functions of degree $d = 3$ with a second-order difference penalty and $m_s = 6$ interior knots. The smoothing parameter was determined by generalized cross-validation (see Wood 2006).

It is seen that founders with little working experience ($<$10 years) tend to have smaller survival rates than founders with 10 or more years of working experience. Also, the model with non-smoothed intercepts (upper panel of Fig. 5.3) yields estimated survival functions that are close to a smooth function, which is due to the relatively large number of equally spaced time points (corresponding to 1-month intervals). Figure 5.4 shows the estimates of the transformed intercept parameters γ_{0t}, as well as their smoothed versions. It is seen that there is a large variation between the non-smooth coefficient estimates of γ_{0t}. By applying smoothing (gray line in Fig. 5.4), one sees a clear trend in the baseline: The baseline risk of failure increases up to a time point of approximately 15 months. After this time point, the baseline risk gradually decreases. □

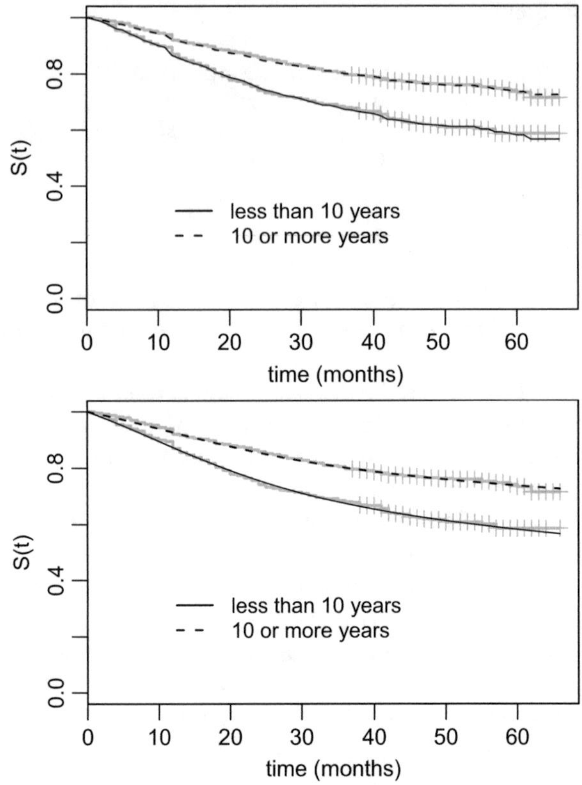

Fig. 5.3 Munich Founder Study. The two plots show the estimated survival functions for the time to failure (obtained from fitting a continuation ratio model). The predictor "working experience of the founder" was considered without smoothing (*upper panel*) and smoothing (*lower panel*). *Gray lines* represent Kaplan–Meier estimates

5.1.2 Smooth Life Table Estimates

If one fits data from a homogeneous population without including any covariates, the smooth baseline hazard is equivalent to a smoothed life table estimator. Therefore, if one applies the methods described in the previous sections to life table data, one obtains a smoothed life table estimator with smoothing based on the expansion in basis functions.

An alternative approach that can be used for life tables is *local smoothing*. Local smoothing borrows strength from the neighborhood of a target value by including observations that are close to the target value. The latter observations are included with weights that decrease with the distance between target value and observation.

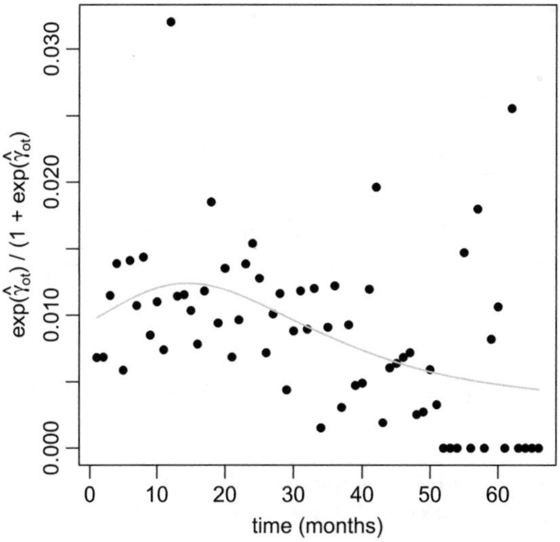

Fig. 5.4 Munich Founder Study. The plot shows the unsmoothed (*dots*) and smoothed (*curve*) estimates of the baseline hazard $\exp(\gamma_0(t))/(1+\exp(\gamma_0(t)))$ obtained from a continuation ratio model. Estimates represent the hazard rate for the reference group (founders with less than 10 years of working experience)

Let t denote the target value, that is, the value at which the hazard rate $\lambda(t|\boldsymbol{x})$ is to be estimated. Then for the estimation of $\lambda(t|\boldsymbol{x})$ one uses not only observations that were collected at t but also observations that were collected in a neighborhood of t.

The weighting of neighborhood observations is obtained by including weights into the binomial log-likelihood given in Eq. (3.25)

$$l = \sum_{i=1}^{n} \sum_{s=1}^{t_i} y_{is} \log \lambda(s) + (1 - y_{is}) \log(1 - \lambda(s)),$$

where y_{is} codes the transition from interval $[a_{s-1}, a_s)$ to $[a_s, a_{s+1})$ in the form

$$y_{is} = \begin{cases} 1 & \text{individual fails in } [a_{s-1}, a_s), \\ 0 & \text{individual survives in } [a_{s-1}, a_s), \end{cases}$$

for $s = 1, \ldots, q$.

With $R_t = \{i : t \leq t_i\}$ denoting the observations at risk at time t, the log-likelihood has the form

$$l = \sum_{s=1}^{q} \sum_{i \in R_s} y_{is} \log \lambda(s) + (1 - y_{is}) \log(1 - \lambda(s)).$$

For fixed target value t one fits a model that assumes in the simplest case that the hazard is constant, $\lambda(s) = \lambda$. Specifically, one maximizes the weighted log-likelihood

$$l = \sum_{s=1}^{q} \sum_{i \in R_s} \{y_{is} \log \lambda + (1 - y_{is}) \log(1 - \lambda)\} \, w_\gamma(t, s),$$

where $w_\gamma(t, s)$ is a weight function that decreases with the distance between t and s, with the decrease depending on a tuning parameter γ. For the extreme weights, i.e., $w_\gamma(t, s) = 1$ if $t = s$ and $w_\gamma(t, s) = 0$ if $t \neq s$, one obtains by maximizing l over λ the expression $\hat{\lambda} = \hat{\lambda}(t) = \sum_{i \in R_t} y_{it}/|R_t|$, which is the number of failures at t divided by the number of individuals at risk. This estimator is the unsmoothed life table estimator. In general one obtains the estimator

$$\hat{\lambda} = \hat{\lambda}(t) = \sum_{s=1}^{q} \left\{ \sum_{i \in R_s} y_{is}/|R_s| \right\} \tilde{w}_\gamma(t, s),$$

where $\tilde{w}_\gamma(t, s) = w_\gamma(t, s)|R_s|/(\sum_{j=1}^{q} w_\gamma(t, j)|R_j|)$ are standardized weights (see Exercise 5.1). It represents a weighted sum of the life table estimates at s, $\sum_{i \in R_s} y_{is}/|R_s|$.

Weight functions that are in common use in localized estimation are built from kernels and have the form $w_\gamma(t, s) \propto K((t - s)/\gamma)$, where the kernel $K(\cdot)$ is a symmetric density function, for example, the Gaussian density. If $\gamma \to 0$, one obtains the unsmoothed life table estimator, whereas for $\gamma \to \infty$ one obtains the ultrasmooth estimates $\hat{\lambda}(1) = \ldots = \hat{\lambda}(q)$.

Fitting a constant function $\hat{\lambda} = \hat{\lambda}(t)$ by using weights yields smooth hazard estimates, but this local constant fitting procedure can suffer from severe bias. Better procedures are often obtained by locally fitting a polynomial. To this purpose, one fits (for fixed target value t) a polynomial that is centered around t. In other words, one fits the model $\lambda_t(s) = h(\beta_o + (s-t)\beta_1 + \ldots + (s-t)^m \beta_m)$, where $h(\cdot)$ is a response function, for example, the logistic distribution function, and the explanatory term is a polynomial of degree m. The subscript t in $\lambda_t(s)$ is used only as a reminder that one wants to estimate the hazard function at the fixed value t. In this case the weighted log-likelihood has the same form as before,

$$l = \sum_{s=1}^{q} \sum_{i \in R_s} \{y_{is} \log \lambda_t(s) + (1 - y_{is}) \log(1 - \lambda_t(s))\} w_\gamma(t, s),$$

but the fitted model now is $\lambda_t(s) = h(\beta_0 + (s-t)\beta_1 + \ldots + (s-t)^m \beta_m)$. Maximization is straightforward by using GLM methodology with weights on the observations. With $\hat{\beta}_0, \ldots, \hat{\beta}_m$ denoting the estimated parameters, the estimated hazard at t is $\hat{\lambda}_t(t)) = h(\hat{\beta}_0)$.

The tuning parameter can be chosen by cross-validation, with the performance measured as in Chap. 4. Typical choices for the degree of the polynomial are 1 and 3. More details on local smoothing are found in Hastie and Loader (1993), Loader (1999), and Fan and Gijbels (1996). For an application to the German unemployment data, see Exercise 5.3.

For heterogeneous intervals weights can be modified to include the distances in continuous time. With $m_i = (a_i - a_{i-1})/2$ again denoting the middle of the intervals, the weights $w_\gamma(t, s)$ are replaced by $w_\gamma(m_t, m_s)$.

5.2 Additive Models

In the previous section only the baseline hazard was modeled as a smooth function over time whereas the effect of the explanatory variables was still captured by a linear predictor. In *additive discrete hazard models* this assumption is weakened by assuming that the predictor has the additive form

$$\eta_{it} = f_0(t) + f_1(x_{i1}) + \ldots + f_p(x_{ip}),$$

where the functions $f_0(\cdot), \ldots, f_p(\cdot)$ are unknown and are to be determined by the data. The function $f_0(t)$ corresponds to the time-varying baseline hazard $\gamma_0(t)$ considered in the previous section.

One approach to estimate the functional form of the predictors is again to assume that they can be expanded as a sum of basis functions

$$f_j(x_j) = \sum_{s=1}^{m_j} \gamma_{js} \phi_{js}(x_j),$$

where the basis functions may depend on the covariate x_j. For example, the basis functions $\phi_{j1}(\cdot), \ldots, \phi_{jm_j}(\cdot)$ represent the basis functions for the jth covariate and have to be defined on the corresponding domain.

The weight parameters γ_{js} are again estimated by maximizing a penalized log-likelihood. If one uses an equally spaced grid for the basis functions, one can again use a difference penalty for all covariates. For example, with differences of order δ one uses the penalty

$$J_\delta = \sum_{j=0}^{p} \sum_{s=\delta+1}^{m_j} (\Delta^\delta \gamma_{js})^2 = \sum_{j=0}^{p} \boldsymbol{\gamma}_j^T \boldsymbol{K}_j \boldsymbol{\gamma}_j = \boldsymbol{\beta}^T \boldsymbol{K} \boldsymbol{\beta}, \tag{5.7}$$

where $\boldsymbol{\gamma}_j^T = (\gamma_{j1}, \ldots, \gamma_{jm_j})$ and $\boldsymbol{\beta}^T = (\boldsymbol{\gamma}_0^T, \ldots, \boldsymbol{\gamma}_p^T)$. The matrices $\boldsymbol{K}_j$ are constructed easily from the differences of parameters for the jth predictor.

Maximization of the penalized log-likelihood uses modified GLM methodology. After transforming the original data into binary data one can use the fitting methods for binary additive models, as implemented in the R package *mgcv*. For details when the functions are expanded in basis functions, see Marx and Eilers (1998), and Wand (2000). Alternatively one can use the framework of smoothing splines (Gu and Wahba 1993; Gu 2002) or backfitting procedures (Hastie and Tibshirani 1990).

Example 5.2 Time Between Cohabitation and First Childbirth

We analyze the data collected for the Second National Survey on Fertility that was introduced in Example 4.1. In Chap. 4 we fitted a proportional continuation ratio model with logistic link function to investigate the effects of various predictor variables on the time between the beginning of cohabitation and first childbirth (measured in years). By specification of the model, all predictors were assumed to have linear effects on the logit-transformed hazard rate. A highly significant covariate was the age at the beginning of cohabitation (measured in years), which had a negative effect on the "hazard" of giving birth to a child (parameter estimate -0.0499, p-value < 0.0001, see Table 4.2).

We now investigate whether the linearity assumption of this effect is justified. To this purpose, we fitted another proportional continuation ratio model to the data, this time allowing for a smooth nonlinear effect of the age at the beginning of cohabitation on the logit-transformed hazard. For estimation we used P-spline basis functions of degree $d = 3$ with second-order difference penalty and six interior knots. Smoothing parameters were determined by generalized cross-validation, as implemented in the R package *mgcv*. All other covariates entered the model in a linear fashion, in the same way as in Example 4.1. The coefficient estimates for these covariates are shown in Table 5.1. Obviously, there are only small differences between the estimates and the original estimates presented in Table 4.2.

The estimated smooth effect of the covariate "age at the beginning of cohabitation" is shown in Fig. 5.5. The P-spline estimate suggests that the chance of giving birth to a child increased within the interval where the women's age at the beginning of cohabitation was between 15 and approximately 18 years. This is an intuitive result if one assumes that the study participants tended to wait until they attained the age of legal majority before they got children. For women aged older than 18 years at the beginning of cohabitation chances of giving birth to a child started to decrease and became almost constant after approximately 25 years. For women aged older than 35 years at the beginning of cohabitation the estimated effect tended to minus infinity, implying that the chance of giving birth to a child tended to zero (which is biologically meaningful).

Obviously, the estimated effect shown in Fig. 5.5 is distinctly nonlinear. This nonlinearity is not captured by the linear structure of the model specified in Example 4.1. A likelihood ratio test on the difference between the models (linear effect vs. P-spline effect) showed that the deviations from nonlinearity were highly significant (p-value = 0.0007). This suggests that modeling age at the beginning of cohabitation in a nonlinear fashion significantly improved the model fit. □

Table 5.1 Time between cohabitation and first childbirth. The table shows the parameter estimates and estimated standard deviations that were obtained from fitting a logistic discrete-time hazard model to the data (edu = educational attainment, area = geographic area, cohort = cohort of birth, occ = occupational status, sibl = number of siblings, time measured in years). In contrast to Table 4.2, a smooth nonlinear effect was specified for the "covariate age at the beginning of cohabitation." The respective effect estimate is not included here but is visualized in Fig. 5.5

Covariate	Parameter estimate	Est. std. error
edu First stage basic (Ref. category)		
edu Second stage basic	0.0351	0.0747
edu Upper secondary	−0.1960	0.0793
edu Degree	−0.2787	0.1099
cohort 1946–1950 (Ref. category)		
cohort 1951–1955	−0.0421	0.0767
cohort 1956–1960	−0.2638	0.0787
cohort 1961–1965	−0.3112	0.0794
cohort 1966–1975	−0.7682	0.0908
area North (Ref. category)		
area Center	0.2957	0.0626
area South	0.6784	0.0621
occ worker (Ref. category)		
occ non-worker	0.2272	0.0529
sibl	0.0548	0.0269

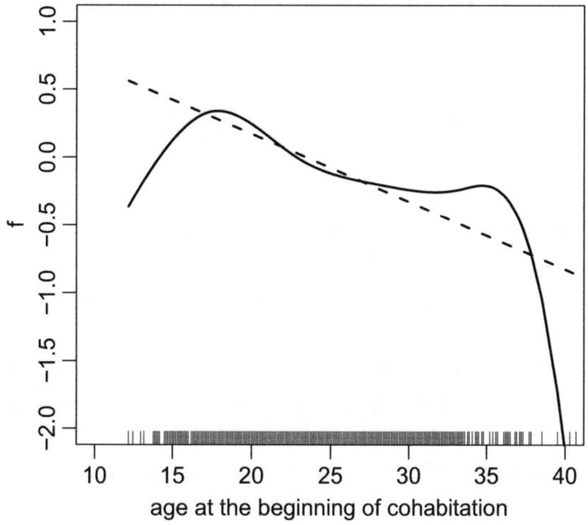

Fig. 5.5 Time between cohabitation and first childbirth. The *solid line* shows the P-spline estimate of the effect of the covariate "age at beginning of cohabitation" that was obtained from a proportional continuation ratio model. The smoothing parameter was obtained via generalized cross-validation. The *dashed line* corresponds to the respective estimate that was obtained when including the covariate in a linear fashion (Example 4.1). Both effect estimates were centered such that the fitted values computed from the data had zero mean

5.3 Time-Varying Coefficients

In the previous sections it has been assumed that the effect of the covariates is the same for all transitions from category t to $t+1$, that is, it has been assumed that the predictor in the model $\lambda(t|\boldsymbol{x}_i) = h(\eta_{it})$ has the form $\eta_{it} = \gamma_0(t) + \boldsymbol{x}_i^T\boldsymbol{\gamma}$ with fixed parameter $\boldsymbol{\gamma}$. But in many applications it has to be assumed that the effects vary over time. In particular when the covariates code some initial condition, for example, the type of treatment at the beginning of the study, the effect on the hazard at earlier times is expected to be stronger than at later times during the study.

A more general approach lets the effects vary over time,

$$\eta_{it} = \gamma_0(t) + \boldsymbol{x}_i^T\boldsymbol{\gamma}(t), \tag{5.8}$$

where $\boldsymbol{\gamma}(t) = (\gamma_1(t), \ldots, \gamma_p(t))$ is a vector-valued function of time with $\gamma_j(t)$ representing the time-varying coefficients of the jth covariate.

It is quite natural to assume that the effects for one covariate vary smoothly over time. Within the basis functions approach one assumes that the functions can be represented by

$$\gamma_j(t) = \sum_{s=1}^{m} \gamma_{js}\phi_s(t). \tag{5.9}$$

It can be assumed that the basis functions are the same for all variables since they all are defined on the same time domain. With $x_{i0} = 1$ the basis functions yield the predictor

$$\eta_{it} = \sum_{j=0}^{p} x_{ij}\gamma_j(t) = \sum_{j=0}^{p}\sum_{s=1}^{m} x_{ij}\phi_s(t)\gamma_{js},$$

which again is linear. More specifically,

$$\eta_{it} = (x_{i0}\phi_1(t), x_{i0}\phi_2(t), \ldots, x_{ip}\phi_m(t))\,\boldsymbol{\beta},$$

where $\boldsymbol{\beta}$ collects all the parameters to be estimated. The penalty is the same as for additive models, only the values of the predictors differ from that of the additive model.

The penalty for smooth effects is the same as for additive models, i.e.,

$$J_\delta = \sum_{j=0}^{p}\sum_{s=\delta+1}^{m} (\Delta^\delta \gamma_{js})^2 = \sum_{j=0}^{p} \boldsymbol{\gamma}_j^T\boldsymbol{K}_j\boldsymbol{\gamma}_j = \boldsymbol{\beta}^T\boldsymbol{K}\boldsymbol{\beta}, \tag{5.10}$$

where $\boldsymbol{\gamma}_j^T = (\gamma_{j1}, \ldots, \gamma_{jm})$ and $\boldsymbol{\beta}^T = (\boldsymbol{\gamma}_0^T, \ldots, \boldsymbol{\gamma}_p^T)$. Since the predictor is linear one uses software for the fitting of binary models that account for a quadratic penalty term.

5.3.1 Penalty for Smooth Time-Varying Effects and Selection

The penalty $\boldsymbol{\gamma}_j^T \boldsymbol{K}_j \boldsymbol{\gamma}_j$ only enforces smoothness of the estimated function but not selection of covariates. Moreover, when using B-splines, the penalty does not penalize all parameters but shrinks the estimate towards a polynomial. For example, if $\boldsymbol{K}_j$ represents first order differences between adjacent basis functions, a constant term is not penalized, and the parameters are shrunk towards a constant. Therefore, to obtain selection of covariates alternative penalties have to be used.

For simplicity, let us consider first order differences with difference vector $\boldsymbol{\gamma}_j^\delta = (\gamma_{j2} - \gamma_{j1}, \ldots, \gamma_{jm} - \gamma_{j,m-1})^T$. A penalty that enforces variable selection is

$$J = \lambda_0 \boldsymbol{\gamma}_0^T \boldsymbol{K}_0 \boldsymbol{\gamma}_0 + \lambda_1 \sum_{j=1}^{p} \|\boldsymbol{\gamma}_j^\delta\| + \lambda_2 \sum_{j=1}^{p} \|\boldsymbol{\gamma}_j\|, \tag{5.11}$$

where the tuning parameters are already included. The first term of the penalty is a simple smoothing penalty, which enforces the smoothness of the baseline hazard, with the amount of smoothing determined by λ_0. The second term simultaneously penalizes the vector of differences. By using the norm of $\boldsymbol{\gamma}_j^\delta$ rather than the squared norm (which would mean smoothing) the components in the difference vector are simultaneously shrunk towards zero. The term is strongly related to the group lasso, which is designed to simultaneously select sets of variables, see Yuan and Lin (2006). For $\lambda_1 \to \infty$ all differences are set to zero and one obtains for each variable a constant term in the linear predictor. The third term penalizes the weight parameter itself. It enforces that also constant effects are set to zero and enforces selection of variables.

The use of basis functions together with tailored penalty terms has the advantage that one can distinguish between effects that vary over time and effects that are constant. In alternative approaches that use localization techniques, where the effects are estimated by using weights on the observations in the neighborhood of the time for which one wants to estimate the effect, all effects are estimated as time-varying. We refer to Kauermann et al. (2005) for an application of localization methods in discrete survival.

Example 5.3 Munich Founder Study

For illustration we use the Munich Founder study introduced in Example 1.2 and use the penalty (5.11) to determine which of the variables have time-varying coefficients. For all coefficient functions cubic B-splines with ten interior knots were used. The tuning parameter for the baseline effect was fixed at 0.001, the tuning parameters for the other terms in the penalty were determined by fivefold cross-validation. The discrete survival model used the complementary log-log link.

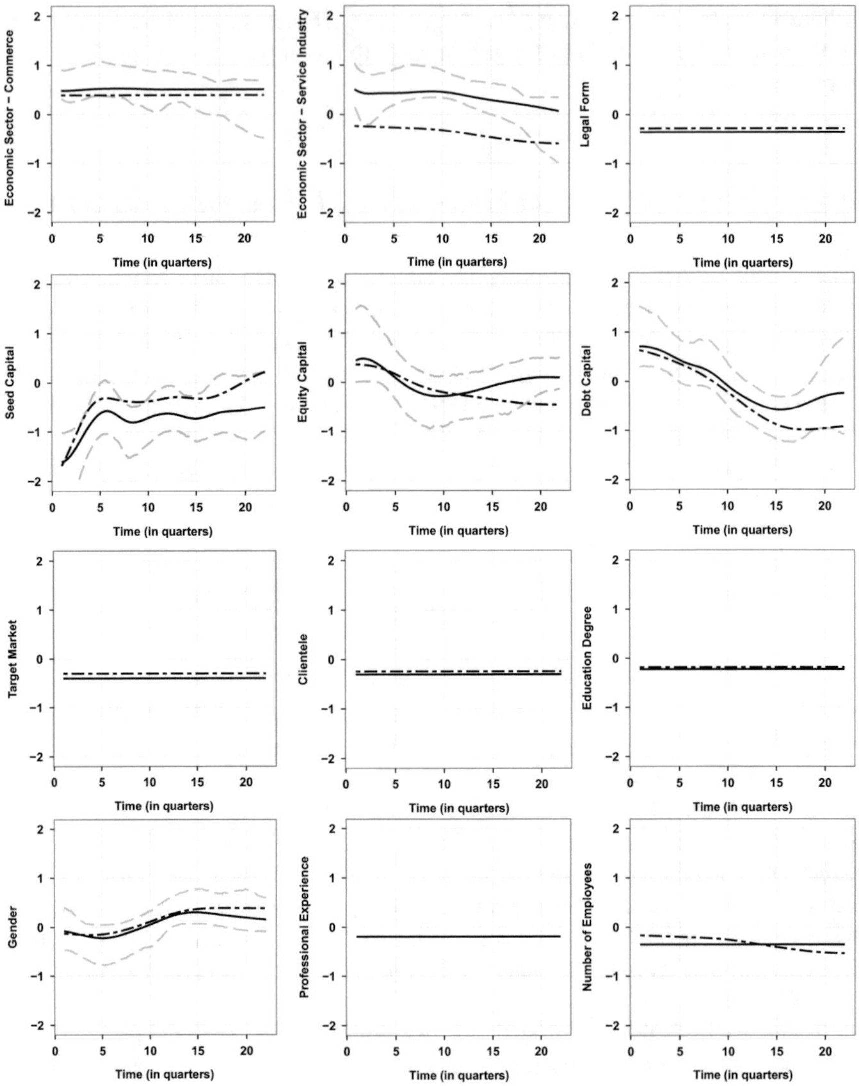

Fig. 5.6 Smooth effect estimates for the Munich Founder Study. The *bold curves* represent the estimates resulting from the use of cubic B-splines with penalty (5.11). *Dashed-dotted curves* stand for the estimates from *mgcv*. *Dashed lines* represent 95 % bootstrap confidence intervals

Figure 5.6 shows the estimated time-varying coefficients. The curves represent the estimates resulting from use of penalty (5.11). Dashed-dotted curves stand for the estimates when using the R package *mgcv* (Wood 2015), which also offers an option to select variables. The dashed lines represent 95 % bootstrap confidence intervals for the estimates obtained by use of (5.11). The coefficient curve for age is omitted because age was estimated to have no impact on the survival of firms. The resulting curves for (5.11) and *mgcv* are rather similar for most of the effects, although *mgcv* has several internal constraints. For example, it enforces the inclusion of a main effect if a variable is categorical and selects only metric covariates. It is seen that some variables show distinct variation of the effects over time while others can be considered as constant over time. For example, the effect of debt capital (1 = yes, 0 = no) is decreasing over time while the legal form (1 = partnership, 0 = small trade) has a negative but time-constant effect. For more details, see Möst (2014). □

5.3.2 Time-Varying Effects and Additive Models

Models with time-varying coefficients are more flexible by allowing for the variation of the effect size over time. However, one should be careful when interpreting these effects because time-varying effects can also be found when the link between response and covariate is misspecified. This may be seen from a simple example where the effect of a covariate is quadratic, that is, the predictor has the form $\eta_{it} = x_i^2$ for positive values of the covariate, which is measured at time $t = 0$. If one fits a linear model with time-varying effects, $\eta_{it} = \gamma_0(t) + x_i^T\gamma(t)$, one obtains very misleading estimates. As shown in Fig. 5.7 one obtains an increasing function for $\hat{\gamma}_0(t)$ and a decreasing function for $\hat{\gamma}(t)$. Since the linear term $x_i^T\gamma(t)$ tries to fit the nonlinear effect x_i^2, the estimated effect $\hat{\gamma}(t)$ is larger in the beginning where all the subjects are in the study but decreases if the subjects with high risk are no longer in the study. One also obtains biased estimates of the baseline hazard. It is constant over time but estimated as an increasing function.

The confusion of nonlinear and time-varying effects can be avoided by simultaneous modeling of flexible covariate effects and time variation. A general model uses the predictor

$$\eta_{it} = f_0(t) + f_1(x_{i1}, t) + \ldots + f_p(x_{ip}, t),$$

where $f_j(x_{ij}, t), j = 1, \ldots, p$, are unknown two-dimensional functions of time and the covariates. In a similar way as for additive models one can expand the unknown functions in basis functions by using tensor products,

$$f_j(x_j, t) = \sum_{s=1}^{m_j} \sum_{l=1}^{m} \gamma_{jsl}\, \phi_{js1}(x_j)\, \phi_{jl2}(t),$$

where $\phi_{j11}(.), \ldots, \phi_{jm_j1}(.)$ denote the basis functions for variable x_j, and $\phi_{j12}(.), \ldots, \phi_{jm2}(.)$ denote the basis functions for time. Since many parameters are involved, penalty terms are needed that restrict the variation over time and covariates. Penalties for differences $\gamma_{j,s+1,l} - \gamma_{jsl}$ and $\gamma_{js,l+1} - \gamma_{jsl}$ were considered by Eilers and Marx (2003) and Currie et al. (2004). In continuous time survival modeling the general hazard regression model (HARE) of Kooperberg et al. (1995) uses the tensor-product approach.

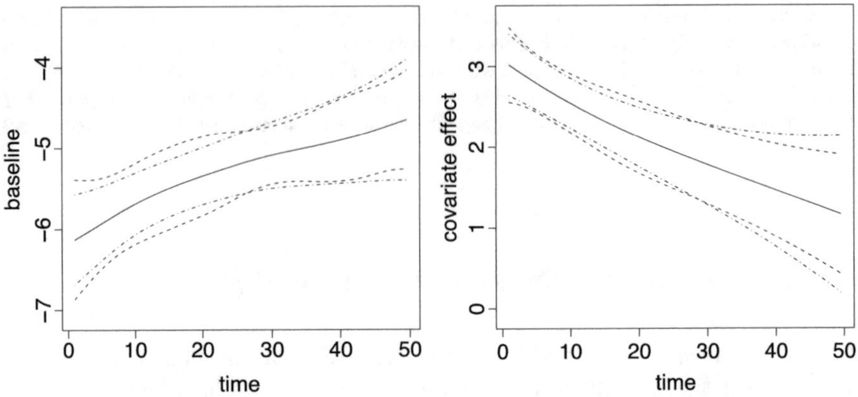

Fig. 5.7 Mean estimates of $\gamma_0(t)$ (*left panel*) and $\gamma(t)$ (*right panel*) when fitting a model with time-varying effects $\eta_{it} = \gamma_0(t) + x_i^T\gamma(t)$ to data generated from a model with quadratic effect $\eta_{it} = x_i^2$ (*dashed lines*: empirical confidence bands, *dashed-dotted lines*: estimated confidence bands)

The model is very flexible by allowing effects of covariates and time to vary freely but yields as many two-dimensional surfaces as variables are available. A more restrictive form has been considered by Tutz and Binder (2004). The predictor

$$\eta_{it} = f_0(t) + \gamma_{t1}f_1(x_{i1}) + \ldots + \gamma_{tp}f_p(x_{ip}) \tag{5.12}$$

assumes that the basic form of the jth predictor, $f_j(.)$, is the same but the strength of the effect varies over time. For example, if γ_{tj} decreases over time, the effect of the jth predictor is damped. Since the model includes multiplicative effects, alternative fitting methods have to be used, see Tutz and Binder (2004). Similar models were considered by Abrahamowicz and MacKenzie (2007) for continuous time data. For an application, see Example 5.4.

5.4 Inclusion of Calendar Time

In studies that cover a long time period, calendar time may have an additional effect on the hazard function. For example, in the analysis of the duration of unemployment the hazard might not only be determined by the time a person is unemployed, but also by calendar time (which contains the economic conditions under which an unemployed person is looking for a job).

Calendar time can be incorporated into discrete hazard models as follows: Let the time of duration as well as calendar time be measured on the same discrete scale, representing, for example, weeks or months. The linear predictor, which determines the hazard for person i after t units of time, can be specified by

$$\eta_{it} = \gamma_0(t) + \gamma_c(c_i + t) + \boldsymbol{x}_i^T\boldsymbol{\gamma}, \tag{5.13}$$

where c_i is the calendar time at the beginning of the duration time that is to be investigated. For example, when modeling the duration of unemployment, c_i is the calendar time when unemployment started, $\gamma_0(t)$ is the effect on the hazard after t months of unemployment, and $\gamma_c(c_i + t)$ is the effect on the hazard at the corresponding calendar time. Both functions $\gamma_0(\cdot)$ and $\gamma_c(\cdot)$ are unknown and are assumed to be smooth functions. Estimates of the unknown functions can be obtained by expanding them in basis functions and using penalty methods as in additive models. Of course it is necessary that there is enough variation in the sample; if unemployment for most of the observations starts at about the same time, there is not enough information to distinguish between the two time scales.

Example 5.4 Psychiatric Hospital Data

For illustration of the semiparametric model (5.12) and the inclusion of calendar time we give an application that was considered by Tutz and Binder (2004). For 1922 patients of a German psychiatric hospital with diagnosis "schizophrenic disorder of paranoid type" the modeled response was the time spent in hospital measured in days. The covariates that were modeled as smooth functions were age at admission, calendar time between January 1, 1995 and December 31, 1999 (measured in days), and the GAF (Global Assessment of Functioning) score at admission, which evaluates the patient's level of functioning. Large values indicate high levels of functioning. Categorical predictors that were included as 0–1 variables were gender ("Male," 1 = male), education ("Edu," 1 = above high school level), partner situation ("Part," 1 = has a permanent partner), job situation ("Job," 1 = full/part time job at admission), first hospitalization ("First," 1 = first admission in a psychiatric hospital), and suicidal action ("Sui," 1 = suicidal act previous to admission). The total predictor of the model had the form

$$\eta_{it} = f_0(t) + f_T(\text{calendar time}) + \text{Male} \cdot \beta_{\text{Male}} + \text{Edu} \cdot \beta_{\text{Edu}} + \text{Part} \cdot \beta_{\text{Part}}$$
$$+ \text{Job} \cdot \beta_{\text{Job}} + \text{First} \cdot \beta_{\text{First}} + \text{Sui} \cdot \beta_{\text{Sui}} + f_{\text{A}}(\text{Age}) + \gamma_t \cdot f_{\text{G}}(\text{GAF score})$$

with smooth functions $f_{\text{T}}, f_{\text{A}}$, and f_{G}. Table 5.2 shows the parameter estimates of the parametric terms. The strongest effect is found for the variable "partner situation," all others can be neglected. Figure 5.8 shows the smooth estimates for the continuous variables. It is seen that there is a tendency that younger people stayed longer in the hospital. The effect of calendar time signals that the time spent in hospital decreases almost continuously with calendar time. The GAF score, which is an assessment score at admission, indicates that a lower level of functioning resulted in a lower probability of dismissal. It seems that there is an essential difference between low and high GAF score, with the effect changing only between 30 and 50 points. The estimates of the modifying factors γ_t (right lower panel of Fig. 5.2) show that the effect of the GAF score at admission vanishes over time, indicating that the predictive power of the initial score diminishes. □

Table 5.2 Estimates of the parametric terms of the model for psychiatric hospital data

Covariates	Estimates	Standard deviations
Male (male)	−0.0525	0.0550
Edu (above high school)	−0.0387	0.0716
Part (has a permanent partner)	0.2619	0.0654
Job (full/part time job at admission)	0.0428	0.0731
First (first admission in a psychiatric hospital)	0.0845	0.0680
Sui (suicidal act previous to admission)	−0.0828	0.1145

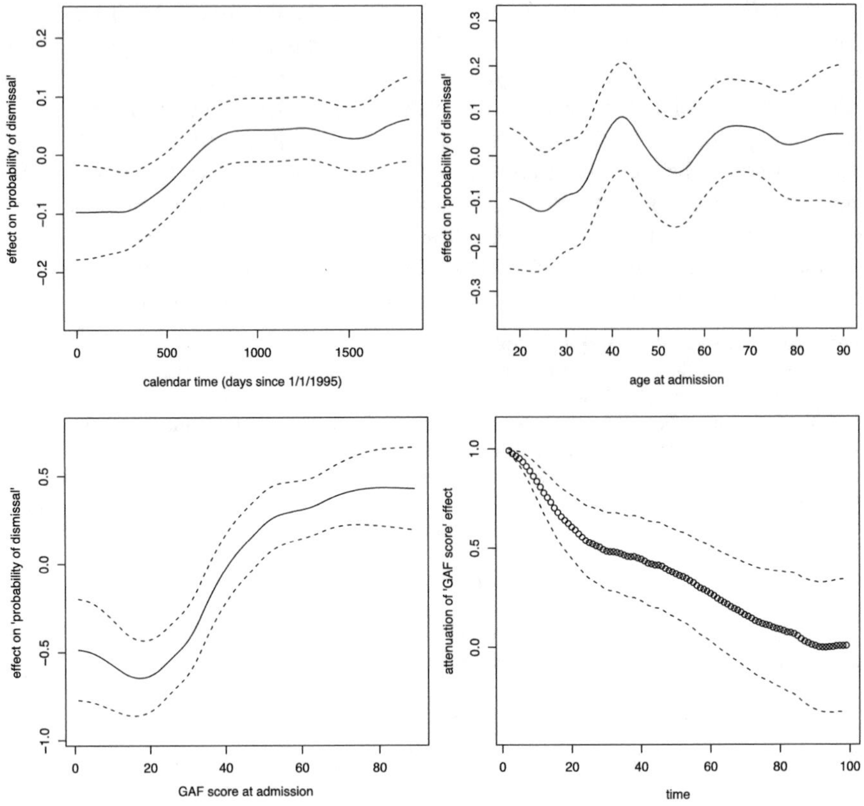

Fig. 5.8 Estimated smooth effects for the psychiatric hospital data (estimates: *solid lines*; confidence bands: *dashed lines*)

5.5 Literature and Further Reading

Local Polynomial Regression. For the general properties of local polynomial regression and the advantages of odd degrees, see Hastie and Loader (1993) and Loader (1999). Asymptotic results are found in Fan and Gijbels (1996). An earlier reference is Cleveland (1979).

Smoothing with Basis Functions and Additive Models. Generalized additive models are treated extensively in Hastie and Tibshirani (1990) and Wood (2006). Penalized regression splines were proposed by Marx and Eilers (1998); selection procedures for the tuning parameters based on the mixed model were proposed by Wand (2000). Asymptotic properties for P-splines were given by Li and Ruppert (2008), Claeskens et al. (2009), and Kauermann et al. (2009).

Time-Varying Coefficients. Fahrmeir (1994) considered the simultaneous estimation of baseline hazard functions and of time-varying covariate effects based on the maximization of posterior densities. Time-varying effects in competing risks models have been considered by Fahrmeir and Wagenpfeil (1996).

5.6 Software

After transforming the original data into binary data for coding transitions over intervals, one can fit smooth baseline hazards and additive models by using software packages for binary regression. For example, an efficient implementation of additive models is contained in the *gam* function of the add-on package *mgcv* (Wood 2015). The *mgcv* package contains a variety of options for the specification of basis functions (specified via the *bs* argument in the model formula). In particular, it is possible to estimate nonlinear predictor effects via cubic regression splines and P-splines. The *method* argument of *gam* provides several algorithms to estimate smoothing parameters (e.g., generalized cross-validation and restricted maximum likelihood estimation). For details, we refer to Wood (2015).

5.7 Exercises

5.1 Locally constant life table estimators use for fixed target value t the weighted log-likelihood

$$l = \sum_{s=1}^{q} \sum_{i \in R_s} \{y_{is} \log \lambda + (1 - y_{is}) \log(1 - \lambda)\}\, w_\gamma(t, s).$$

(a) Derive the estimator $\hat{\lambda}$ by maximizing the log-likelihood.
(b) Derive $\hat{\lambda}$ for the extreme weights given by $\bar{w}_\gamma(t, s) = 1$ if $t = s$ and $\bar{w}_\gamma(t, s) = 0$ if $t \neq s$.

5.2 Consider the difference penalty J_δ given in Eq. (5.5). Show that J_δ can be written in the form

$$J_\delta = \boldsymbol{\gamma}_0^T \boldsymbol{K}_0 \boldsymbol{\gamma}_0 = \boldsymbol{\beta}^T \boldsymbol{K} \boldsymbol{\beta}$$

for $\gamma_0^T = (\gamma_{01}, \ldots, \gamma_{0q})$ and calculate the entries k_{ij} of the matrix $\boldsymbol{K}$ explicitly for $\delta = 1, 2$.

5.3 Apply local polynomial fitting to the German unemployment data introduced in Example 2.1.

(a) Convert the data to a set of augmented data with binary response.
(b) Consider the fixed target value $t = 18$ and calculate the hazard function $\hat{\lambda}(18)$ by using a Gaussian kernel with bandwidth $\gamma = 1$.
(c) Next consider local polynomial smoothing by fitting the hazard $\lambda_t(s) = h(\beta_0 + \cdots + (s - t)^m \beta_m)$ with degree $m = 3$. For each of the bandwidths $\gamma = 0.01, 0.1, 0.2, 0.3, 0.4, 0.5, 1, 3, 10, 50$ estimate the hazard rate at $t = 18$.
(d) Compare the resulting estimates to the raw hazard estimates in Table 2.1.

5.4 In this exercise we consider additive models with smooth baseline hazard and smooth covariate effects. To this purpose, the data set on promotions in rank for biochemists (Example 4.2) is considered.

(a) Convert the data to a set of augmented data with binary response.
(b) Fit a discrete hazard model with logistic link function and a smooth baseline hazard. Consider the prestige of the Ph.D. institution (smooth effect), the cumulative number of published articles, and the cumulative number of citations as covariates. Use penalized B-splines to estimate smooth effects and determine the smoothing parameters via generalized cross-validation. Which covariates have a significant effect (at level $\alpha = 0.05$) on the time to event?
(c) Plot the estimated spline functions for the baseline hazard and the effect of the prestige of the Ph.D. institution. How does the prestige of the Ph.D. institution affect the hazard?

5.5 The aim is to fit a discrete survival model to a set of echocardiogram data that was collected for analyzing the survival behavior of patients after heart attack. The data, which were originally collected at The Reed Institute (Miami), are stored in the UCI Machine Learning Repository (Lichman 2013) and are publicly available at https://archive.ics.uci.edu/ml/datasets/Echocardiogram. All patients contained in the data ($n = 130$) suffered a heart attack at some point in the past; the survival time after heart attack was measured in months. The event of interest is death of the patients. The median time of observed patient survival was 24.5 months; 32.3 % of the observations were censored. A description and summary of the covariates are given in Tables 5.3 and 5.4, respectively.

(a) Prepare the data set for analysis:
    (i) Delete observations with missing values in the response.
    (ii) Generate an event indicator (1 = observed death, 0 = still alive).
    (iii) Impute missing values in the continuous covariates by inserting the respective sample means.

Table 5.3 Description of the covariates contained in the echocardiogram data (Exercise 5.5)

Variable	Description
AHA	Age at heart attack (measured in years)
PE	Indicator if pericardial effusion is fluid (= 1) or not (= 0)
FS	A measure of contractility around the heart; lower numbers are increasingly abnormal
epss	e-point septal separation; another measure of contractility; larger numbers are increasingly abnormal
lvdd	Left ventricular end-diastolic dimension; measures the size of the heart at end-diastole
WMI	Wall-motion-score; measures how the segments of the left ventricle are moving; standardized by the number of segments seen

Table 5.4 Descriptive analysis of the covariates contained in the echocardiogram data (Exercise 5.5)

Variable	Categories/unit	Sample proportion/median (range)
AHA	Years	62 (35–86)
PE	Fluid	18.5 %
	Otherwise	81.5 %
FS	Score/continuous	0.22 (0.01–0.61)
epss	Score/continuous	12 (0–40)
lvdd	Score/continuous	12 (0–40)
WMI	Score/continuous	1.22 (1–3)

(iv) Randomly generate a training sample (containing 75 % of the observations) and a test sample (containing 25 % of the observations).
(v) Convert both samples to sets of augmented data with binary response and construct an event indicator for the censoring process.

(b) Fit a discrete hazard model with logistic link function and consider penalized B-spline basis expansions of various dimensions ($m = 4, 5, \ldots, 15$). Estimate the smoothing parameters via generalized cross-validation. Investigate the effect of the number of basis functions on the shape of the smooth function estimates.
(c) Calculate the integrated PE curve for all basis dimension configurations from the test data. Is there an effect of the basis dimension on prediction accuracy?

Chapter 6
Tree-Based Approaches

The modeling techniques described in Chaps. 3 and 5 are based on the assumption that the predictor is an additive function of the covariates. Although this assumption is intuitive and facilitates interpretation of the models, it often happens in practice that additive predictors may not capture the true data structure very well. This is, for example, the case when interactions between categorical covariates are present, i.e., when the combination of two (or more) levels of some covariates affects the survival in more than just an additive way.

In principle, interaction terms (being the products of two or more covariates) may be easily incorporated into discrete hazard models. However, the necessary specification of the model formula requires data analysts to know about the respective interactions *in advance*. In other words, unknown interactions between covariates, especially if they involve more than two variables, cannot be automatically detected by the models presented in Chaps. 3 and 5. Although, in principle, one could apply traditional stepwise variable selection techniques (known from linear regression) to build models that contain both main effects and interaction terms, this strategy is often unfeasible because of the large number of possible interaction terms. Moreover, backward selection strategies face the problem that estimation becomes numerically unstable or that estimators do not even exist if the number of parameters is large relative to the sample size. This issue is particularly cumbersome when the covariate space contains a set of categorical variables with large numbers of categories, or when the number of predictors is high-dimensional ("small n, large p").

Recursive partitioning techniques (also termed "tree-based" techniques) are a popular method to address these problems. The method has its roots in automatic interaction detection (AID), proposed by Morgan and Sonquist (1963). A modern version is due to Breiman et al. (1984) and is known by the name of *classification and regression trees*, often abbreviated as CART. In this chapter we consider versions of recursive partitioning that are useful in discrete survival modeling.

G. Tutz, M. Schmid, *Modeling Discrete Time-to-Event Data*,
Springer Series in Statistics, DOI 10.1007/978-3-319-28158-2_6

6.1 Recursive Partitioning

The idea of recursive partitioning is to subdivide the covariate space into a set of rectangles and then fit a covariate-free model to the observations in each of them. For example, if the outcome variable is a continuous event time, a covariate-free estimate of the survival function is obtained by applying the Kaplan–Meier estimator. The most popular algorithm for recursive partitioning is the classification and regression tree (CART) algorithm (Breiman et al. 1984), which is defined by the following procedure: Starting with the "root node" (referring to the unpartitioned covariate space and containing the complete set of observations), partitioning is done in a hierarchical way by recursively applying binary splits to the data (see Fig. 6.1 for an illustration). In each node (i.e., in each rectangle), the idea is to

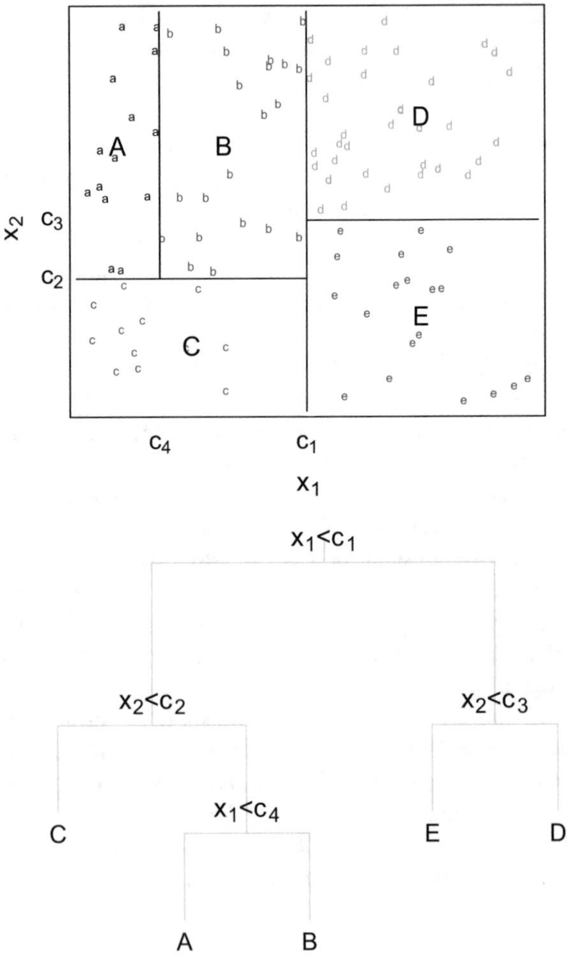

Fig. 6.1 Illustration of recursive partitioning. The *upper figure* shows an example partition of a covariate space with two continuous predictor variables x_1 and x_2. In the first step, x_1 is used to subdivide the covariate space into two rectangles at threshold c_1. In the second step, x_2 is used to subdivide the left rectangle into two more rectangles referring to "$x_2 \leq c_2$" and "$x_2 > c_2$". Two more splits are carried out at thresholds c_3 and c_4, so that the whole covariate space is subdivided into five rectangles. The resulting tree with five terminal nodes (referring to the five rectangles) is visualized in the *lower figure*

select a single covariate x_k, $k \in \{1, \ldots, p\}$, and a binary splitting rule $R(x_k)$ that is obtained by the optimization of a pre-defined splitting criterion. For example, if x_k is continuous or ordinal, the splitting rule $R(x_k)$ is of the form "$x_k \leq c_k$ vs. $x_k > c_k$" with threshold c_k (Fig. 6.1). Consequently, the covariate space is subdivided into two rectangles (termed "children nodes") according to $R(x_k)$. If x_k is a categorical predictor with categories $\mathcal{C}_k = \{c_{k1}, \ldots, c_{kq_k}\}$, the idea is to subdivide $\mathcal{C}_k$ into two mutually exclusive sets $\mathcal{C}_{k1}$ and $\mathcal{C}_{k2}$ with $\mathcal{C}_{k1} \cup \mathcal{C}_{k2} = \mathcal{C}_k$, and the splitting rule $R(x_k)$ becomes "$x_k \in \mathcal{C}_{k1}$ vs. $x_k \in \mathcal{C}_{k2}$". Of course x_k, c_k, $\mathcal{C}_{k1}$ and $\mathcal{C}_{k2}$ may vary across the nodes.

The choice of the splitting criterion depends on the scale of the outcome variable Y. For example, if Y is a binary variable, a popular strategy is to construct a *classification tree*. An often used splitting criterion for binary Y is the Gini impurity measure, which is computed as follows: Assume that a node has to be split into two children nodes using covariate x_k. Denote the children nodes by $\mathcal{N}_m(x_k, R(x_k))$, $m = 1, 2$, and let $p_m(x_k, R(x_k))$ be the proportions of ones in the children nodes. The Gini impurity measure is defined as $G_m(x_k, R(x_k)) := 2p_m(x_k, R(x_k))$ $(1 - p_m(x_k, R(x_k)))$, so that it attains its minimum value 0 in pure nodes with $p_m \in \{0, 1\}$. The optimization problem in each split is then given by minimizing the weighted sum of the Gini coefficients in the children nodes

$$\min_{x_k, R(x_k)} \left\{ |\mathcal{N}_1(x_k, R(x_k))| \cdot G_1(x_k, R(x_k)) + |\mathcal{N}_2(x_k, R(x_k))| \cdot G_2(x_k, R(x_k)) \right\}, \quad (6.1)$$

where $|\mathcal{N}_1|$ and $|\mathcal{N}_2|$ denote the cardinalities of the sets of observations contained in the nodes $\mathcal{N}_1$ and $\mathcal{N}_2$, respectively. Similarly, if Y is a continuous survival time, a *survival tree* can be constructed by maximizing the log-rank statistic obtained from the survival times in the children nodes (Bou-Hamad et al. 2011b). The result of a recursive partitioning procedure is a set of "terminal nodes," each containing a subset of the observations of the data. Tree estimates are given by fitting covariate-free models to the observations in the terminal nodes.

In the literature, many types of recursive partitioning methods have been proposed. These methods mainly differ in the algorithm that is used to determine the optimal covariate x_k, and also in the choice of splitting criteria and techniques for determining the optimal tree size. Apart from the CART algorithm, popular methods are C4.5 (Quinlan 1993) and conditional inference trees (Hothorn et al. 2006). Overviews of the various methods are given, e.g., in Hastie et al. (2009), Tutz (2012), and Strobl et al. (2009). In the following we consider two recursive partitioning methods that are specifically designed for discrete-time survival outcomes.

6.2 Recursive Partitioning Based on Covariate-Free Discrete Hazard Models

An algorithm for discrete failure times that extends the CART approach to discrete-time survival data has been developed by Bou-Hamad et al. (2009). The approach uses the log-likelihood of a discrete survival model given by

$$l \propto \sum_{i=1}^{n} \sum_{s=1}^{t_i} y_{is} \log \lambda(s|\boldsymbol{x}_i) + (1 - y_{is}) \log(1 - \lambda(s|\boldsymbol{x}_i)) \tag{6.2}$$

to define a splitting criterion for tree construction. In each child node one fits a covariate-free discrete hazard model of the simple form $\lambda(t|\boldsymbol{x}_i) = h(\gamma_{0t})$, which contains only intercepts. Splits are obtained by maximizing the sum of the two observed log-likelihoods in the children nodes. More specifically, the optimization problem in each split is given by

$$\max_{x_k, R(x_k)} \left\{ l_1(x_k, R(x_k)) + l_2(x_k, R(x_k)) \right\}, \tag{6.3}$$

where l_1 and l_2 refer to the log-likelihood functions of the intercept models in the children nodes $\mathcal{N}_1$ and $\mathcal{N}_2$, respectively.

After having grown the tree, the hazard functions of the covariate-free model with intercepts γ_{0t} only are estimated in each of the terminal nodes. These functions constitute the tree estimate of the hazard $\lambda(t|\cdot)$ conditional on covariate combinations $\boldsymbol{x}$.

A problem of recursive partitioning methods is their tendency to overfit the data if the number of terminal nodes becomes too large. For example, growing the largest possible tree with exactly one observation in each terminal node is not a good strategy, as the estimation of the hazard functions would be based on only one observation each. For this reason, classification and regression trees are usually "pruned" after tree construction. Starting with the terminal nodes of the full tree, a cost-complexity criterion (governing the trade-off between classification accuracy and tree size) is successively evaluated by collapsing the nodes that result in the smallest decrease of classification accuracy. The optimal subtree is given by the tree with the minimum value of the cost-complexity criterion.

Bou-Hamad et al. (2009) adapted this strategy to discrete-time survival trees as follows: After tree construction, pruning is accomplished by minimizing the information criterion

$$-2 \cdot l_T + \xi \cdot q \cdot Q, \tag{6.4}$$

where l_T is the sum of the log-likelihood functions in the terminal nodes and Q is the number of terminal nodes. The tuning parameter ξ governs the trade-off between model fit (measured by l_T) and model complexity (measured by Q). Popular values are $\xi = 2$ (giving rise to Akaike's information criterion) and $\xi = \log(n)$ (giving rise to the Bayesian information criterion). The optimal tree is then given by the subtree with minimum value of (6.4).

The tree method described above follows the same rationale as recursive partitioning techniques for continuous survival data. But for continuous time one uses the Kaplan–Meier estimate instead of a model that contains intercepts only to obtain covariate-free estimates in the terminal nodes. In fact, the two methods are not so different because the Kaplan–Meier estimator presented in Chap. 2 is strongly related to the life table estimator. Also, continuous survival trees are often based on the maximum value of the log-rank statistic for obtaining splits of covariates (LeBlanc and Crowley 1993). Because this measure is sensitive to the differences between the (covariate-free) Kaplan–Meier estimates in the children nodes, it follows the same principle as the sum of the covariate-free discrete log-likelihood functions in (6.3).

Because of these similarities, survival trees for continuous failure times might also work when applied to discrete failure time data, especially when the number of time points is large and intervals are equidistant. Nevertheless, splitting criteria such as the log-rank statistic are problematic when data are grouped and when the number of ties is large. These issues are avoided when using the recursive partitioning techniques for discrete survival times that are presented in this chapter.

6.3 Recursive Partitioning with Binary Outcome

An alternative way to obtain trees for discrete failure times is to explicitly use the binary variables in the representation of the log-likelihood function given in (6.2) and to fit a classification tree to the augmented learning data (Schmid et al. 2016). Basically one uses trees for binary responses. Since one uses the augmented data in this case, the approach comprises the following steps:

Step 1: Specification of the Data Structure

By definition of the log-likelihood function (6.2), it is obvious that the values of the binary outcome variable are given by the first columns of the augmented data matrices

Binary observations	Design variables					
0	1	0	0	...	0	$\boldsymbol{x}_i^T$
0	0	1	0	...	0	$\boldsymbol{x}_i^T$
0	0	0	1	...	0	
$\vdots$						
1	0	0	0	...	1	$\boldsymbol{x}_i^T$

and

Binary observations	Design variables					
0	1	0	0	...	0	$\boldsymbol{x}_i^T$
0	0	1	0	...	0	$\boldsymbol{x}_i^T$
0	0	0	1	...	0	
$\vdots$						
0	0	0	0	...	1	$\boldsymbol{x}_i^T$

for uncensored and censored observations, respectively. The same matrices have already been used to estimate the parametric discrete-time hazard models in Chap. 3. Also, the definition of the hazard function

$$\lambda(t|\boldsymbol{x}) = P(T = t \,|\, T \geq t, \boldsymbol{x}), \quad t = 1, 2, \ldots$$

implies that one can condition on both the covariate values $\boldsymbol{x}$ and the event "$T \geq t$". To account for the ordinal structure of T, the dummy variables for the baseline hazard in the design matrices above are replaced by the column vector $(1, 2, \ldots)^\top$. The input data for individual observations are thus given by

Binary observations	Design variables	
0	1	$\boldsymbol{x}_i^T$
0	2	$\boldsymbol{x}_i^T$
0	3	
$\vdots$		
1	t_i	$\boldsymbol{x}_i^T$

and

Binary observations	Design variables	
0	1	$\boldsymbol{x}_i^T$
0	2	$\boldsymbol{x}_i^T$
0	3	
$\vdots$		
0	t_i	$\boldsymbol{x}_i^T$

for uncensored and censored observations, respectively. The augmented data set for tree construction is obtained by combining the above matrices. By definition, the resulting design matrix has $\tilde{n} := \sum_{i=1}^{n} t_i$ rows. This data structure, which implies that T is treated as an ordinal covariate during tree construction, represents a much more flexible form than the specification of the time trend γ_{0t} in a discrete hazard model.

Step 2: Tree Construction and Estimation of the Hazard Function

Because of the binomial structure of the log-likelihood function (6.2), recursive partitioning methods for binary outcomes can be applied to the augmented data specified in Step 1. Assuming that an appropriate splitting criterion has been defined (for details see below), this strategy results in a set of terminal nodes that are represented by binary outcome values $y_j \in \{0, 1\}, j \in \{1, \ldots, \tilde{n}\}$ each. These binary values can be used to obtain an estimate of the hazard function as follows: Because T is also a candidate splitting variable for tree construction, the terminal nodes of the tree correspond to values of $\boldsymbol{x}$ and to time intervals $T_{(1)} \cup T_{(2)} \cup \ldots \cup T_{(Q)} = \{1, \ldots, q\}$ (each being a subset of $\{1, \ldots, q\}$), see Fig. 6.2 for an illustration. Consequently, for each combination of the predictor variables $\boldsymbol{x}$, estimates of $\lambda(t \in T_{(\cdot)}|\cdot)$ are available by the proportions of ones in the respective terminal nodes. Denoting these estimates by $\hat{\lambda}_1, \ldots, \hat{\lambda}_Q$, estimates of the conditional survival function $S(t|\boldsymbol{x})$ are obtained by applying

$$S(t|\boldsymbol{x}) = P(T > t \,|\, \boldsymbol{x}) = \prod_{i=1}^{t} (1 - \lambda(i|\boldsymbol{x}))$$

to $\hat{\lambda}_1, \ldots, \hat{\lambda}_Q$.

Concerning the choice of an appropriate splitting criterion, discrete-time survival trees do not focus on the correct classification of the individual values $y_j \in \{0, 1\}$ but on the accurate estimation of the *probabilities* $\lambda_1, \ldots, \lambda_Q$ ("probability estimation tree," Provost and Domingos 2003). Therefore, the aim is to minimize the deviations of the true node probabilities from the estimated probabilities in each node during tree construction. Denoting by $\mathcal{N}$ the set of observations in some arbitrary node, a natural measure of node impurity is given by the Brier score

$$\begin{aligned} BS_{\mathcal{N}} &:= \frac{1}{|\mathcal{N}|} \sum_{j \in \mathcal{N}} \Big[\Big(\hat{\mathrm{P}}(y_j = 1 \,|\, j \in \mathcal{N}) - \mathrm{I}(y_j = 1) \Big)^2 \\ &\quad + \Big(\hat{\mathrm{P}}(y_j = 0 \,|\, j \in \mathcal{N}) - \mathrm{I}(y_j = 0) \Big)^2 \Big] \\ &= \frac{1}{|\mathcal{N}|} \sum_{j \in \mathcal{N}} \Big[\Big(\hat{\lambda}_{\mathcal{N}} - \mathrm{I}(y_j = 1) \Big)^2 + \Big((1 - \hat{\lambda}_{\mathcal{N}}) - \mathrm{I}(y_j = 0) \Big)^2 \Big], \end{aligned} \tag{6.5}$$

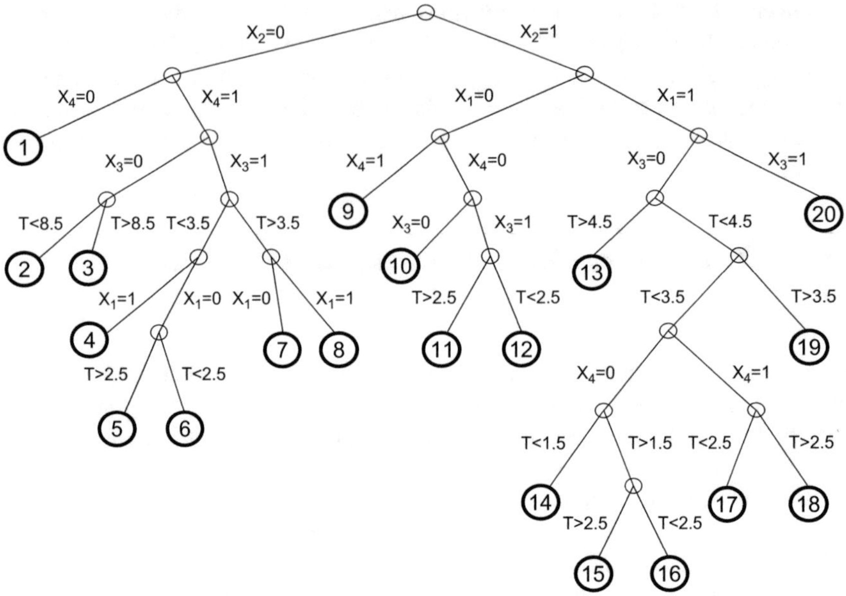

Fig. 6.2 Illustration of the tree building approach with binary outcome. The tree was constructed by applying the CART algorithm to a simulated data set with four binary predictor variables $x_1, \ldots, x_4$. Tree construction resulted in 20 terminal nodes, with the terminal nodes defining time intervals $T_{(1)}, \ldots, T_{(Q)} \subset \{1, \ldots, 20\}$. For example, the time interval corresponding to the first node (referring to observations with $x_2 = 0$ and $x_4 = 0$) is $T_{(1)} = \{1, \ldots, 20\}$ because T was not used in the construction of node 1. Consequently, the estimated hazard for the respective observations is time-constant. Conversely, the time interval for nodes 7 and 8 is given by $T_{(7)} = T_{(8)} = \{4, 5, \ldots\}$ because T was used as a splitting variable in the construction of the two nodes

which quantifies the squared distance between the "observed" hazards $y_j \in \{0, 1\}$, $j \in \mathcal{N}$, and the estimated hazards $\hat{\lambda}_{\mathcal{N}} := \sum_j y_j / |\mathcal{N}|$. The Brier score is a "proper" measure in the sense that (6.5) becomes minimal if the true probabilities $P(y_j = 1 | j \in \mathcal{N})$ are used instead of $\hat{\lambda}_{\mathcal{N}}$ (Gneiting and Raftery 2007).

Because the outcome values y_j are binary, the Brier score as a measure of node impurity is equivalent to the Gini impurity measure defined above (Exercise 6.2). Consequently, the traditional CART algorithm based on the Gini criterion can be used for survival tree construction, and the hazard $\lambda(t|\cdot)$ can be estimated from the terminal nodes as described previously.

Step 3: Selection of Tuning Parameters

Similar to classification and regression trees, probability estimation trees may overfit the data if they involve too many terminal nodes. For example, growing the largest possible tree with exactly one observation in each terminal node is not desirable, as the "probability" estimates $\hat{\lambda}_q$ would all be either 0 or 1 in this case. Moreover, the variance of $\hat{\lambda}_{\mathcal{N}}$ is inversely related to the node size, implying that larger nodes lead to more accurate estimates of $\mathrm{P}(y_j = 1 | j \in \mathcal{N})$.

In view of these considerations, tree construction for discrete survival times can be optimized by using the minimum number of observations in the terminal nodes as the main tuning parameter of the algorithm ("cardinality pruning"). This strategy implies that tree construction is stopped when further splitting of any of the current nodes would result in children nodes that contain less observations than the minimum node size. In practice, the optimum minimum node size can either be determined by means of information criteria or by means of cross-validation techniques. Similar to (6.4), information criteria can be defined by

$$-2l + \xi \cdot (Q-1) , \tag{6.6}$$

where l is the binomial log-likelihood (6.2) evaluated at $\hat{\lambda}_1, \ldots, \hat{\lambda}_Q$, and where $(Q-1)$ is the estimated complexity of the tree (measured by the number of binary splits). Specifying $\xi = 2$ and $\xi = \log(\tilde{n})$ gives rise to the AIC and BIC criteria, respectively. Because the complexity term $(Q-1)$ ignores the search of the covariate space in each split of the tree and therefore underestimates its true complexity, an alternative strategy is to consider cross-validated values of l or of the integrated prediction error curve $\widehat{\mathrm{PE}}_{\mathrm{int}}$ described in Chap. 4. The optimum minimum node size is obtained from the tree that optimizes the chosen performance criterion.

It should be emphasized that cardinality pruning is different from the cost-complexity pruning techniques that are usually applied to classification and regression trees. While cost-complexity pruning usually produces accurate trees for classification, the technique is suboptimal when the aim is to estimate class probabilities from the terminal nodes. This is because trees that optimize classification accuracy are often smaller than trees that are optimal for probability estimation (see Provost and Domingos 2003 for examples and an in-depth discussion). In view of these considerations, cardinality pruning is a compromise between too small trees (obtained from cost-complexity pruning) and too large trees (having too little observations in the terminal nodes).

Step 4: Estimation of Conditional Survival Functions

The final step is to obtain an estimate of the conditional survival function $S(t|\boldsymbol{x}_j^{\mathcal{T}})$ for a new observation that is contained in a test sample $(\tilde{t}_j^{\mathcal{T}}, \delta_j^{\mathcal{T}}, \boldsymbol{x}_j^{\mathcal{T}}), j = 1, \ldots, n^{\mathcal{T}}$. This is done as follows: First, the new covariate values $\boldsymbol{x}_j^{\mathcal{T}}$ are combined with every possible time point t, yielding a set of vectors $((\boldsymbol{x}_j^{\mathcal{T}})^\top, 1), \ldots, ((\boldsymbol{x}_j^{\mathcal{T}})^\top, t_{\max})$, $j = 1, \ldots, n^{\mathcal{T}}$. These vectors are dropped down the tree, and the estimates $\hat{\lambda}_q$

Input: Learning data $(t_i, \delta_i, \boldsymbol{x}_i)$, $i = 1, \ldots, n$.

Step 1 (data augmentation): Generate the set of augmented data by constructing matrices with binary outcome values y_{is} and ordinal representation of T.

Step 2 (tree construction): Apply the CART algorithm with Gini impurity measure to the augmented data.

Step 3 (tuning): Determine the optimum minimum node size via cardinality pruning (either by using information criteria or by means of cross-validation of l or $\widehat{PE}_{\text{int}}$).

Step 4 (estimation of the conditional survival function): Predict the hazard and survival functions by combining a new set of observations $(t_j^{\mathcal{T}}, \delta_j^{\mathcal{T}}, \boldsymbol{x}_j^{\mathcal{T}}), j = 1, \ldots, n^{\mathcal{T}}$, with every possible time point and by dropping the resulting vectors down the tree.

Fig. 6.3 Schematic overview of recursive partitioning with binary outcome

in the respective terminal nodes form the estimated hazard function $\hat{\lambda}(t|\boldsymbol{x}_j^{\mathcal{T}})$. By definition of the survival function (3.2), a prediction of $S(t|\boldsymbol{x}_j^{\mathcal{T}})$ (denoted by $\hat{S}(t|\boldsymbol{x}_j^{\mathcal{T}})$) is obtained.

A schematic overview of Steps 1–4 is given in Fig. 6.3.

Remark A key feature of the method is that the estimated hazard rate of an observation may depend on different sets of predictor variables at different time points. Also, the method allows for a flexible modeling of the baseline hazard. In particular, the method includes a data-driven detection of time-constant hazards (because T is treated in the same way as the other covariates and does not necessarily have to be selected as a splitting variable for tree construction).

Example 6.1 Copenhagen Stroke Study

We illustrate the two recursive partitioning algorithms by fitting survival trees to a learning sample of size $n = 345$ that was drawn randomly from the complete data set. Because the complete data set included 518 observations, the learning sample contained approximately two thirds of the observations of the complete data set. Survival time was grouped into 1-year intervals. All covariates listed in Table 1.3, i.e., sex, hypertension, ischemic heart disease, previous stroke, other disabling disease, alcohol intake, diabetes, smoking behavior, atrial fibrillation, hemorrhage, age, Scandinavian stroke score, and cholesterol level, were used for tree construction. For the first method (recursive partitioning based on covariate-free discrete hazard models) we used the AIC-type criterion with $\xi = 2$ to determine the optimal tree. Figure 6.4 shows the AIC values for various pruning steps. The structure of the resulting survival tree is shown in Fig. 6.5.

For the second method (recursive partitioning with binary outcome) the optimum minimum node size was determined by drawing five random samples of size 230 from the learning data (i.e., two thirds of the learning data) and by evaluating the integrated prediction error $\widehat{\text{PE}}_{\text{int}}$ on the five remaining sets containing 115 observations each. The average value of $\widehat{\text{PE}}_{\text{int}}$ obtained from the five samples is shown in Fig. 6.6. It is seen that the minimum node size with smallest prediction error was 80. Note that this minimum node size does not refer to the original survival data but to the augmented data which contained 2022 data lines. The structure of the resulting survival tree (fitted to the complete augmented learning sample with minimum node size 80) is shown in Fig. 6.7.

Figures 6.5 and 6.7 show that both methods selected the Scandinavian stroke score first, indicating that this covariate was of high importance for the prediction of survival. Note that the thresholds (48 and 50.5 for Methods 1 and 2, respectively) were very similar. Another important covariate is age, which was selected in the second steps of both methods. In case of Method 2,

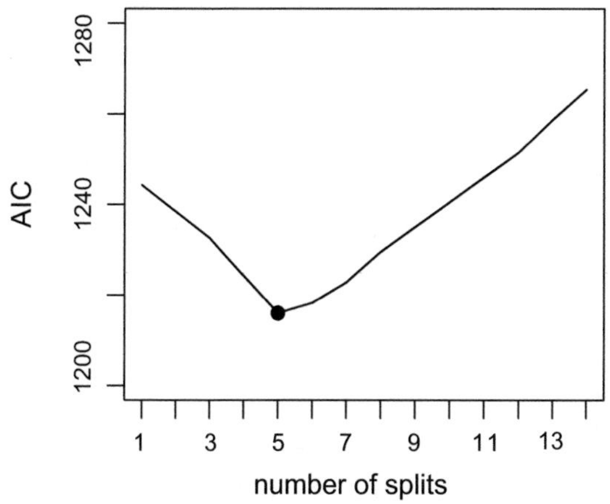

Fig. 6.4 Copenhagen stroke study. The panel shows the AIC values that were obtained from Method 1 (recursive partitioning based on covariate-free discrete hazard models). Estimation was based on a random sample of size $n = 345$. The *black dot* indicates the optimal number of splits, which was estimated to be equal to 5

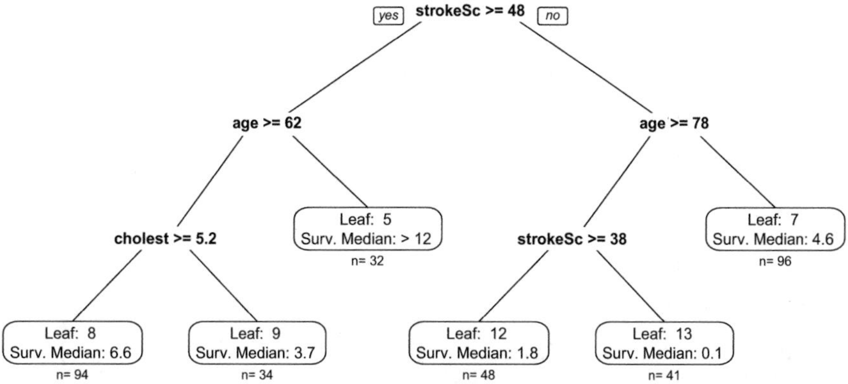

Fig. 6.5 Copenhagen stroke study. The figure shows the survival tree that was estimated via Method 1 (recursive partitioning based on covariate-free discrete hazard models) from a random sample of size $n = 345$. Each node contains an estimate of the median survival time, i.e., of the time point for which $\hat{S}(t|\boldsymbol{x}) = 0.5$

the survival time T was used in addition to the covariates to construct the 13 terminal nodes. For example, there was a change in the estimated hazard rate after 3 years ("time.interval < 3.5"), as this splitting rule was implemented in the second step of Method 2. The numbers below the terminal nodes in Fig. 6.7 are the estimates of the hazard rates. Figure 6.8 shows two examples of survival functions that were obtained by averaging the predictions obtained from Method 2 for patients with Scandinavian stroke score below and above median (which was equal to 46 in the learning data). As shown in the figure, patients with a stroke score below the median had smaller survival probabilities on average. □

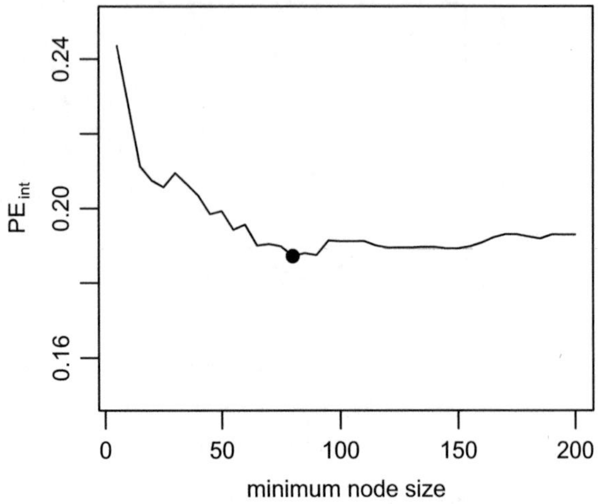

Fig. 6.6 Copenhagen stroke study. The panel shows the prediction error $\widehat{\text{PE}}_{\text{int}}$ that was obtained from applying Method 2 (recursive partitioning with binary outcome) to five sets of learning and evaluation data (of sizes 230 and 115, respectively, each) that were drawn from a random sample of size $n = 345$. The *black dot* indicates the optimum minimum node size for the augmented data (2022 data lines), which was estimated to be 80

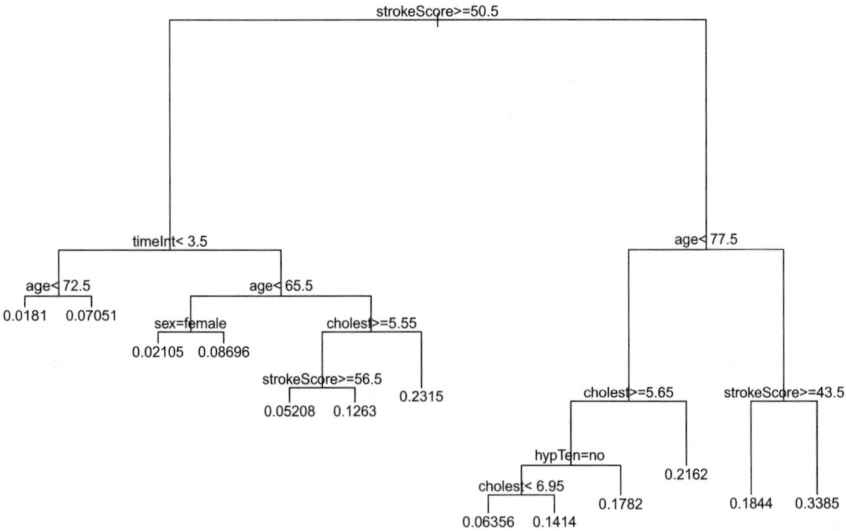

Fig. 6.7 Copenhagen stroke study. The figure shows the survival tree with minimum node size 80 that was estimated via Method 2 (recursive partitioning with binary outcome) from a random sample of size $n = 345$. The numbers below the terminal nodes are the estimated hazards $\hat{\lambda}_1, \ldots, \hat{\lambda}_{13}$ (timeInt = time interval, strokeScore = Scandinavian stroke score, cholest = cholesterol level, hypTen = hypertension)

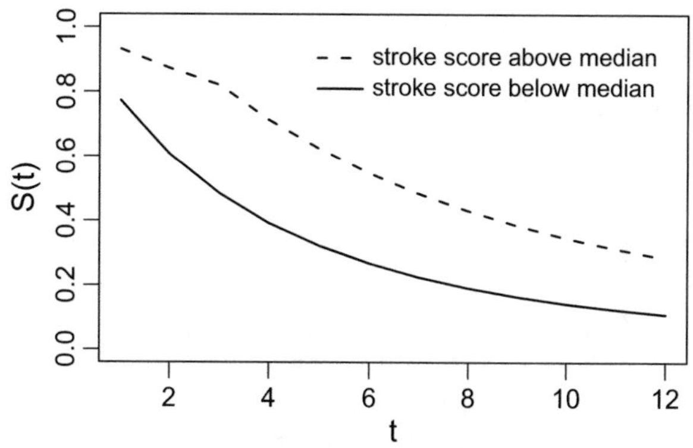

Fig. 6.8 Copenhagen stroke study. The figure shows the survival functions that were obtained by averaging the predictions for patients with Scandinavian stroke score below and above the median (= 46). Estimates were obtained via Method 2 (recursive partitioning with binary outcome). It is seen that patients with below median score values tend to have an increased risk of dying at all time points

6.4 Ensemble Methods

A drawback of recursive partitioning methods is that the resulting tree estimators usually suffer from a large variance. This means that small variations in the data can result in completely different trees. Therefore, when the focus is not on interpretability but on prediction accuracy, it is a convenient strategy to stabilize the results obtained from single trees by applying *ensemble methods* to the data. Briefly spoken, the idea of ensemble methods is to apply recursive partitioning not only to a single training sample but to a larger number of samples that are generated from the original data. Often these samples are generated via bootstrapping, i.e., via drawing random samples of size n from the original data with replacement. The ensemble estimate is then given by the average of the individual estimates, and the variability in the predictions is thereby reduced. Here we consider *bagging* and *random forests*, which are among the most popular ensemble techniques.

6.4.1 Bagging

The idea of bagging (Breiman 1996) is to generate a fixed number of samples from the original data and to apply recursive partitioning techniques to each of the samples. Prediction accuracy typically increases as the number of bootstrap samples (denoted by B) gets larger; in practice, $100 \leq B \leq 500$ samples are usually considered sufficient. In the case of a discrete failure time outcome, bagging can either be carried out by drawing bootstrap samples from the original data set and by applying Method 1 to the samples or by augmenting the data first and by applying

Method 2 to bootstrap samples drawn from the augmented data. The bagged hazard and survival function estimates are then given by the averages of the B individual hazard and survival function estimates, respectively.

6.4.2 *Random Forests*

While bagging reduces the variance of a single tree, the variance of the bagged estimate may still be large if the B individual trees are very similar (i.e., if the B tree estimates resemble each other despite being constructed from different input data). It may therefore be of interest to *decorrelate* the B trees, i.e., to reduce their similarity in order to obtain a smaller variance. This approach is implemented in the *random forest* algorithm (Breiman 2001), which artificially reduces the number of covariates that are available for splitting in each node. Similar to bagging, random forests apply recursive partitioning methods to B bootstrap samples. The main difference between the two methods is that random forests only use a small number of covariates (denoted by $mtry$, where $mtry \ll p$) that are sampled randomly from the whole set of covariates in each node. With the random forest approach, $mtry$ is an additional tuning parameter that needs to be determined using cross-validation methods. Usually, optimization of $mtry$ is performed in a highly efficient way by using the out-of-bootstrap observations (i.e., those observations that are not contained in the bootstrap samples) as test data for each of the B trees. Similar to bagging, random forests can be adapted to discrete failure time outcomes by either applying Method 1 to bootstrap samples from the original data or by applying Method 2 to bootstrap samples from the augmented data. The random forest estimates are then given by the averages of the B individual hazard and survival function estimates.

Compared to single trees, bagging and random forests have the advantage that predictions are usually more accurate (see Hastie et al. 2009). On the other hand, interpretability of the model (which is simple and intuitive in case of a single tree) is lost. Despite the high prediction accuracy of bagging and random forest methods, this may be considered as a disadvantage, especially when the aim is to build an easy-to-interpret prediction formula and to quantify the effect of a specific predictor variable on survival. Overviews of the bagging and random forest algorithms are given in Fig. 6.9.

Example 6.2 Copenhagen Stroke Study
Here we consider Method 2 (recursive partitioning with binary data). In Example 6.1 we fitted a discrete-time survival tree with minimum node size 80 to the augmented data of 345 observations ("learning" sample) that were drawn randomly from the complete data. The value of the summary measure $\widehat{\text{PE}}_{\text{int}}$ that was computed from the remaining 173 "test" observations is shown in Fig. 6.10. Figure 6.10 also shows the values of $\widehat{\text{PE}}_{\text{int}}$ that were obtained from applying bagging and random forests to the learning sample. The number of trees (with minimum node size 80 each) that was used for both bagging and random forests was 500. The value of $mtry$ was set to 3, which is the default value of the R package *randomForest* (Breiman et al. 2015). It is seen that both bagging and random forests improved the prediction accuracy of the single tree. Also, both the single tree and the ensemble methods performed better than a null model without covariate information (that was

Bagging.

Step 1: Generate a fixed number B of bootstrap samples (with replacement) from the complete data set.

Step 2: Apply the recursive partitioning algorithms described in Sections 6.2 and 6.3 to each of the B samples. In case of Method 2, the minimum node size can be optimized using the complete augmented data, and this minimum node size can be used for each of the B trees.

Step 3: Calculate the average of the B outputs (i.e., of the individual hazard estimates) to obtain the bagging estimate.

Random Forests.

Step 1: Generate a fixed number B of bootstrap samples (with replacement) from the complete data set.

Step 2: Apply recursive partitioning techniques to each of the B samples. In each split only a randomly chosen subset of size $mtry \ll p$ of the covariates is considered. In case of Method 2, the minimum node size can be optimized using the complete augmented data, and this minimum node size can be used for each of the B trees.

Step 3: Calculate the average of the B outputs (i.e., of the individual hazard estimates) to obtain the random forest estimate.

Fig. 6.9 Overview of bagging and random forests

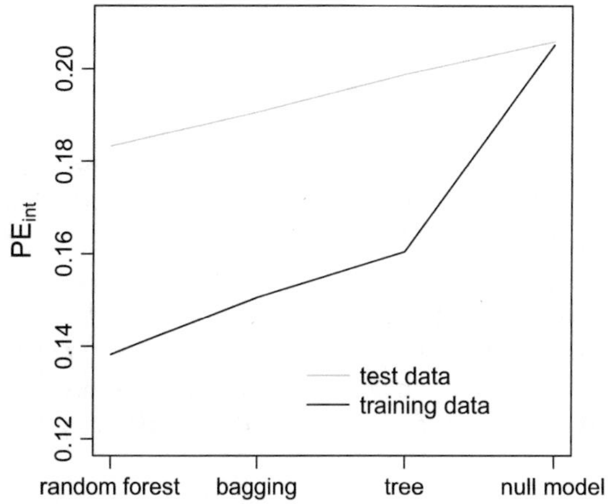

Fig. 6.10 Copenhagen stroke study. The figure shows the values of the summary measures $\widehat{\text{PE}}_{\text{int}}$ that were obtained from the learning and test data sets (of sizes 345 and 173, respectively)

obtained by fitting a discrete-time survival tree with T as the only splitting variable). In addition to the values of $\widehat{\text{PE}}_{\text{int}}$ computed from the test data, Fig. 6.10 also shows the "in-sample" values of $\widehat{\text{PE}}_{\text{int}}$ that were obtained by computing $\widehat{\text{PE}}_{\text{int}}$ from the learning data. As expected, the in-sample values of $\widehat{\text{PE}}_{\text{int}}$ (which can be considered as a measure of deviation from perfect model fit) were smaller for all methods than the estimates of prediction error that were computed from the test data. Regarding the comparison of estimation techniques, however, a similar pattern was observed in both situations: random forests had the smallest prediction error, followed by bagging and by the single survival tree. □

6.5 Literature and Further Reading

Various splitting criteria for tree construction have been proposed for continuous survival outcomes. A review of early approaches is given in LeBlanc and Crowley (1995); for an overview of more recent approaches, see Bou-Hamad et al. (2011b). An extension of Method 1 to time-dependent covariates has been proposed by Bou-Hamad et al. (2011a). Method 2 can be extended by using alternative techniques for the estimation of the hazards in the terminal nodes (such as the Laplace correction and the m-estimate, see, e.g., Ferri et al. (2003) or Broström (2007) for a discussion of various node probability estimators). A bagging method for continuous survival outcomes has been proposed by Hothorn et al. (2004); random survival forests for continuous outcomes were first considered in Ishwaran et al. (2008). For recent developments in this field, especially with regard to variable selection, see Ishwaran et al. (2011).

6.6 Software

Method 1 (recursive partitioning based on covariate-free discrete hazard models) is implemented in the R package *DStree* (Mayer et al. 2014). This package also contains a function for bagging via Method 1. Method 2 (recursive partitioning with binary outcome) can be applied by using the R add-on package *rpart* (Therneau et al. 2015). Bagging is implemented in the *bagging* function of the *ipred* package. The *randomForest*package (functions *randomForest* and *tuneRF*) can be used to obtain random forest estimates via Method 2. Prediction error curves can be obtained via the *predErrDiscShort* function that is contained in the *discSurv* package.

6.7 Exercises

6.1 Construct a tree from the partition of the covariate space shown below (analogous to Fig. 6.1).

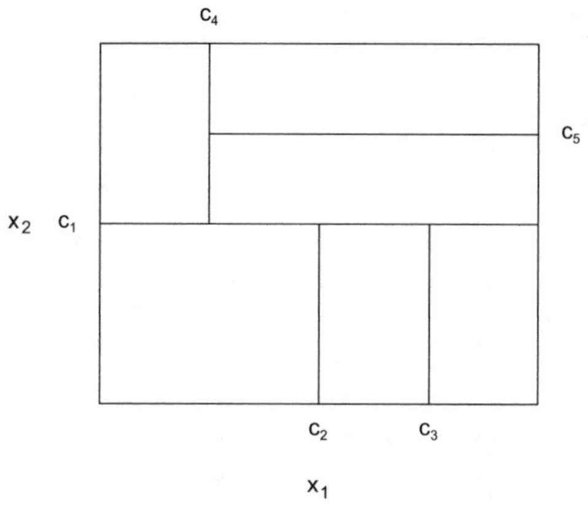

Table 6.1 Description of the covariates contained in the stage C prostate cancer data

Variable	Description
age	Age of patients in years
eet	Was an early endocrine therapy conducted (yes/no)?
g2	Percent of cells in G2 phase, as found by flow cytometry
grade	Grade of the tumor, Farrow system
gleason	Grade of the tumor, Gleason system
ploidy	Ploidy status of the tumor, from flow cytometry

6.2 Show that—up to constant terms—the Gini impurity measure defined by $G_m(x_k, R(x_k)) = 2p_m(x_k, R(x_k))(1 - p_m(x_k, R(x_k)))$ is equal to the Brier score given in (6.5).

6.3 The aim is to apply recursive partitioning techniques to a data set that consists of $n = 146$ Stage C Prostate Cancer patients. The data are publicly available as part of the R add-on package *rpart* (Therneau et al. 2015). The outcome of interest is the time to progression of prostate cancer. The median observed survival time is 5.9 years; 63 % of the observations are censored. Covariates include age, grade, and information from flow cytometry (see Tables 6.1 and 6.2).

1. Round the progression times to years and remove observations with missing values.
2. Subdivide the data into fivefolds and generate learning and test samples for fivefold cross-validation.
3. Convert all learning and test samples to sets of augmented data with binary outcome values y_{is}.

Table 6.2 Summary of the covariates contained in the stage C prostate cancer data

Variable	Categories/unit	Sample proportion/median (range)
age	Years	63 (47–75)
eet	Yes	76 %
	No	24 %
g2	Percent	13 % (2–55 %)
grade	1	2 %
	2	40 %
	3	54 %
	4	4 %
gleason	3	2 %
	4	4 %
	5	25 %
	6	24 %
	7	27 %
	8	13 %
	9	3 %
	10	2 %
ploidy	diploid	48 %
	tetraploid	48 %
	aneuploid	4 %

4. Estimate the conditional survival function by applying Method 2 (recursive partitioning with binary outcome) to the five learning samples. Use the covariates *age*, *eet*, *grade*, *g2*, and *gleason* and consider the following grid of values for the minimum node size: $\{i = 10, 20, \ldots, 600\}$.
5. Estimate the survival function of the censoring process by fitting a covariate-free continuation ratio model with events $1 - \delta_i$, $i = 1, \ldots, n$, to the complete data.
6. For each minimum node size calculate the integrated prediction error curves from the five test samples.
7. Fit the model with optimum minimum node size to the complete data and display the final tree graphically. Which covariates have an effect on progression-free survival?
8. Compare the results to those obtained from Method 1 (recursive partitioning based on covariate-free discrete hazard models).

6.4 Consider the *pneumon* data that are contained in the R-package *KMsurv* (Klein et al. 2012). The outcome of interest is the time to hospitalized pneumonia (measured in months). Data were obtained from $n = 3470$ children, with 97.9 % of the observations being censored. Observed event times ranged from 0.5 months to 12 months (median 12 months). In addition to the outcome variable, the data contain various risk factors such as the age, smoking status and poverty level of the mother (see Tables 6.3 and 6.4).

1. Delete observations with missing values and convert the data into a set of augmented data with binary outcome y_{is}.
2. Fit random forests with 500 trees to the augmented data, i.e., apply Method 2 to 1000 bootstrap samples with replacement. Consider all available covariates and vary the number of randomly selected covariates in each split from 1 to 10.
3. Choose the model with lowest prediction error on the data that were not included in the bootstrap samples ("out-of-bag data").
4. Inspect the Gini variable importance coefficients. Which variables have a strong effect on the time to hospitalized pneumonia?
5. Fit a single survival tree (using Method 2 based on the Gini splitting criterion) to the data. Are the covariates with high random forest Gini variable importance also contained in the first splits of the single tree?
6. Compare the Gini variable importance and the permutation-based variable importance coefficients of the random forest. Can the differences be explained?

Table 6.3 Description of the covariates contained in the pneumon data set

Variable	Description
alcohol	Alcohol use by mother during pregnancy
bweight	Indicator for normal birthweight of the child (>5.5 lbs.)
education	Education of the mother, measured in years
mthage	Age of the mother in years
nsibs	Number of siblings of the child
poverty	Indicator for the mother living at poverty level
race	Race of the mother
region	Geographic region
sfmonth	Month the child was ready for solid food
smoke	Indicator for cigarette smoking during pregnancy
urban	Does the mother live in an urban environment?
wmonth	Month the child was weaned

Table 6.4 Summary of the covariates contained in the pneumon data set

Variable	Categories/unit	Sample proportion/median (range)
alcohol	Alcohol	21 %
	No	79 %
bweight	Weight > 5.5 lbs	35 %
	Weight $\leq$ 5.5 lbs	65 %
education	Years	12 (0–19)
mthage	Years	21 (14–29)
nsibs	Counts	0 (0–6)
poverty	Poverty	92 %
	No poverty	8 %
race	White	52 %
	Black	29 %
	Other	19 %
region	Northeast	14 %
	North central	24 %
	South	41 %
	West	21 %
sfmonth	Months	0 (0–18)
smoke	Cigarette smoker	23 %
	Non-smoker	77 %
urban	Urban environment	76 %
	Non-urban environment	24 %
wmonth	Months	0 (0–28)

Chapter 7
High-Dimensional Models: Structuring and Selection of Predictors

In this chapter we consider strategies to select the relevant variables in cases where many explanatory variables are available. It is important to select the relevant ones in order to obtain a reduced model that is easier to interpret than a big model with a multitude of variables. Moreover, prediction performance typically suffers if many irrelevant variables are included in the model. Variable selection even becomes the central issue in applications where the number of predictors exceeds the number of observations, for example, when the effects of genes are to be investigated. Typical data of this type are microarray data, where the expressions of thousands of predictors (genes) are observed and only some hundred samples are available. In these cases the maximum likelihood estimates for the full model do not exist, and alternatives are needed. In the following we will consider a data set on breast cancer, which contains information on clinical variables as well as on a pre-selected number of gene expression levels.

Example 7.1 Breast Cancer
Breast cancer is the most common invasive cancer in women worldwide. In the Western World breast cancer accounts for approximately 20 % of all cancers diagnosed in female patients. Although 5-year survival rates are larger than 80 % in most OECD countries, breast cancer is still the most common cause of cancer-related death in women. Depending on a variety of risk factors (such as age and disease stage), response rates of patients to breast cancer treatment vary considerably. It is therefore essential to analyze the effect of clinical and genetic variables on breast cancer prognosis.

We consider a data set collected by the Netherlands Cancer Institute to validate predictions for breast cancer in $n = 144$ lymph node positive women (van de Vijver et al. 2002). The outcome of the study was the time to the development of distant metastases, which is an important measure of treatment response. Clinical predictor variables included the age of the patients (median: 45 years, range: 26–53 years), the grade of the tumor, the number of affected lymph nodes, the tumor diameter, and the estrogen receptor status (indicating whether estrogen receptor proteins were over-expressed in breast cancer cells, see Table 7.1). In addition to the clinical predictor variables, the data contain expression measurements of 70 genes (measured on a continuous scale using cDNA microarray technology). Observed metastasis-free survival times ranged from 0.05 months to 17.66 months, with two thirds of the observations being censored. Details on the clinical variables

G. Tutz, M. Schmid, *Modeling Discrete Time-to-Event Data*,
Springer Series in Statistics, DOI 10.1007/978-3-319-28158-2_7

Table 7.1 Clinical explanatory variables for the breast cancer data (*nki70* data set in R package *penalized*)

Variable	Category	Sample proportion (%)
Tumor diameter	≤2 cm	50.69
	>2 cm	49.31
Number of pos. lymph nodes	1–3	73.61
	≥4	26.39
Estrogen receptor status	Negative	18.75
	Positive	81.25
Tumor grade	Poorly differentiated	33.33
	Intermediate	38.19
	Well differentiated	28.47

are given in Table 7.1. The data are publicly available as part of the R add-on package *penalized* (Goeman et al. 2014).

The aim of our analysis is to quantify the effects of the predictor variables on metastasis-free survival. An important issue in this regard is whether the expression values of the 70 genes can be used to build a prediction model for the time to development of distant metastases. Specifically, the question is whether all 70 genes need to be included into the model, or whether it is sufficient to include only a small number of informative genes. When building a prediction model, one also has to take into account that measuring gene expression values is relatively expensive; on the other hand, the clinical variables in Table 7.1 are well-established predictors for survival that are readily available. The task therefore is to investigate the predictive value of the genes *in addition* to the clinical predictors. In this situation, one wants to identify only those genes that improve the survival predictions derived from the clinical variables. □

The issue of variable selection was traditionally addressed by applying stepwise procedures in the form of forward, backward, or forward/backward ("stepwise") selection. However, these types of variable selection procedures are very variable with respect to the input data. In particular, the results can be affected even by very small changes in the data, leading to a poor performance, see, for example, Frank and Friedman (1993).

An alternative to stepwise selection are *regularization methods*, which have been studied extensively during the past years. Two of the main regularization approaches are *penalty methods*, which select variables simultaneously via optimizing a penalized likelihood and *boosting techniques*, which originate in the machine learning field but also serve as regularization methods in structured regression. We will consider penalty methods in Sect. 7.1 and boosting methods in Sect. 7.2.

7.1 Penalized Likelihood Approaches

We consider the hazard model with linear predictor from Chap. 3, which is given by

$$\lambda(t|\boldsymbol{x}) = h(\gamma_{0t} + \boldsymbol{x}^T\boldsymbol{\gamma}). \tag{7.1}$$

The maximum likelihood methods for estimation of γ_{0t} and $\boldsymbol{\gamma}$ discussed in Chap. 3 have the property that all parameter estimates are different from zero with probability 1. Consequently, classical maximum likelihood estimation is not useful if variable selection is desired.

In penalized likelihood approaches, the idea is therefore to replace the usual log-likelihood by

$$l_p(\boldsymbol{\gamma}) = l(\boldsymbol{\gamma}) - \frac{\lambda}{2}J(\boldsymbol{\gamma}), \tag{7.2}$$

where $l(\boldsymbol{\gamma})$ is the usual log-likelihood function, λ is a tuning parameter, and $J(\boldsymbol{\gamma})$ is a penalty that puts restrictions on $\boldsymbol{\gamma}$ that enforce variable selection. Note that the tuning parameter λ should not be confused with the hazard function $\lambda(t|\boldsymbol{x})$. We will denote both terms by λ, as this is standard notation that is commonly used in the literature. Penalized likelihood approaches have already been considered in Chap. 5, but with the focus on smoothing and not on variable selection. A penalty that distinctly enforces variable selection is the L_1 or lasso penalty (for "least absolute shrinkage and selection operator")

$$J(\boldsymbol{\gamma}) = \sum_{j=1}^{p} |\gamma_j|, \tag{7.3}$$

which was proposed by Tibshirani (1996). The penalty contains the sum over the absolute values of all the parameters. When used in (7.2), in the extreme case $\lambda = 0$ one obtains the maximum likelihood estimate, whereas if $\lambda \to \infty$ all parameters are set to zero. The most interesting case is therefore the intermediate case with appropriately chosen tuning parameter λ between 0 and ∞. In this case all coefficients are shrunk toward zero and, depending on λ, few or many parameters are set to zero. The latter property of the lasso method effectively implies variable selection. Generally, the lasso tends to avoid the high variability of stepwise selection while producing a sparse model that shows good prediction performance.

Example 7.2 Breast Cancer
We used a penalized likelihood approach to investigate the effects of the 70 genes on metastasis-free survival. To this purpose, we subdivided the data into a learning data set containing 96 observations (i.e., two thirds of the complete data set) and a test data set containing 48 observations. Survival times were grouped into 3-month intervals (with the last interval being defined as ">18 months"). This grouping pattern was chosen because the focus in cancer research is often on a small number of survival probabilities at distinct time points (e.g., 3-month survival, 6-month survival, etc.).

In the first step, we built a prediction model using the clinical covariates only. To this purpose we fitted a continuation ratio model to the learning data that contained the covariates "tumor diameter," "number of affected lymph nodes," "estrogen receptor status," "tumor grade," and "age at diagnosis." The coefficient estimates obtained from this model (in the following termed "clinical model") are presented in Table 7.2. These estimates reflect often observed effects in cancer research: For example, a large number of affected lymph nodes increase the risk of developing distant metastases. The same is true for patients with negative estrogen receptor status.

Table 7.2 Breast cancer data. The table shows the coefficient estimates obtained from two continuation ratio models fitted to a learning data set of size 96 (clinical model = continuation ratio model with the clinical variables only, combined model = L_1 penalized continuation ratio model with unpenalized clinical covariates). Abbreviations of covariates are as follows: Diam = tumor diameter, N = number of affected lymph nodes, ER = estrogen receptor status

	Coefficient estimates	
	Clinical model	Combined model
Gene name		
TSPYL5		−0.4755
QSCN6L1		0.9312
Contig32125_RC		1.4342
RUNDC1		1.2185
GPR180		−1.0926
ZNF533		−0.1447
COL4A2		0.1205
ORC6L		0.3014
LOC643008		−0.9720
IGFBP5.1		0.9958
NMU		−0.1133
LGP2		1.8194
PRC1		1.3828
Contig20217_RC		−0.2920
NM_004702		0.0165
Variable name		
Diam ≤2 cm	0.0000	0.0000
Diam >2 cm	0.4217	0.3936
N ≥4	0.0000	0.0000
N 1–3	−0.9769	−0.8368
ER negative	0.0000	0.0000
ER positive	−0.7032	−1.5282
Grade poorly diff.	0.0000	0.0000
Grade intermediate	−0.3974	−0.2073
Grade well diff.	−0.3252	−0.3697
Age	−0.0278	−0.0237

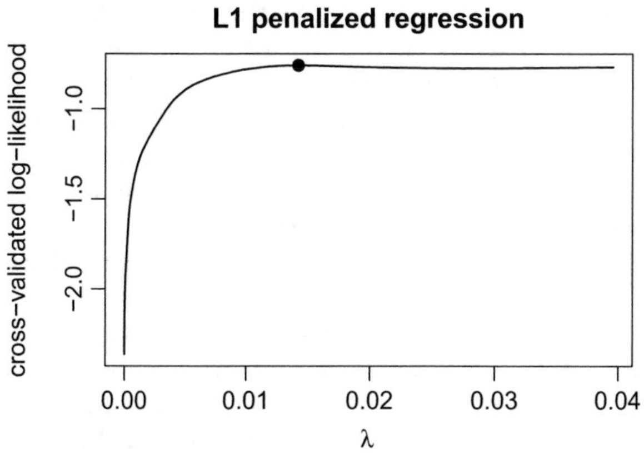

Fig. 7.1 Breast cancer data. The figure shows the cross-validated log-likelihood of an L_1 penalized continuation ratio model that was obtained by applying fivefold cross-validation to a learning sample of size 96. The *curve* corresponds to the average over the fivefolds. Note that the values of λ only refer to the 70 genes but not to the clinical covariates. The latter covariates entered the model in an unpenalized fashion to ensure their inclusion in the model. The *black dot* indicates the cross-validated log-likelihood at the optimal value of $\lambda = 0.014$

In the next step, we investigated the predictive value of the 70 genes in addition to the available clinical covariates. To this purpose we fitted a penalized continuation ratio model with L_1 penalty ("lasso") to the learning data. This model contains both the clinical covariates and the expression values of the 70 genes. In contrast to the values of the 70 genes, the clinical covariates (and also the dummy variables for the baseline hazard) entered the model in an unpenalized fashion, i.e. their coefficients were not included in the penalty in (7.3). In contrast, the coefficients of the 70 genes were penalized, and the tuning parameter of the lasso penalty was determined by fivefold cross-validation. This strategy implied that the 70 genes were subject to variable selection whereas all clinical covariates were "forced" a priori to enter the model. Consequently, only those genes that increased the predictive power of the clinical variables were selected.

The results of fivefold cross-validation are presented in Fig. 7.1. As seen from Fig. 7.1, the optimal value of λ was estimated to be $\lambda = 0.014$. From Table 7.2 it is seen that only 15 of the 70 genes entered the model. This result suggests that part of the predictive power contained in the 70 genes is already contained in the clinical covariates.

In the final step, we compared the predictive power of the clinical model using the clinical covariates only and the combined model containing the unpenalized clinical covariates and the penalized expression values of the 15 selected genes. The integrated prediction error curves for the two models (evaluated on the test data) resulted in $\widehat{\mathrm{PE}}_{\mathrm{int}} = 0.187$ for the model with clinical variables and $\widehat{\mathrm{PE}}_{\mathrm{int}} = 0.157$ for the combined model. This indicates that the combined model (incorporating both genetic and clinical information) had a larger predictive power than the clinical model. □

The basic lasso has the disadvantage that the selection procedure is not consistent in terms of variable selection. Therefore, Zou (2006) proposed the *adaptive lasso*, which is an extended version of the lasso for which the penalty has the form

$$J(\boldsymbol{\gamma}) = \sum_{j=1}^{p} w_j |\gamma_j|, \tag{7.4}$$

where w_j are known weights. He showed that for appropriately chosen data-dependent weights the adaptive lasso is consistent. One choice of weights is based on a root-n consistent estimator $\tilde{\boldsymbol{\gamma}}$ of $\boldsymbol{\gamma}$, for example, the maximum likelihood estimate. In this case weights are defined by $w_j = 1/|\tilde{\gamma}_j|^\delta$ for fixed chosen $\delta > 0$. For growing sample size the weights for zero-coefficients get inflated, whereas the weights on non-zero-coefficients converge to a finite constant. Further results on optimality of the adaptive lasso were given by Zou (2006).

One restriction of the lasso in the form considered so far is that all coefficients enter the penalty term in an unweighted fashion. Hence all coefficients are penalized in the same way, and it is recommended to standardize variables before analysis to avoid problems with covariates that are measured on different scales. Another problem occurs when a categorical covariate enters the model in the form of a set of dummy variables. Then the lasso has no information that the coefficients of these dummy variables are linked together, and it may happen that some of the categories end up with zero-coefficients while others do not.

A procedure that enforces selection of whole groups of parameters is the *group lasso* proposed by Yuan and Lin (2006). Let the p-dimensional predictor be structured as $\boldsymbol{x}_i^T = (\boldsymbol{x}_{i1}^T, \dots, \boldsymbol{x}_{i,G}^T)$, where $\boldsymbol{x}_{ij}$ corresponds to the jth group of variables. A group of variables typically refers to the dummy variables of one categorical predictor, with df_j denoting the number of the variables in the jth group. But it also can contain only one parameter if the variable is a continuous variable that enters the model as a main effect. Let the parameter vector be partitioned into the corresponding subvectors $\boldsymbol{\gamma}^T = (\boldsymbol{\gamma}_1^T, \dots, \boldsymbol{\gamma}_G^T)$. Then the group lasso uses the penalty

$$J(\boldsymbol{\gamma}) = \sum_{j=1}^{G} \sqrt{df_j} \|\boldsymbol{\gamma}_j\|_2, \tag{7.5}$$

where $\|\boldsymbol{\gamma}_j\|_2 = (\gamma_{j1}^2 + \cdots + \gamma_{j,df_j}^2)^{1/2}$ is the L_2-norm of the parameters of the jth group. The penalty encourages sparsity in the sense that either $\hat{\boldsymbol{\gamma}}_j = \boldsymbol{0}$ or $\hat{\gamma}_{js} \neq 0$ for $s = 1, \dots, df_j$. For a geometrical interpretation of the penalty, see Yuan and Lin (2006). Meier et al. (2008) showed that under sparsity the resulting estimates are consistent even when the number of predictors is larger than the sample size.

Although the lasso and its extensions are the most widely used methods for variable selection by penalization, modifications and alternatives with good performance are available. One should mention the elastic net, which is a combination of lasso and ridge penalties (Zou and Hastie 2005), SCAD for smoothly clipped absolute derivation penalty (Fan and Li 2001), and the Dantzig selector (Candes and Tao 2007; James and Radchenko 2009).

7.2 Boosting

Another popular technique for simultaneous model fitting and variable selection is boosting. Similar to the lasso, boosting is especially useful in high-dimensional settings where the number of available covariates exceeds the number of observations ($p > n$). In the literature, several approaches to construct boosting algorithms have been proposed. Historically, the first boosting method (the so-called AdaBoost algorithm, Freund and Schapire 1996) originated in the machine learning community and was designed for the prediction of binary outcome variables, without explicitly focussing on variable selection. Later, boosting algorithms were adapted to become an optimization method for building a wide range of regression models with many possible types of outcomes and predictor effects (see Mayr et al. 2014a,b for a review). Often used boosting algorithms include *gradient boosting* (Friedman 2001; Bühlmann and Hothorn 2007) and *likelihood-based boosting* (Tutz and Binder 2006). Since both approaches often yield similar results, we only present gradient boosting here.

The aim is again to estimate the coefficient vector $\boldsymbol{\gamma}$ of the discrete-time hazard model

$$\lambda(t|\boldsymbol{x}) = h(\gamma_{0t} + \boldsymbol{x}^T\boldsymbol{\gamma}). \tag{7.6}$$

In addition, one wants to select the relevant predictor variables. As will be demonstrated in the following, gradient boosting can be used to accomplish model fitting and variable selection simultaneously. We start with a general description of gradient boosting algorithms for arbitrary outcome variables and will discuss their application to discrete failure time data later.

7.2.1 *Generic Boosting Algorithm for Arbitrary Outcomes*

Definition of the Optimization Criterion In their most general form, gradient boosting algorithms start with an outcome variable y, a set of predictors $\boldsymbol{x}$, and a loss function $\rho(y, f(\boldsymbol{x}))$ that quantifies the deviation between the outcome and the prediction function f. For example, in Gaussian regression, ρ is usually defined as the squared error loss $(y - f(\boldsymbol{x}))^2$. In the same way as in Chaps. 3 and 5, the prediction function is unknown and has to be estimated from the data. As in Chap. 3, we assume that f is linear in the covariates, i.e., $f(\boldsymbol{x}) = \boldsymbol{x}^T\boldsymbol{\gamma}$ with a set of unknown coefficients $\boldsymbol{\gamma}$ that has to be estimated. Note that the restriction to linear prediction functions is purely for convenience here; boosting algorithms also allow for more flexible types of effects such as the smooth effects discussed in Chap. 5 (cf. Bühlmann and Yu 2003; Schmid and Hothorn 2008; Schmid et al. 2011). The loss function ρ is assumed to be differentiable with respect to f. For example, in case of the squared error loss the derivative is given by $\partial\rho/\partial f = -2\,(y - f(\boldsymbol{x}))$.

In the generic boosting framework with arbitrary outcome variable y, the aim is to estimate the "optimal" prediction function f^* in terms of minimization of the expected loss

$$f^* := \text{argmin}_f \, \mathrm{E}_{y,x}\left[\rho(y, f(\boldsymbol{x}))\right] . \tag{7.7}$$

The idea is hence to minimize a risk function that is given by the expectation of the loss function ρ. For example, in Gaussian regression, this approach corresponds to minimizing the theoretical mean $\mathrm{E}(y - f(\boldsymbol{x}))^2$ over f.

In practice, the true data-generating process (and hence the theoretical mean in (7.7)) is usually unknown. Instead, one has a data set $(y_i, \boldsymbol{x}_i)$, $i = 1, \ldots, n$, that contains realizations of the random variables y and $\boldsymbol{x}$. Consequently, one does not minimize the theoretical risk in (7.7) but replaces it by the *empirical risk*

$$\mathcal{R} := \frac{1}{n} \sum_{i=1}^{n} \rho(y_i, f(\boldsymbol{x}_i)) , \tag{7.8}$$

which is the empirical mean of the individual deviations between y_i and $\boldsymbol{x}_i$ (and hence is an unbiased estimator of the theoretical risk). For example, in Gaussian regression with the squared error loss, the empirical risk is defined by $\mathcal{R} = \sum_{i=1}^{n} (y_i - f(\boldsymbol{x}_i))^2 / n$, which is the well-known residual sum of squares used in linear regression.

Non-Gaussian Loss Functions If the outcome variable is not normally distributed, a common strategy is to define ρ as the negative probability density function of the outcome distribution. Then, if the distribution of the outcome belongs to the exponential family of distributions, the empirical risk is equivalent to the negative log-likelihood function of a generalized linear model:

$$\mathcal{R} = -\frac{1}{n} \sum_{i=1}^{n} \varphi(y_i, f(\boldsymbol{x}_i)) , \tag{7.9}$$

where φ denotes the probability density of y_i. In (7.9), $f(\boldsymbol{x}_i)$ is a linear predictor that is associated with the conditional mean of $y_i | \boldsymbol{x}_i$ via a known link function (which is implicitly assumed to be incorporated into φ). In other words, minimizing the empirical risk in (7.9) over f is equivalent to maximum likelihood estimation of the linear predictor f in a generalized linear model.

Specification of the Gradient Boosting Algorithm Having defined the optimization problem, a gradient boosting algorithm is used to estimate f^*. The idea is to begin with an n-dimensional vector of starting values (which represents the starting values for the predicted values of the n observations in the data) and to update this vector iteratively. The updates are carried out by the so-called set of *base-learners*, which are defined as simple linear regression models with one input variable and one output variable. Their role will become clear below. Gradient boosting is formally defined as follows:

1. Initialize the n-dimensional vector $\hat{\boldsymbol{f}}^{[0]} = (\hat{f}_1^{[0]}, \ldots, \hat{f}_n^{[0]})^T$ with starting values. For example, start with the same constant value (denoted by $\hat{\boldsymbol{\gamma}}^{[0]}$) for each of the n elements of $\hat{\boldsymbol{f}}^{[0]}$. This constant value can, e.g., be obtained by minimizing the empirical risk of a covariate-free model numerically over $\boldsymbol{f}$.
2. For each of the predictor variables specify a *base-learner*, i.e., a simple linear regression model with the respective predictor variable as input variable and one output variable (which will be defined below). Set the iteration counter m to 0.
3. Increase m by 1.
4. (a) Compute the negative gradient $-\frac{\partial \mathcal{R}}{\partial f}$ and evaluate at $\left(y_i, \hat{f}_i^{[m-1]}\right)$, $i = 1, \ldots, n$. This yields the negative gradient vector

$$\boldsymbol{U}^{[m]} = \left(\boldsymbol{U}_i^{[m]}\right)_{i=1,\ldots,n} := \left(-\frac{\partial}{\partial f}\mathcal{R}\left(y_i, \hat{f}_i^{[m-1]}\right)\right)_{i=1,\ldots,n}. \tag{7.10}$$

   (b) Fit the negative gradient vector $\boldsymbol{U}^{[m]}$ to each of the p covariates separately by using the p base-learners specified in Step 2. Hence the negative gradient $\boldsymbol{U}^{[m]}$, whose values are measured on a continuous scale, becomes the output variable of the base-learners. Since the base-learners are simple linear models, ordinary least squares estimation is carried out to estimate $\boldsymbol{U}^{[m]}$. This procedure yields p vectors of predicted values (one vector per base-learner), where each vector is an estimate of the negative gradient vector $\boldsymbol{U}^{[m]}$.
   (c) Select the base-learner that fits $\boldsymbol{U}^{[m]}$ best according to the R^2 goodness-of-fit criterion. Set $\hat{\boldsymbol{U}}^{[m]}$ equal to the fitted values of the best model.
   (d) Update $\hat{\boldsymbol{f}}^{[m]} \leftarrow \hat{\boldsymbol{f}}^{[m-1]} + \nu\, \hat{\boldsymbol{U}}^{[m]}$, where $0 < \nu \leq 1$ is a real-valued step length factor.
5. Iterate Steps 3 and 4 until the stopping iteration m_{stop} is reached. The choice of m_{stop} will be discussed below.

From Step 4 it is seen that the algorithm descends the gradient of the empirical risk $\mathcal{R}$: in each iteration, an estimate of the true negative gradient of $\mathcal{R}$ is added to the current estimate of f^*. Moreover, as seen from Steps 4(c) and 4(d), the gradient boosting additionally carries out variable selection, as only one base-learner (and therefore only one covariate) is selected for updating $\hat{\boldsymbol{f}}^{[m]}$ in each iteration. Due to the additive update in Step 5, the final boosting estimate at iteration m_{stop} can be interpreted as an additive prediction function. Importantly, it can be shown that the update in Step 5 results in an additive update of the estimated coefficient vector $\hat{\boldsymbol{\gamma}}$ in each iteration (for details see Example 7.3).

7.2.2 Application to Discrete Hazard Models

Definition of the Risk Function Having defined a generic gradient boosting algorithm for arbitrary outcomes, the task is to specify a suitable loss function for the discrete hazard model. Keeping in mind that the log-likelihood function of model (7.6) is equivalent to the log-likelihood function of a binary regression model (cf. Chap. 3), a convenient choice is to set $\mathcal{R}$ equal to the negative binomial log-likelihood function, i.e.,

$$\mathcal{R} = -\sum_{i=1}^{n}\sum_{s=1}^{t_i} y_{is} \log \lambda(s|\boldsymbol{x}_i) + (1 - y_{is}) \log(1 - \lambda(s|\boldsymbol{x}_i)), \tag{7.11}$$

where the y_{is}'s code the transition to the next period. As in Sect. 3.4 we use the linear predictor $f(\boldsymbol{x}_{it}) := \boldsymbol{x}_{it}^T\boldsymbol{\beta}$ with $\boldsymbol{x}_{it}^T = (0, \ldots, 0, 1, 0, \ldots, 0, \boldsymbol{x}_i^T)$ and $\boldsymbol{\beta}^T = (\gamma_{01}, \ldots, \gamma_{0q}, \boldsymbol{\gamma}^T)$. Then the generic boosting algorithm defined in the previous subsection can be applied to the augmented data. As before the base-learners that are used consist of only one predictor variable, that is, one component of $\boldsymbol{x}$. The corresponding intercept parameters are estimated without penalization in the first step of the algorithm, and the resulting estimates are used as offset values for gradient boosting.

Interpretation of the Model Fit The interpretation of the model fit is directly related to the choice of simple linear models as base-learners in Step 2. In fact, the linearity of the base-learners directly results in the linearity of the whole estimated prediction function. This can be easily seen from the following example, which for simplicity ignores the parameters γ_{0t} that are linked to the baseline hazard.

Example 7.3 A Simple Example with Three Covariates
Assume that there are three predictor variables x_1, x_2, x_3. Then, if predictor variable $x_j, j \in \{1, 2, 3\}$, is chosen in boosting iteration m, a simple linear model is fitted to the negative gradient, and there is a coefficient estimate $\hat{\gamma}_j^{[m]}$ resulting from this model. Further suppose that the number of boosting iterations is $m_{\text{stop}} = 5$, and that x_1 was selected in iterations 1, 2, and 5. For iterations 3 and 4 we assume that x_3 was selected. Keeping in mind the additive structure of the update Step 4(d), the estimated prediction function can be written as follows:

$$\begin{aligned}
\hat{f}^{[m_{\text{stop}}]} &= \hat{f}^{[0]} + \nu\,\hat{U}^{[0]} + \nu\,\hat{U}^{[1]} + \nu\,\hat{U}^{[2]} + \nu\,\hat{U}^{[3]} + \nu\,\hat{U}^{[4]} \\
&= \hat{\gamma}^{[0]} + \nu\,\hat{\gamma}_1^{[0]}x_1 + \nu\,\hat{\gamma}_1^{[1]}x_1 + \nu\,\hat{\gamma}_3^{[2]}x_3 + \nu\,\hat{\gamma}_3^{[3]}x_3 + \nu\,\hat{\gamma}_1^{[4]}x_1 \\
&= \hat{\gamma}^{[0]} + \nu\left(\hat{\gamma}_1^{[0]} + \hat{\gamma}_1^{[1]} + \hat{\gamma}_1^{[4]}\right)x_1 + \nu\left(\hat{\gamma}_3^{[2]} + \hat{\gamma}_3^{[3]}\right)x_3 \\
&= \hat{\gamma}^{[0]} + \hat{\gamma}_1^{*}x_1 + \hat{\gamma}_3^{*}x_3
\end{aligned}$$

with $\hat{\gamma}_1^* := \nu\left(\hat{\gamma}_1^{[0]} + \hat{\gamma}_1^{[1]} + \hat{\gamma}_1^{[4]}\right)$ and $\hat{\gamma}_3^* := \nu\left(\hat{\gamma}_3^{[2]} + \hat{\gamma}_3^{[3]}\right)$. Hence it is clear that the linearity of the base-learners implies the linearity of the estimated prediction function. Also, it is now clear how an estimate of the coefficient vector $\boldsymbol{\gamma}$ is obtained. The main difference between gradient boosting and the standard maximum likelihood techniques in Chap. 3 is the variable selection mechanism in Step 4(c). While standard maximum likelihood techniques typically result in non-zero estimates for all elements of $\boldsymbol{y}$, gradient boosting uses only a subset of the covariates for estimating f^*. For example, x_2 is not included in the estimated prediction function above. □

Tuning Parameters The remaining issue is to specify appropriate values for the tuning parameters m_{stop} and ν. Generally, if the stopping iteration becomes too large, overfits resulting in a suboptimal out-of-sample prediction accuracy are likely (see Bühlmann and Hothorn 2007). In particular, the number of selected covariates—and hence the sparsity of the prediction function—is directly related to the number of iterations. Consider, e.g., the above example: If the algorithm had stopped after the second iteration, only one covariate would have been included in the prediction function). On the other hand, if the stopping iteration m_{stop} is too large, then it might happen that a large number of non-informative predictors are included in the estimate of f^*. The solution to this problem is to stop the algorithm before convergence ("early stopping") and to choose m_{stop} such that out-of-sample prediction accuracy becomes optimal. To determine the optimal values of m_{stop}, cross-validation is a natural choice. In Example 7.4 below, we will use fivefold cross-validation, implying that m_{stop} is the iteration with lowest predictive empirical risk averaged over the fivefolds.

The choice of the step length factor ν is usually of minor importance for the predictive performance of a boosting algorithm. It might be optimized in each iteration (as suggested by Friedman 2001), but this will often not improve prediction accuracy but just increase the number of boosting iterations. An important requirement, however, is that the value of ν is "small," such that a stagewise adaption of the prediction function is possible (see Schmid and Hothorn 2008). Common choices are $\nu = 0.1$ or $\nu = 0.01$.

Example 7.4 Breast Cancer

The aim is again to investigate the added predictive value of the 70 genes. In contrast to Sect. 7.1, we now use gradient boosting instead of L_1-penalized regression to investigate the effects of the 70 genes on metastasis-free survival. To this purpose, we use the same learning data set (containing 96 observations) and the same test data set (containing 48 observations) as in Example 7.2. Metastasis-free survival times were again grouped into 3-month intervals. The negative log-likelihood function of the continuation ratio model was used as risk function for gradient boosting. The step length factor ν was chosen to be $\nu = 0.1$, and the optimal stopping iteration m_{stop} was determined by fivefold cross-validation on the learning data.

To investigate the predictive value of the 70 genes in addition to the readily available clinical covariates, we first fitted a continuation ratio model using the covariates "tumor diameter," "number of affected lymph nodes," "estrogen receptor status," "tumor grade," and "age at diagnosis" to the learning data by using the maximum likelihood estimation techniques described in Chap. 3. The coefficient estimates obtained from this model (in the following termed "clinical model") are presented in Table 7.3; by definition, they are the same as those presented in Table 7.2.

In the next step, we applied gradient boosting with the expression values of the 70 genes to the learning data. To ensure that the clinical covariates were "forced" into the model and were not subject to variable selection, we used the predictions of the clinical model as offset values for gradient boosting. In other words, the offset vector $\hat{f}^{[0]}$ was set equal to the predictions of the clinical model, and the set of covariates for gradient boosting comprised the 70 genes.

Table 7.3 Breast cancer data. The table shows the coefficient estimates obtained from two continuation ratio models fitted to a learning data set of size 96 (clinical model = continuation ratio model with the clinical variables only, combined model = gradient boosting with the 70 genes as covariates and the clinical covariates as offset values). Abbreviations of covariates are as follows: Diam = tumor diameter, N = number of affected lymph nodes, ER = estrogen receptor status

	Coefficient estimates	
	Clinical model	Combined model
Gene name		
TSPYL5		−0.6008
QSCN6L1		0.3378
GPR180		0.8991
IGFBP5.1		−1.4568
LGP2		0.8382
PRC1		1.5119
NUSAP1		1.7227
Variable name		
Diam ≤2 cm	0.0000	0.0000
Diam >2 cm	0.4217	0.4217
N ≥4	0.0000	0.0000
N 1–3	−0.9769	−0.9769
ER negative	0.0000	0.0000
ER positive	−0.7032	−0.7032
Grade poorly diff.	0.0000	0.0000
Grade intermediate	−0.3974	−0.3974
Grade well diff.	−0.3252	−0.3252
Age	−0.0278	−0.0278

The results of fivefold cross-validation are presented in Fig. 7.2. As seen from Fig. 7.2, the optimal stopping iteration was estimated to be $m_{\text{stop}} = 84$. At $m_{\text{stop}} = 84$, 7 of the 70 genes entered the model (Table 7.3). Again this result suggests that part of the predictive power contained in the 70 genes is already contained in the clinical covariates.

In the final step we compared the predictive power of the clinical model and the combined model. The integrated prediction error curves for these models (evaluated on the test data) resulted in $\widehat{\text{PE}}_{\text{int}} = 0.186$ and $\widehat{\text{PE}}_{\text{int}} = 0.157$, respectively. This result indicates that the combined model (incorporating both genetic and clinical information) had a larger predictive power than the clinical model, and that incorporating genetic information into the survival model may increase prediction accuracy. Note that the values of $\widehat{\text{PE}}_{\text{int}}$ are almost identical to those obtained from L_1-penalized regression in Sect. 7.1. In addition, 6 of the 7 genes selected for boosting are also included in the L_1-penalized model, highlighting the similarities between the two methods (cf. Table 7.2). □

Example 7.5 Stage II Colon Cancer
In this example we apply L_1 penalized regression and gradient boosting to develop a gene signature for the prediction of metachronous metastases after surgery in stage II colon cancer patients. Such signatures may help to improve individual patient prognosis and to also identify patients for which postoperative adjuvant chemotherapy might be beneficial. Our analysis was based on a set of mRNA tumor gene expression data that was collected by Barrier et al. (2006). The sample consisted

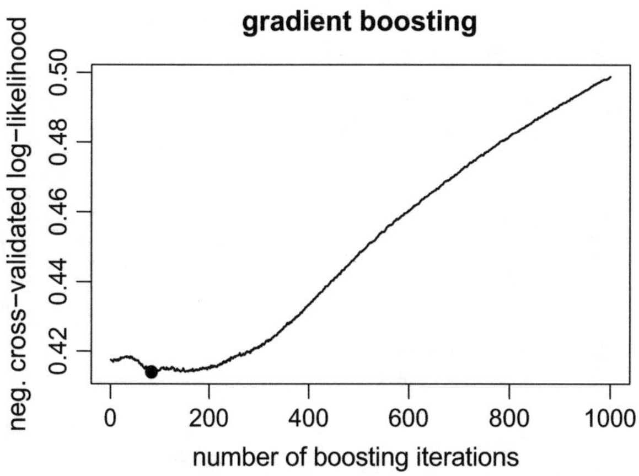

Fig. 7.2 Breast cancer data. The figure shows the cross-validated negative log-likelihood of a continuation ratio model that was obtained by applying fivefold cross-validation to a learning sample of size 96. The *curve* corresponds to the average over the fivefolds. Gradient boosting with the 70 genes as covariates was used to fit continuation ratio models to the data in the fivefolds. The fitted values of the clinical model were used as offset values to ensure that all clinical covariates were included the model. The *black dot* indicates the cross-validated negative log-likelihood at the optimal boosting iteration m_{stop}, which was found to be 84

of 50 patients who underwent surgery due to stage II colon cancer and did not receive postoperative adjuvant chemotherapy; we thank Sandrine Dudoit for providing us with the data. Times to the development of metachronous metastases were grouped by the authors according to the criterion "$t < 60$ months," so that only two time intervals ($[0, 60)$ and $[60, \infty)$) were considered. Twenty-five patients developed metachronous metastases within the first 60 months after surgery ($t < 60$), and another 25 patients remained disease free for at least 60 months ($t \geq 60$). Gene expression levels of $p = 22{,}283$ genes (measured with the Affymetrix® HGU133A GeneChip) were available. Unlike for the analysis of the breast cancer data in Example 7.2, clinical covariates were not used in the predictive analysis by Barrier et al. (2006).

In the same way as in Examples 7.2 and 7.4, we used L_1 penalized regression and gradient boosting to carry out variable selection and to investigate the effects of the 22,283 genes on the development of metachronous metastases. The results of fivefold cross-validation for the continuation ratio model with logistic link function are presented in Fig. 7.3. The optimal value of λ for the L_1 penalized regression model was $\lambda = 0.1331$. For gradient boosting (with step length $\nu = 0.1$) the optimal stopping iteration was found to be $m_{\text{stop}} = 13$. From Table 7.4 it is seen that 10 of the 22,283 genes entered the L_1 penalized regression model, whereas 9 genes were selected by gradient boosting.

It is remarkable that the sets of genes that were selected by L_1 penalized regression and gradient boosting almost coincide. In fact, all 9 genes that were selected by gradient boosting were also contained in the set of genes selected by L_1 penalized regression. In addition, the signs of the respective coefficient estimates coincide. It is also noteworthy that 8 of the 10 genes selected by L_1 penalized regression are also contained in the 30-gene prognosis predictor that was identified in the original publication by Barrier et al. (2006) with quite different methods. □

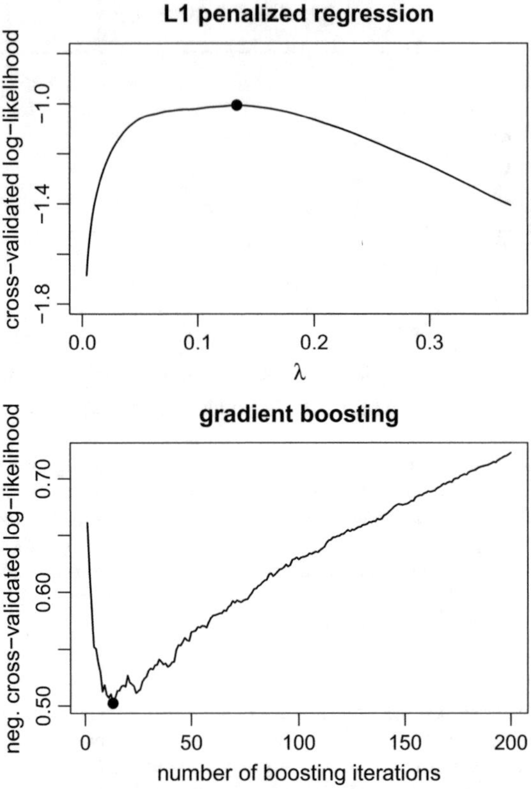

Fig. 7.3 Stage II colon cancer data. The *upper panel* shows the cross-validated log-likelihood of an L_1 penalized continuation ratio model that was obtained by applying fivefold cross-validation to the data. The *lower panel* shows the cross-validated negative log-likelihood of a continuation ratio model that was fitted via gradient boosting. The *curves* correspond to the averages over the fivefolds. The *black dots* refer to the optimal values of λ and m_{stop}

7.3 Extension to Additive Predictors

The variable selection methods considered in the previous sections refer to models with a linear predictor. It is straightforward to extend the methods to the case of additive predictors, where the model has the form $\lambda(t|\boldsymbol{x}_i) = h(\eta_{it})$ with predictor

$$\eta_{it} = f_0(t) + f_1(x_{i1}) + \cdots + f_p(x_{ip}),$$

where the functions $f_0(\cdot), \ldots, f_p(\cdot)$ are unknown and will be determined by the data. As in Sect. 5.2 let the functional form of the predictors be determined by an

Table 7.4 Stage II cancer data. The table shows the coefficient estimates obtained from two continuation ratio models that were fitted to the data via L_1 penalized regression (lasso) and gradient boosting. It is seen that 10 genes were selected by the L_1 penalized regression model, whereas 9 genes were selected by gradient boosting. Eight of these genes were also identified in the original publication by Barrier et al. (2006)

	Coefficient estimates		Identified by
	lasso	boosting	Barrier et al. (2006)
Gene name			
X200630_x_at	−0.0553	−0.1100	×
X202739_s_at	0.1031	0.1472	
X203815_at	0.0162		
X205550_s_at	0.9767	0.8206	×
X209221_s_at	0.4894	0.5351	×
X210243_s_at	0.2572	0.3246	×
X213893_x_at	0.1119	0.2244	×
X218157_x_at	−0.0632	−0.1691	×
X219038_at	0.1840	0.1677	×
X221943_x_at	−0.5061	−0.4157	×

expansion in basis functions

$$f_j(x_j) = \sum_{s=1}^{m_j} \gamma_{js}\phi_{js}(x_j),$$

where the basis functions depend on the covariate x_j. Let $\boldsymbol{\gamma}_j^T = (\gamma_{j1}, \dots, \gamma_{jm_j})$ represent the vector of parameters linked to the jth predictor.

Then one can use lasso-type selection procedures by penalizing the parameter vectors $\boldsymbol{\gamma}_j$ in the form of the group lasso (7.5). Alternative penalty terms for variable selection in additive models were used by Cantoni et al. (2011) and Marra and Wood (2011). In boosting procedures one can use blockwise boosting, which means that the group of parameters linked to one variable is updated simultaneously (Bühlmann and Yu 2003; Tutz and Binder 2006; Schmid and Hothorn 2008). In this case the base learner is a linear model with the basis functions of the corresponding variable as input. It has been shown in particular by Tutz and Binder (2006) that the method selects additive predictors efficiently also in very high-dimensional settings.

7.4 Literature and Further Reading

Variable Selection by Penalized Estimation Variable selection by using penalty terms was proposed in the seminal paper on the lasso (Tibshirani 1996). Various extensions have been developed, in particular the adaptive lasso (Zou 2006), the elastic net (Zou and Hastie 2005), and the group lasso (Yuan and Lin 2006; Meier et al. 2008).

Boosting Statistical concepts of boosting were propagated by Friedman (2001), Friedman et al. (2000), Bühlmann and Yu (2003) and Bühlmann (2006). An overview on gradient boosting was given by Bühlmann and Hothorn (2007);

likelihood-based boosting was considered by Tutz and Binder (2006). More recently, an overview on boosting techniques with discussion was given by Mayr et al. (2014a,b), and Bühlmann et al. (2014). An extension of gradient boosting to rank-based time-to-event analysis, which can also be used to model discrete survival data, has been proposed by Mayr and Schmid (2014).

Added Predictive Value Further details and considerations on how to investigate the added predictive value of molecular data are provided in Boulesteix and Hothorn (2010) and Boulesteix and Sauerbrei (2011). For likelihood-based boosting, this issue has been treated in Bender and Schumacher (2008).

7.5 Software

L_1-penalized regression techniques are implemented in the versatile R package *glmnet* (Friedman et al. 2015), which also contains an option for fitting group lasso models. Another package is *penalized* (Goeman et al. 2014). Methods to fit group lasso models are contained in the R packages *grplasso* (Meier 2015) and *grpreg* (Breheny 2015), where the latter package additionally contains options for using other penalties such as SCAD. Gradient boosting methods are implemented in the R package *mboost* (Hothorn et al. 2015), which contains a large variety of loss functions, especially for binary outcome values. The *gamboost* function in *mboost* implements a blockwise boosting algorithm that allows for specifying nonlinear predictor effects, giving rise to additive hazard models with variable selection.

7.6 Exercises

7.1 Consider the gradient boosting algorithm for discrete hazard models and derive the negative gradient vector $-\frac{\partial \mathcal{R}}{\partial f}$ for the case where the risk function is given by (7.11). Derive the negative gradient separately for the logistic, probit, Gompertz, and Gumbel link functions.

7.2 A popular approach to illustrate penalized regression and gradient boosting methods is to draw *coefficient path plots*. With this technique, coefficient estimates (on the y-axis) are plotted against different values of the respective tuning parameter (on the x-axis). The behavior of the coefficient estimates can thus be analyzed for varying levels of regularization.

1. Generate a coefficient path plot for the L_1 penalized regression model of Example 7.2 and visualize the relationship between the tuning parameter λ (in decreasing order on the x-axis) and the resulting coefficient estimates (on the y-axis). Which is the first gene to enter the model as λ starts to decrease?

2. Similarly, generate a coefficient path plot for the gradient boosting model of Example 7.4 and visualize the relationship between the number of boosting iterations (on the x-axis) and the resulting coefficient estimates (on the y-axis). Compare the plot to the respective plot for L_1 penalized regression model and analyze the orders in which the genes enter the model.

7.3 In Sect. 7.1 the adaptive lasso and the group lasso were introduced. It is possible to use the advantages of both methods simultaneously by penalizing categorical variables together and by adaptively choosing the weights of each variable. Wang and Leng (2008) showed that this method is able to consistently identify the true underlying model. Apply the adaptive group lasso to the SOEP data and use the time until drop-out as outcome variable:

1. Estimate the initial weights $w_j = 1/|\gamma_j|^\delta$ of a discrete hazard model with logistic link using $\delta = 1$. For illustration purposes and for numerical reasons exclude the following variables from the model (but include all other variables in the SOEP data):

   - *HID, HGTYP1HH, HGNUTS1, HGRSUBS, HGOWNER, HGACQUIS.*

2. Based on the specified weights fit the adaptive group lasso to the data and estimate the optimal value of the tuning parameter λ via fivefold cross-validation. Hint: Use the function *cv.glmnet (..., penalty.factor, type.multinomial = "grouped").*
3. Refit the survival model by using all observations of the SOEP data as well as the optimal λ. Draw the coefficient paths. Do any variables have coefficients with zero values?

7.4 Again consider the SOEP data. The aim is to analyze the data by using gradient boosting techniques with smooth nonlinear predictor effects and by considering the same covariates as in the previous exercise.

1. For all continuous covariates specify penalized B-spline base-learners (using the default implementation in the *bbs* function of R package *mboost*). For categorical variables use linear base-learners (*bols* function in R package *mboost*, see Hofner et al. 2014 for details on the implementation of base-learners in *mboost*).
2. Fit a discrete survival model with logistic link function and determine an appropriate number of boosting iterations using the *cvrisk* function in *mboost*. Visualize the effect of each selected covariate on the linear predictor and interpret the partial effects of the variables.
3. What are the relative frequencies of the selected variables across the boosting iterations?

Chapter 8
Competing Risks Models

In the previous chapters we have considered various statistical techniques that model the time to a particular event of interest. There are applications, however, where these models do not apply because the interest is in several distinct types of target events. For example, in survival analysis the events may refer to several causes of death. Similarly, when modeling duration of unemployment one often distinguishes between full-time and part-time jobs that end the unemployment spell. Models for this type of data are often referred to as *competing risks models*. In this chapter we will first consider parametric competing risks models for discrete time-to-event data and then show how the estimation can be embedded into the framework of GLMs.

8.1 Parametric Models

In simple time-to-event models with one target event the dynamics of the process were described by one hazard function. In the case of several target events it is useful to define several hazard functions, one for each type of event. Let in the following $R \in \{1, \ldots, m\}$ denote the distinct target events. For discrete time $T \in \{1, \ldots, q+1\}$, the *cause-specific hazard function* resulting from cause or risk r is defined by

$$\lambda_r(t|\boldsymbol{x}) = P(T = t, R = r \mid T \geq t, \boldsymbol{x}),$$

where $\boldsymbol{x}$ is a vector of time-independent covariates. The m hazard functions $\lambda_1(t|\boldsymbol{x}), \ \ldots, \lambda_m(t|\boldsymbol{x})$ can be combined into one hazard function that describes the process regardless of the type of target event. The resulting *overall hazard function* is defined by

$$\lambda(t|\boldsymbol{x}) = \sum_{r=1}^{m} \lambda_r(t|\boldsymbol{x}) = P(T = t \mid T \geq t, \boldsymbol{x}).$$

G. Tutz, M. Schmid, *Modeling Discrete Time-to-Event Data*,
Springer Series in Statistics, DOI 10.1007/978-3-319-28158-2_8

The survival function and unconditional probability of an event in period t have the same form as in the simple case of one target event, i.e.,

$$S(t|x) = P(T > t \,|\, \boldsymbol{x}) = \prod_{i=1}^{t}(1 - \lambda(i|\boldsymbol{x}))$$

and

$$P(T = t \,|\, \boldsymbol{x}) = \lambda(t|\boldsymbol{x})S(t-1|\boldsymbol{x}).$$

For an individual reaching interval $[a_{t-1}, a_t)$, there are m possible outcomes, namely the end of the duration in one of the m target events, or survival beyond $[a_{t-1}, a_t)$. The corresponding conditional response probabilities are given by

$$\lambda_1(t|\boldsymbol{x}), \ldots, \lambda_m(t|\boldsymbol{x}), 1 - \lambda(t|\boldsymbol{x}),$$

where $1 - \lambda(t|\boldsymbol{x})$ is the probability of survival. Natural models for these $m + 1$ events are multi-category models that are used in the modeling of categorical data. An overview of the basic concepts for competing risks models is given in Fig. 8.1. In the following we will consider (among others) the frequently used *multinomial model*, and also a discretized version of a competing risks model for continuous time.

Cause-specific discrete hazard

$$\lambda_r(t|\boldsymbol{x}) = P(T = t, R = r \,|\, T \geq t, \boldsymbol{x})$$

Overall hazard

$$\lambda(t|\boldsymbol{x}) = \sum_{r=1}^{m} \lambda_r(t|\boldsymbol{x}) = P(T = t \,|\, T \geq t, \boldsymbol{x})$$

Survival function

$$S(t|\boldsymbol{x}) = P(T > t \,|\, \boldsymbol{x}) = \prod_{i=1}^{t}(1 - \lambda(i|\boldsymbol{x}))$$

Event probability

$$P(T = t, R = r \,|\, \boldsymbol{x}) = \lambda_r(t|\boldsymbol{x})S(t-1|\boldsymbol{x})$$

Fig. 8.1 Basic concepts for competing risks models in discrete time

8.1.1 Multinomial Logit Model

The multinomial logit model is the most widely used model for categorical responses, see, for example, Tutz (2012) or Agresti (2013). In discrete survival the responses are either the target events or survival. The corresponding model is given by

$$\lambda_r(t|\boldsymbol{x}) = \frac{\exp(\gamma_{0tr} + \boldsymbol{x}^T\boldsymbol{\gamma}_r)}{1 + \sum_{i=1}^{m} \exp(\gamma_{0ti} + \boldsymbol{x}^T\boldsymbol{\gamma}_i)} \tag{8.1}$$

for $r = 1, \ldots, m, t = 1, \ldots, q$. The parameters $\gamma_{01j}, \ldots, \gamma_{0qj}$ represent the cause-specific baseline hazard function, and $\boldsymbol{\gamma}_r$ is the cause-specific vector of coefficients. It should be noted that, although $m + 1$ response categories can occur, it suffices to specify the conditional probability of the target events $1, \ldots, m$. The reference category is conditional survival, and its probability is simply given by

$$P(T > t \mid T \geq t, \boldsymbol{x}) = 1 - \sum_{r=1}^{m} \lambda_r(t|\boldsymbol{x}) = \frac{1}{1 + \sum_{j=1}^{m} \exp(\gamma_{0tj} + \boldsymbol{x}^T\boldsymbol{\gamma}_j)}.$$

Thus the conditional model that is used is the multinomial logit model for $m + 1$ categories. With $R \in \{0, 1, \ldots, m\}$, where $R = 0$ denotes conditional survival, the conditional probabilities that sum up to 1 are given by $\lambda_0(t|\boldsymbol{x}) = P(T > t \mid T \geq t, \boldsymbol{x}), \lambda_1(t|\boldsymbol{x}), \ldots, \lambda_m(t|\boldsymbol{x})$.

For the interpretation of parameters it is useful to consider the model in the form

$$\log\left(\frac{\lambda_r(t|\boldsymbol{x})}{\lambda_0(t|\boldsymbol{x})}\right) = \gamma_{0tr} + \boldsymbol{x}^T\boldsymbol{\gamma}_r.$$

It is seen that the linear predictor determines the cause-specific log-odds, that means the logarithm of the proportion $\lambda_r(t|\boldsymbol{x})/\lambda_0(t|\boldsymbol{x})$, which compares the conditional probability of the target event $R = r$ to conditional survival. With parameter vector $\boldsymbol{\gamma}_r^T = (\gamma_{r1}, \ldots, \gamma_{rp})$ one obtains

$$\frac{\lambda_r(t|\boldsymbol{x})}{\lambda_0(t|\boldsymbol{x})} = \exp(\gamma_{0tr})\exp(\gamma_{r1})^{x_1} \cdots \exp(\gamma_{rp})^{x_p}.$$

Thus the increase of x_j by one unit increases the cause-specific odds by the factor $\exp(\gamma_{rj})$. While γ_{rj} gives the additive effect of variable x_j on the log-odds, the transformed parameter $\exp(\gamma_{rj})$ shows the multiplicative effect on the odds, which is often more intuitive.

As in the single-event case, the baseline hazard function may be simplified by assuming a smooth function, and the weight $\boldsymbol{\gamma}_r$ may depend on time.

8.1.2 Ordered Target Events

The multinomial logit model can be used for any number of risk categories but contains many parameters. For each category of the risk one has to estimate the risk-specific baseline hazard γ_{0tr} as a function in t and the parameter vector $\boldsymbol{\gamma}_r$. If the causes or risks are ordered, sparser parameterizations can be found. For example, in a study on unemployment, the target events $R \in \{1, \ldots, m\}$ can represent "part-time job" or "full-time job" as alternatives to remaining unemployed, where the latter category can be denoted by $R = 0$. In cases like this one can consider R as an *ordered* categorical response given that a specific time point is reached.

If R has a natural order, one can use classical ordinal response models as proposed by McCullagh (1980) to model the cause-specific hazards. The cumulative-type model uses cumulative probabilities, which in the case of discrete hazards are given by

$$\lambda_r(t|\boldsymbol{x}) = \sum_{j=1}^{r} \lambda_j(t|\boldsymbol{x}) = P(T = t, R \leq r \,|\, T \geq t, \boldsymbol{x}).$$

The so-called *cumulative model for ordered responses* assumes

$$\lambda_r(t|\boldsymbol{x}) = F(\gamma_{0tr} + \boldsymbol{x}^T\boldsymbol{\gamma}), \tag{8.2}$$

where $F(.)$ is a fixed cumulative distribution function, and the intercepts must satisfy $\gamma_{0tr} \leq \gamma_{0t,r+1}$ for all r. Specifically, if $F(\cdot)$ is the logistic distribution function, one obtains McCullagh's proportional odds model for responses R given by

$$\log\left(\frac{\lambda_r(t|\boldsymbol{x})}{1 - \lambda_r(t|\boldsymbol{x})}\right) = \gamma_{0tr} + \boldsymbol{x}^T\boldsymbol{\gamma}.$$

Given that the model fits the data well, the advantage of the model over the multinomial logit model is that one needs only one parameter vector $\boldsymbol{\gamma}$ instead of one parameter vector $\boldsymbol{\gamma}_r$ for each category. For an application and further discussion, see Tutz (1995).

8.1.3 General Form

The models considered above all have a common form. They can be written as

$$\lambda_r(t|\boldsymbol{x}) = h_r(\boldsymbol{X}_t\boldsymbol{\beta}), \tag{8.3}$$

where h_r is a response function for responses in interval $[a_{t-1}, a_t)$ and $\boldsymbol{X}_t$ is a design matrix composed of $\boldsymbol{x}$ and depending on time t. For example, the multinomial model uses the logistic response function

$$h_r(\eta_1, \ldots, \eta_m) = \frac{\exp(\eta_r)}{1 + \sum_{i=1}^{m} \exp(\eta_i)}$$

and design matrix

$$X_t = \begin{bmatrix} 0 & \ldots & 1 & & & \ldots & 0 & x^T & & & \\ 0 & \ldots & & 1 & & \ldots & 0 & & x^T & & \\ 0 & \ldots & & & \ddots & \ldots & 0 & & & \ddots & \\ 0 & \ldots & & & 1 & \ldots & 0 & & & & x^T \end{bmatrix}, \tag{8.4}$$

where a 1 in rth row of X_t is at the $(t + r)$th position. The parameter vector in this case is then given by

$$\boldsymbol{\beta}^T = (\gamma_{011}, \ldots, \gamma_{01m}, \gamma_{021}, \ldots, \gamma_{0qm}, \boldsymbol{\gamma}_1^T, \ldots, \boldsymbol{\gamma}_m^T).$$

If the covariates are time-dependent stochastic processes $\boldsymbol{x}_{i1}, \ldots, \boldsymbol{x}_{it}$, cause-specific and global hazard functions have the forms

$$\lambda_r(t|\boldsymbol{x}_i(t)) = P(T_i = t, R_i = r \mid T_i \geq t, \boldsymbol{x}_i(t)),$$

$$\lambda(t|\boldsymbol{x}_i(t)) = \sum_{r=1}^{m} \lambda_r(t|\boldsymbol{x}_i(t)),$$

where $\boldsymbol{x}_i(t)^T = (\boldsymbol{x}_{i1}, \ldots, \boldsymbol{x}_{it})$ is the sequence of observations until time t. The model for the hazard function has the form (8.3), where the design matrix X_t is a function of t and $\boldsymbol{x}(t)$.

8.1.4 Separate Modeling of Single Targets

In competing risks models multiple target events are modeled *simultaneously*. One might be tempted to use a simpler modeling approach by focussing on one target event and considering the occurrence of other targets as censored observations. Then, for fixed r_0 one would use the hazard function

$$\lambda_{r_0}(t|\boldsymbol{x}) = \lambda(t|\boldsymbol{x}) = P(T = t, R = r_0 \mid T \geq t, \boldsymbol{x}).$$

Let the data for the competing risks again be given by $(t_i, r_i, \delta_i, \boldsymbol{x}_i)$, where $r_i \in \{1, \ldots, m\}$ indicates the target event. When focussing on this event, one considers the transformed data

$$(t_i, \delta_i^{(r_0)}, \boldsymbol{x}_i), \text{ where } \delta_i^{(r_0)} = 0 \text{ if } \delta_i = 0 \text{ or } r_i \neq r_0.$$

The indicator function $\delta_i^{(r_0)}$ denotes censoring in the single-cause model for the r_0th target event.

Although this approach seems attractive because simple binary models are used, it has severe disadvantages. In particular, estimation can be strongly biased. This is because when fitting simple discrete survival models, it is assumed that censoring and survival are independent (the so-called random censoring property). Thus, when the underlying survival times for the competing events are correlated, the censoring process in the simplified model for separate single targets is correlated with the survival time. If correlation between survival time and censoring is ignored, the estimated hazards will be biased. As a consequence, if survival times are correlated, separate modeling of single targets cannot be recommended. Since in practice the correlation structure is usually unknown, competing risks modeling is often the better choice.

8.2 Maximum Likelihood Estimation

Let the data be given by $(t_i, r_i, \delta_i, \boldsymbol{x}_i)$, where $r_i \in \{1, \ldots, m\}$ indicates the target event. We again assume random censoring at the end of the interval with $t_i = \min\{T_i, C_i\}$, where events are defined by the indicator function

$$\delta_i = \begin{cases} 1, & T_i \leq C_i, \text{i.e., the event of interest occurred in interval } [a_{t_i-1}, a_{t_i}), \\ 0, & T_i > C_i, \text{which refers to censoring in interval } [a_{t_i-1}, a_{t_i}). \end{cases}$$

In the following it is shown how estimates of competing risks models can be obtained using maximum likelihood estimation in multivariate GLMs.

The likelihood contribution of the ith observation for the general model (8.3) is

$$L_i = P(T_i = t_i, R_i = r_i)^{\delta_i} P(T_i > t_i)^{1-\delta_i} P(C_i \geq t_i)^{\delta_i} P(C_i = t_i)^{1-\delta_i}.$$

Under the assumption of random censoring, the factor $P(C_i \geq t_i)^{\delta_i} P(C_i = t_i)^{1-\delta_i}$ can be omitted, and the likelihood reduces to

$$\begin{aligned} L_i &= P(T_i = t_i, R_i = r_i \,|\, \boldsymbol{x}_i)^{\delta_i} \; P(T_i > t_i \,|\, \boldsymbol{x}_i)^{1-\delta_i} \\ &= \lambda_{r_i}(t_i|\boldsymbol{x}_i)^{\delta_i} (1 - \lambda(t_i|\boldsymbol{x}_i))^{1-\delta_i} \prod_{t=1}^{t_i-1} \left(1 - \lambda(t|\boldsymbol{x}_i)\right). \end{aligned} \tag{8.5}$$

Analogous to Chap. 3, embedding model (8.3) into the GLM framework uses the representation by binary indicators for the transition to the next time period. Therefore one specifies indicator variables in the following way: For each observation one defines for $t < t_i$

$$\boldsymbol{y}_{it}^T = (y_{it0}, y_{it1}, \ldots, y_{itm}) = (1, 0, \ldots, 0),$$

which encodes survival for all time points before t_i. For $t = t_i$ one defines for $\delta_i = 1$

$$\boldsymbol{y}_{it_i}^T = (y_{it_i0}, y_{it_i1}, \ldots, y_{it_im}) = (0, \ldots, 1, \ldots, 0)$$

with $y_{it_ir_i} = 1$ and all other entries zero, and for $\delta_i = 0$

$$\boldsymbol{y}_{it_i}^T = (y_{it_i0}, y_{it_i1}, \ldots, y_{it_im}) = (1, 0, \ldots, 0).$$

With these indicator variables the likelihood for the ith observation can be written in the form

$$\begin{aligned} L_i &= \prod_{t=1}^{t_i} \{\prod_{r=1}^{m} \lambda_r(t|\boldsymbol{x}_i)^{y_{itr}}\}\{1 - \lambda(t|\boldsymbol{x}_i)\}^{y_{it0}} \\ &= \prod_{t=1}^{t_i} \{\prod_{r=1}^{m} \lambda_r(t|\boldsymbol{x}_i)^{y_{itr}}\}\{1 - \sum_{r=1}^{m} \lambda_r(t|\boldsymbol{x}_i)\}^{y_{it0}}. \end{aligned}$$

This means that the likelihood for the ith observation is the same as the likelihood for the t_i observations $\boldsymbol{y}_{i1}, \ldots, \boldsymbol{y}_{it_i}$ of a multinomial response model. The indicator variables actually represent the distributions given that a specific interval is reached. Given that an individual reaches interval $[a_{t-1}, a_t)$, the response is multinomially distributed with $\boldsymbol{y}_{it}^T = (y_{it0}, y_{it1}, \ldots, y_{itm}) \sim M(1,\ 1-\lambda(t|\boldsymbol{x}_i), \lambda_1(t|\boldsymbol{x}_i), \ldots, \lambda_m(t|\boldsymbol{x}_i))$. The dummy variable $y_{it0} = 1 - y_{it1} - \ldots - y_{itm}$ has value 1 if individual i does not fail in interval $[a_{t-1}, a_t)$ and $y_{it0} = 0$ if individual i fails in $[a_{t-1}, a_t)$.

As a consequence, the likelihood is that of the multi-categorical model $P(Y_{it} = r) = h_r(\boldsymbol{X}_t\beta)$, where $Y_{it} = r$ if $y_{itr} = 1$. As in the single-cause model, maximum likelihood estimates may be calculated within the framework of multivariate generalized linear models after augmenting the design matrices. For the ith observation, the response and design matrices are given by

$$\begin{bmatrix} \boldsymbol{y}_{i1} \\ \vdots \\ \boldsymbol{y}_{i,t_i} \end{bmatrix}, \begin{bmatrix} \boldsymbol{X}_1 \\ \vdots \\ \boldsymbol{X}_{t_i} \end{bmatrix},$$

and the total log-likelihood is given by

$$\begin{aligned} l &= \sum_{i=1}^{n} \sum_{t=1}^{t_i} \left(\sum_{r=1}^{m} y_{itr} \log \lambda_r(t|\boldsymbol{x}_i) + y_{it0} \log \left(1 - \sum_{r=1}^{m} \lambda_r(t|\boldsymbol{x}_i)\right) \right) \\ &= \sum_{t=1}^{q} \sum_{i \in R_t} \left(\sum_{r=1}^{m} y_{itr} \log \lambda_r(t|\boldsymbol{x}_i) + y_{it0} \log \left(1 - \sum_{r=1}^{m} \lambda_r(t|\boldsymbol{x}_i)\right) \right), \end{aligned} \quad (8.6)$$

where in the latter form $R_t = \{i \,|\, t_i \geq t\}$ is the number of individuals at risk in the interval $[a_{t-1}, a_t)$. Details on the maximization of the log-likelihood of a multinomial distribution are given in Tutz (2012).

Example 8.1 Duration of Unemployment of U.S. Citizens
We consider the unemployment data described in Example 1.1 with two competing events: re-employed at full-time job and re-employed at part-time job. Event times were measured in two-week intervals. The censoring event, which in our analysis constituted the reference category, was "still jobless."

To account for competing risks, a multinomial logit model with covariates *age*, *filed UI claim*, and *log weekly earnings in lost job* was fitted to the data. Baseline hazards were fitted by using cubic smoothing splines with four degrees of freedom (which is the default implementation in the R package *VGAM*). Figure 8.2 shows the estimated baseline coefficients for the two events. Obviously, the baseline chances of finding a job are very similar to the lifetable estimates shown in Fig. 2.3. In particular, the curves start to increase after 20 weeks and have a peak after 26 weeks, which can be attributed to the fact that benefits from the state-funded unemployment compensation program stop after 26 weeks in some U.S. states. Generally, the baseline risks for the two events are very similar; it is seen, however, that the baseline chance of getting re-employed at a part-time job is higher in the first time period (0–20 weeks) while chances of finding a full-time job tend to become higher after 20 weeks.

Coefficient estimates with 95 % confidence intervals are presented in Table 8.1. As expected, there is a negative effect of age on the chance of re-employment at a full-time job. Conversely, the chances of getting re-employed at a part-time job were largely independent of age. Similar to Example 2.2, filing a UI claim significantly lowered the chances for both events. Possibly these persons are less ambitious in finding a new job. The logarithmic wages have a significant impact (confidence intervals do not include zero) on both events. The higher the former logarithmic wage, the more likely the person will later be re-employed at a full-time job. Conversely, the odds of being re-employed at a part-time job decrease, implying that low wages in former jobs increase the chance of finding a part-time job instead of a full-time job. □

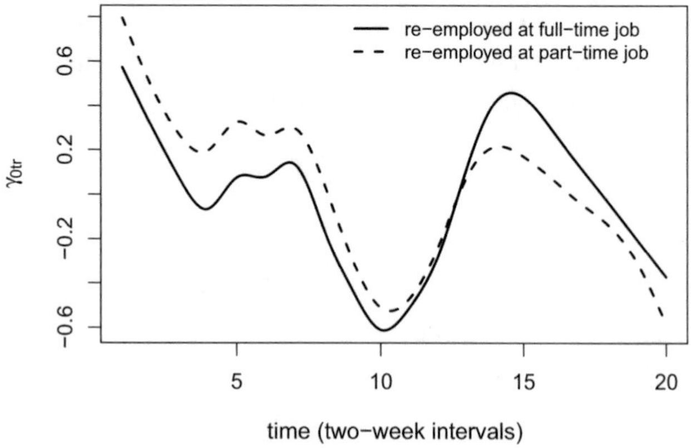

Fig. 8.2 Duration of unemployment of U.S. citizens. The figure shows the smooth baseline hazard estimates that were obtained from a competing risks model with logistic link function. Event times were measured in 2-week intervals

Table 8.1 Duration of unemployment of U.S. citizens. The table shows the effect estimates for the three covariates "age," "filed UI claim?" and "log weekly earnings in lost job." The 95 % interval estimates were obtained from 250 bootstrap samples

Event	Coef. estimate for age	Coef. estimate for UI claim	Coef. estimate for log weekly earnings
Re-employed at ft job	−0.01248 (−0.01895, −0.00617)	−1.14683 (−1.28556, −1.02068)	0.49464 (0.36700, 0.61977)
Re-employed at pt job	0.00119 (−0.00892, 0.01226)	−1.17169 (−1.37452, −0.94198)	−0.30369 (−0.51747, −0.08458)

8.3 Variable Selection

The linear predictor in the multinomial model for the cause-specific hazard $\lambda_r(t|\boldsymbol{x})$ has the form

$$\eta_r = \gamma_{0tr} + \boldsymbol{x}^T\boldsymbol{\gamma}_r,$$

where $\boldsymbol{x}^T = (x_1, \ldots, x_p)$ and $\boldsymbol{\gamma}_r^T = (\gamma_{r1}, \ldots, \gamma_{rp})$. Let in the following all parameters be collected in the vector $\boldsymbol{\gamma}$.

Variable selection in single-cause models can be obtained by using methods that maximize the penalized log-likelihood $l_p(\boldsymbol{\gamma}) = l(\boldsymbol{\gamma}) - \frac{\lambda}{2}J(\boldsymbol{\gamma})$ instead of the usual log-likelihood $l(\boldsymbol{\gamma})$ (cf. Chap. 7). In particular the lasso can be used to identify relevant predictors if many are available (see Sect. 7.1). For the cause-specific model, however, the straightforward use of the lasso has severe disadvantages because the simple lasso penalty

$$J(\boldsymbol{\gamma}) = \sum_{r=1}^{m}\sum_{j=1}^{p} |\gamma_{rj}|$$

enforces the selection of *parameters* but not of *variables*. With appropriate choice of the tuning parameters part of the parameters will be set to zero, but the remaining parameters can be linked to any of the variables. Thus it might occur that all variables have still to be kept in the model.

An alternative method that explicitly enforces variable selection instead of parameter selection uses a penalty that specifies groups of parameters and links them to one covariate each. Let all the effects on the jth variable be collected in $\boldsymbol{\gamma}_{.j}^T = (\gamma_{1j}, \ldots, \gamma_{mj})$ and consider the *grouped penalty*

$$J(\boldsymbol{\gamma}) = \sum_{j=1}^{p} ||\boldsymbol{\gamma}_{.j}|| = \sum_{j=1}^{p} (\gamma_{1j}^2 + \cdots + \gamma_{mj}^2)^{1/2},$$

where $||\boldsymbol{u}|| = ||\boldsymbol{u}||_2 = \sqrt{\boldsymbol{u}^T\boldsymbol{u}}$ denotes the L_2 norm. The penalty enforces variable selection, that is, all the parameters in $\boldsymbol{\gamma}_{.j}$ are simultaneously shrunk toward zero. It is strongly related to the group lasso (Yuan and Lin 2006), see Sect. 7.1. However, in the group lasso the grouping refers to the parameters that are linked to a categorical predictor within a univariate regression model, whereas in the present model grouping arises from the multivariate response structure. It was originally proposed for multinomial responses by Tutz et al. (2015). In discrete survival the penalty should be amended by a term that ensures that the baseline hazard is sufficiently smooth over time. A penalty that enforces structured and effective variable selection and that smooths the baseline hazards over time is given by

$$J_{\zeta_1,\zeta_2}(\boldsymbol{\gamma}) = \zeta_1 \sum_{r=1}^{m} \sum_{t=2}^{q} (\gamma_{0tr} - \gamma_{0,t-1,r})^2 + \zeta_2 \sum_{j=1}^{p} \phi_j \left\| \boldsymbol{\gamma}_{.j} \right\|, \tag{8.7}$$

where $\phi_j = \sqrt{m}$ is a weight that adjusts the penalty level on parameter vectors $\boldsymbol{\gamma}_{.j}$ for their dimension. The importance of the penalty terms is determined by the tuning parameters ζ_1 and ζ_2. Without a penalty, that is with $\zeta_1 = \zeta_2 = 0$, ordinary maximum likelihood estimation is obtained.

Generally, the common penalty level ζ_2 for all $\left\| \boldsymbol{\gamma}_{.j} \right\|$ is not an optimal choice. As was shown by Zou (2006), penalties of the form (8.7) are inconsistent if used with a common penalty parameter. The proposed remedy are so-called *adaptive weights*, which are obtained by replacing the weights ϕ_j by

$$\phi_j^a = \frac{\sqrt{m}}{||\hat{\boldsymbol{\gamma}}_{.j}^{\text{Init}}||},$$

where $\hat{\boldsymbol{\gamma}}_{.j}^{\text{Init}}$ denotes an appropriate initial estimator. For example, the penalized estimator that results from application of penalty (8.7) with $\zeta_2 = 0$ can be used as initial estimator. In this case, the initial estimator uses unpenalized covariate effects, but an active smoothing penalty on the baseline effects. The tuning parameters themselves have to be chosen, for example, by cross-validation. For details, see Möst et al. (2015).

Example 8.2 Congressional Careers

We consider the data on congressional careers described in Example 1.4. The competing risks were defined by the way a career ends, by *retirement*, an alternative office (*ambition*), losing a primary election (*primary*) or losing a general election (*general*). The dependent variable is defined by the transition process of a Congressman from his/her first election up to one of the competing events *general, primary, retirement, or ambition*. The duration until the occurrence of one of the competing events is measured as terms served, where a maximum of 16 terms can be reached. Predictors were described in Example 1.4, and summaries were given in Tables 1.4 and 1.5.

We fitted a penalized multinomial logit model with risks defined by cause 1 (*general*), 2 (*primary*), 3 (*retirement*), and 4 (*ambition*). The effect of covariates is specified by the cause-specific linear predictors $\eta_{itr} = \gamma_{0tr} + \boldsymbol{x}_{it}^T \boldsymbol{\gamma}_r$. All covariates described in Table 1.4 were considered. To be on comparable scales, all covariates were standardized to have equal variance. Moreover, we included all pairwise interactions with the exception of *republican:leader, leader:redist, opengub:scandal, scandal:redist* because the data contained too few observations of the corresponding combinations. Such a high-dimensional interaction model cannot be properly handled by unpenalized maximum likelihood estimation, but stable estimation and efficient variable selection is obtained by using penalization. Since the adaptive version of the penalty (8.7) yielded better cross-validation scores,

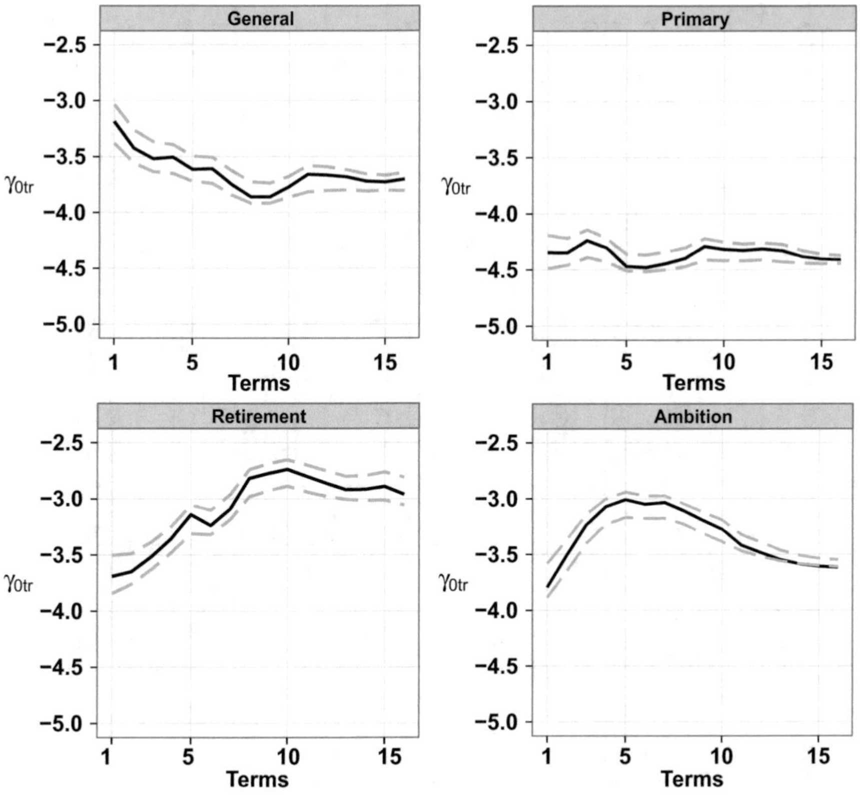

Fig. 8.3 Parameter estimates of the cause-specific time-varying baseline effects for the Congressional careers data. *Dashed lines* represent the 95 % pointwise bootstrap intervals

adaptive weights were included. Tuning parameters ζ_1 and ζ_2 were chosen on a two-dimensional grid by fivefold cross validation with the predictive deviance as loss criterion.

Figure 8.3 shows the parameter estimates for the cause-specific time-varying baseline effects. The corresponding pointwise confidence intervals, marked by light gray dashed lines, were estimated by a nonparametric bootstrap method with 1000 bootstrap replications. It can be seen that cause-specific baseline effects are needed because the shapes are quite different. For retirement the parameters increase over early terms and eventually become stable, while for ambition there is an early peak at about five terms and then a decrease. Due to the penalization of adjacent coefficients, the estimated baseline effects are rather smooth.

Parameter estimates of the covariate effects are summarized in Table 8.2. It shows the ordinary maximum likelihood estimates and the estimates resulting from the penalized competing risk model with their corresponding standard errors. The computation of the standard errors is again based on a nonparametric bootstrap approach with 1000 bootstrap replications. It is immediately seen that the penalization removes a considerable number of effects, that is, only 68 out of 128 parameters remain in the model, leading to a strong reduction of the model complexity. The selection procedure suggests that the main effects *Republican* and *Leader* are not needed in the predictor. Moreover, a large number of interaction effects have been deleted. Concerning

Table 8.2 Parameter estimates for the Congressional careers data. Ordinary maximum likelihood estimates are denoted by "ML"; penalized estimates are denoted by "pen." Estimated standard errors for the penalized model obtained by bootstrapping are given in the columns denoted by "sd"

	General			Primary			Retirement			Ambition		
	ML	pen.	sd	ML	pen.	sd	ML	pen.	sd	ML	pen.	sd
Age	0.069	0.046	0.008	0.071	0.046	0.011	0.070	0.068	0.008	−0.034	−0.037	0.007
Republican	0.255	0	0.005	−0.188	0	0.002	−0.201	0	0.009	0.343	0	0.018
Priorm	−0.078	−0.060	0.005	0.006	0.001	0.005	−0.007	−0.005	0.003	−0.010	−0.004	0.002
Leader	−0.272	0	0.087	−2.779	0	0.081	−0.393	0	0.065	0.033	0	0.080
Opengub	0.815	0.205	0.116	0.598	0.181	0.097	0.227	0.109	0.077	0.528	0.208	0.121
Opensen	−0.638	−0.243	0.125	−0.215	−0.193	0.134	−0.086	0.062	0.125	1.136	0.878	0.134
Scandal	3.750	2.689	0.370	3.215	3.272	0.428	1.921	1.611	0.441	−3.118	−1.532	0.073
Redist	2.548	1.617	0.447	1.465	1.149	0.499	−0.563	0.431	0.251	0.574	0.801	0.309
Age:Republican	0.007	0.011	0.007	−0.045	−0.010	0.007	0.041	0.030	0.009	−0.038	−0.029	0.009
Age:Priorm	0.001	0.000	0.000	−0.001	0.000	0.000	0.000	0.000	0.000	0.000	0.000	0.000
Age:Leader	0.014	0	0.002	−0.117	0	0.002	0.018	0	0.002	−0.269	0	0.001
Age:Opengub	−0.006	0	0	0.034	0	0	−0.016	0	0	−0.011	0	0
Age:Opensen	−0.005	0	0.001	−0.074	0	0.001	−0.039	0	0.004	−0.015	0	0.002
Age:Scandal	−0.106	0	0	0.022	0	0	0.090	0	0	0.009	0	0
Age:Redist	−0.001	0.007	0.016	−0.066	−0.039	0.018	0.174	0.097	0.031	0.037	0.018	0.016
Republican:Priorm	0.016	0.005	0.004	−0.041	−0.016	0.005	−0.008	−0.004	0.004	0.015	0.012	0.004
Republican:Opengub	−0.532	−0.342	0.200	−4.282	−1.337	0.147	−0.147	−0.233	0.201	−0.063	0.294	0.184
Republican:Opensen	0.323	0	0.001	−0.092	0	0.002	0.802	0	0.010	−0.260	0	0.011
Republican:Scandal	0.007	0	0.021	2.121	0	0.054	0.182	0	0.005	−1.418	0	0.001
Republican:Redist	−1.833	0	0.076	0.447	0	0.059	1.247	0	0.050	−0.276	0	0.051

(continued)

Table 8.2 (continued)

	General			Primary			Retirement			Ambition		
	ML	pen.	sd	ML	pen.	sd	ML	pen.	sd	ML	pen.	sd
Priorm:Leader	0.025	0	0	−0.009	0	0	−0.008	0	0.001	0.057	0	0
Priorm:Opengub	0.020	0	0	−0.001	0	0.001	0.008	0	0.001	0.009	0	0.001
Priorm:Opensen	−0.016	0	0.001	−0.019	0	0.002	0.013	0	0.002	0.011	0	0.004
Priorm:Scandal	0.006	0.007	0.005	−0.017	−0.010	0.004	−0.071	−0.019	0.006	−0.028	−0.001	0
Priorm:Redist	0.066	0.037	0.019	0.000	−0.002	0.003	0.030	0.010	0.006	−0.013	−0.009	0.007
Leader:Opengub	−5.168	0	0.117	−1.693	0	0.087	1.054	0	0.359	−5.402	0	0.116
Leader:Opensen	−4.513	0	0	−0.941	0	0	1.001	0	0	−6.053	0	0
Leader:Scandal	−0.213	−0.029	0.594	−4.212	−1.803	0.733	−8.621	−1.925	0.756	−0.897	−0.108	0.047
Opengub:Opensen	−0.436	0	0	0.124	0	0	−0.280	0	0	−0.429	0	0
Openub:Redist	−0.175	0.172	0.663	−4.274	−0.415	0.125	−5.297	−0.666	0.237	2.751	2.126	0.932
Opensen:Scandal	−2.277	0	0.307	−1.482	0	0.206	−8.270	0	0.266	−3.311	0	0.058
Opensen:Redist	0.914	0	0.052	−4.560	0	0.006	−0.522	0	0.031	1.771	0	0.147

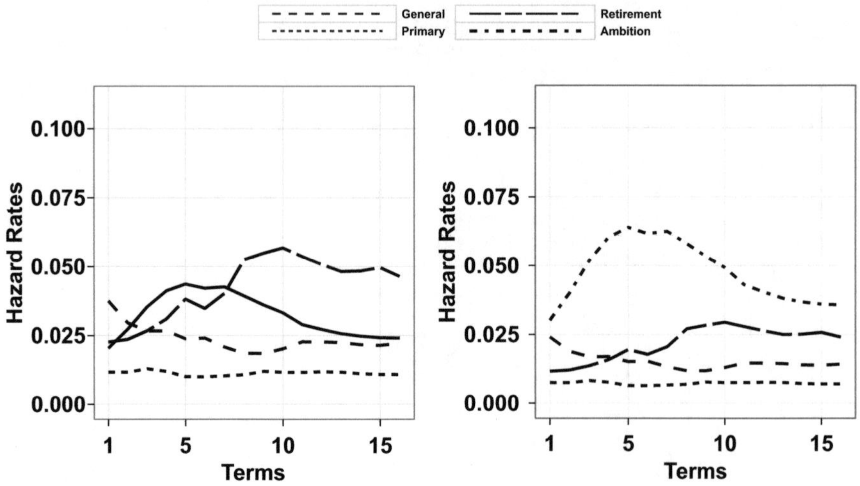

Fig. 8.4 Estimated hazard rates for the Congressional careers data. The following covariate specifications were used: Age = 51 (*left*), Age = 41 (*right*), Prior Margin = 35, no Republican, no Leadership, no open Gubernatorial seat, no open Senatorial seat, no Scandal and no Redistricting

interpretation, for example, the absolute value for the effect of the covariate *Scandal* indicates a strong effect. If a Congressman became embroiled in a scandal it is more likely that he/she loses a primary or general election or that he/she retires. A scandal also decreases the probability of seeking an alternative office as compared to re-election.

In Fig. 8.4 a selection of the resulting hazard rates is depicted. It shows hazard functions for the following covariate specifications: Age = 51 (left) and Age = 41 (right), Prior Margin = 35, no Republican, no Leadership, no open Gubernatorial seat, no open Senatorial seat, no Scandal, and no Redistricting for the transitions to *General*, *Primary*, *Retirement*, and *Ambition*. It can be seen that the probability of retirement tends to increase over early terms and then remains rather stable. The probability of seeking an alternative office as compared to re-election increases for early terms and then decreases. The hazard rate for losing either a primary or a general election is rather constant in the considered group. For more details, in particular on the selection of effects, see Möst (2014) and Möst et al. (2015). □

8.4 Literature and Further Reading

Competing Risks for Continuous Time Most of the literature on competing risks consider the case of continuous time, see, for example, Kalbfleisch and Prentice (2002), Klein and Moeschberger (2003), Beyersmann et al. (2011), and Kleinbaum and Klein (2013).

Discrete Hazards Narendranathan and Stewart (1993) considered discrete competing risks in the modeling of unemployment spells with flexible baseline hazards. Fahrmeir and Wagenpfeil (1996) proposed to estimate smooth hazard functions and time-varying effects by posterior modes. A random effects model of workfare transitions was considered by Enberg et al. (1990), and a general multilevel multistate competing risks model for repeated episodes was considered by Steele et al. (2004). Han and Hausman (1990) considered discretized versions of continuous-time models.

8.5 Software

The *VGAM* package (Yee 2010) can be used to fit multinomial and ordinal additive models. Ordinal models can also be fitted with the R package *ordinal* (Bojesen Christensen 2015). Variable selection can be carried out by use of the *MLSP* package, which is available at http://www.statistik.lmu.de/~poessnecker/software.html. The *data.long.comp.risk* function in R package *discSurv* can be used to convert survival data with competing events to a data frame with multinomial response.

8.6 Exercises

8.1 Assume that for continuous time the specific cause-specific proportional hazard model

$$\lambda_r(t) = \lambda_0(t)\exp(\eta_r), \quad \eta_r = \boldsymbol{x}^T\boldsymbol{\gamma}_r$$

holds. Show that the corresponding discrete hazard model with $T = t$ if failure occurs in interval $[a_{t-1}, a_t)$ has the form

$$\lambda_r(t|\boldsymbol{x}) = \frac{\exp(\eta_r)}{\sum_{j=1}^m \exp(\eta_j)}\Big\{1 - \exp\Big(-\sum_{j=1}^m \exp(\eta_j)\Big)\Big\},$$

where $\gamma_{0t} = \log\left(\int_{a_{t-1}}^{a_t} \lambda_0(t)\right)$.

8.2 Consider the response function h_r given by

$$h_r(\eta_1, \dots, \eta_m) = \frac{\exp(\eta_r)}{\sum_{j=1}^m \exp(\eta_j)}\Big\{1 - \exp\Big(-\sum_{j=1}^m \exp(\eta_j)\Big)\Big\}.$$

Calculate the corresponding design matrix $\boldsymbol{X}_t$ and the parameter vector $\boldsymbol{\beta}$, i.e. rewrite λ_r as

$$\lambda_r(t|\boldsymbol{x}) = h_r(\boldsymbol{X}_t\boldsymbol{\beta}).$$

8.3 In Example 8.1 a multinomial logit model was used to analyze the U.S. unemployment data. This model is best suited for unordered event categories because it allows for estimating a separate coefficient vector for each target event. The aim of this exercise is to investigate whether a cumulative logit model fits the data better (or at least equally well). In principle, fitting a cumulative model is justified by the fact that the target events of the U.S. unemployment data have a natural order ("still jobless," "re-employed at part-time job," "re-employed at full-time job"). On the other hand, Example 8.1 suggested very different effects of some of the covariates on the target events; this would in turn justify the use of a multinomial logit model.

1. Subdivide the U.S. unemployment data randomly into a learning sample (comprising two thirds of the observations) and a validation sample (comprising the remaining third of observations).
2. Convert the learning and validation samples into sets of augmented data.
3. Fit a multinomial logit model with covariates *age*, *filed UI claim* and *log weekly earnings in lost job* to the learning data. In addition, estimate the parameters of a cumulative logit model that contains the same covariates.
4. For both models compute the predictive deviance in the validation sample.
5. Repeat the above steps 100 times. For both logistic models (multinomial and cumulative) compute the means, medians and standard deviations of the predicted deviance values of the 100 validation samples. Which model results in the higher prediction accuracy?

8.4 The aim of this exercise is to investigate how the estimates obtained from competing risks models and the estimates obtained from separate modeling of single targets differ in the case of correlated events. Since the exercise is based on simulated data, it also serves to illustrate how survival data with correlated events can be generated for simulation purposes. It is assumed that there are three events of interest and that the respective event times (denoted by E_1, E_2, and E_3) follow a Weibull distribution each. The correlation structure between the event times is modeled via a Gaussian copula approach (see below). The censoring time (denoted by C) is assumed to follow an exponential distribution. Scale and shape parameters of the distributions are specified as follows:

$$E_1 \sim \text{Weibull}(\text{shape} = 0.5,\ \text{scale} = \exp(\eta_1)) , \tag{8.8}$$

$$E_2 \sim \text{Weibull}(\text{shape} = 1,\ \text{scale} = \exp(\eta_2)) , \tag{8.9}$$

$$E_3 \sim \text{Weibull}(\text{shape} = 2,\ \text{scale} = \exp(\eta_3)) , \tag{8.10}$$

$$C \sim \text{Exp}\left(\lambda = \frac{2}{3}\Big(\Gamma(3) + \Gamma(2) + \Gamma(1.5)\Big)\right) , \tag{8.11}$$

where $\eta_e := (X_1, X_2, X_3)^\top \beta_{E_e}$, $e = 1, 2, 3$, are linear predictors based on three covariates and event-specific vectors of coefficients β_{E_e}. $\Gamma()$ refers to the gamma function.

Regarding the covariates X_1, X_2, X_3 and the coefficient vectors $\beta_{E_1}, \beta_{E_2}, \beta_{E_3}$, the following specifications are made:

$$X_1 \sim \text{Bin}(n = 2,\ \pi = 0.5)\,, \tag{8.12}$$

$$X_2 \sim \text{Gamma}(\text{shape} = 1,\ \text{scale} = 1)\,, \tag{8.13}$$

$$X_3 \sim \text{N}(\mu = 0,\ \sigma^2 = 1)\,, \tag{8.14}$$

$$\beta_{E_1} = (-0.5,\ 1,\ 0.5)\,, \tag{8.15}$$

$$\beta_{E_2} = (1,\ -1,\ 1)\,, \tag{8.16}$$

$$\beta_{E_3} = (-0.5,\ -0.5,\ 2)\,. \tag{8.17}$$

Regarding the correlation structure between the event times, three different correlation matrices are considered. We specify each of the matrices via Kendall's τ rank correlation coefficients:

$$\text{RespCorr}_1 = \begin{bmatrix} 1 & 0 & 0 \\ 0 & 1 & 0 \\ 0 & 0 & 1 \end{bmatrix},\ \text{RespCorr}_2 = \begin{bmatrix} 1 & 0.1 & 0.2 \\ 0.1 & 1 & 0.3 \\ 0.2 & 0.3 & 1 \end{bmatrix},\ \text{RespCorr}_3 = \begin{bmatrix} 1 & 0.3 & 0.4 \\ 0.3 & 1 & 0.5 \\ 0.4 & 0.5 & 1 \end{bmatrix}.$$

The idea of Gaussian copula modeling is to first draw vectors of correlated normally distributed random numbers. Since the population version of Kendall's τ is related to the population version of the Bravais–Pearson correlation coefficient ρ by the equation $\rho = \sin(\tau\frac{\pi}{2})$ (Kruskal 1958), the values of ρ can be used to specify the correlation structure of the normally distributed random variables. In the next step, the normally distributed random numbers are converted into uniformly distributed random numbers via the standard normal cumulative distribution function. Finally, Weibull distributed random numbers are generated by re-transforming the uniformly distributed random numbers via the quantile functions (i.e., the inverse cumulative distribution functions) of the Weibull distributions specified above. Since Kendall's τ is invariant under monotone transformations, the correlation structures specified above do not only apply to the normally distributed random numbers in the first step but also to the Weibull distributed random numbers generated in the last step.

The correlation structure between the three covariates is specified as follows:

$$\text{CovariateCorr} = \begin{bmatrix} 1 & -0.25 & 0 \\ -0.25 & 1 & 0.25 \\ 0 & 0.25 & 1 \end{bmatrix}.$$

1. Specify 100 random seeds and save them to make the results of the simulation study reproducible.

2. Repeat the following steps 100 times for each of the three correlation matrices ($\rightarrow$ 3×100 Monte Carlo samples):

   (a) Express the correlation matrix of the covariates in terms of Bravais–Pearson correlation coefficients. (Hint: Use the function *tauToPearson* or the simulation function for competing risk models *simCompRisk* in the R package *discSurv*.)
   (b) Generate the covariate values via the Gaussian copula approach:

      i. First draw $n = 1000$ random vectors of length 3 each from a multivariate normal distribution with expectation $\mu = (0, 0, 0)$ and the Bravais–Pearson correlation matrix calculated in (a).
      ii. Use the univariate standard normal distribution function to convert the random numbers into sets of uniformly distributed data.
      iii. Insert the uniformly distributed random numbers into the quantile functions of X_1, X_2, X_3.

   (c) In the next step generate the values of the event times E_1, E_2, E_3 via the Gaussian copula approach:

      i. Express the correlation matrix of the event times in terms of Bravais–Pearson correlation coefficients.
      ii. Draw $n = 1000$ random vectors of length 3 each from a multivariate normal distribution with expectation $\mu = (0, 0, 0)$ and the correlation matrix calculated in (i).
      iii. Use the univariate standard normal distribution function to convert the random numbers into sets of uniformly distributed data.
      iv. Use the covariate values generated in (b) and the coefficients β_{E_e} to calculate the linear predictors. Insert the uniformly distributed random numbers into the quantile functions of E_1, E_2, E_3.

   (d) Simulate the censoring process by independently drawing random numbers from the exponential distribution specified above.
   (e) Calculate the observed event times and censoring indicators (assuming right censoring).

3. Discretize all simulated event times using the grid $g = \left\{\frac{i-1}{20}; i = 1, \ldots, 100\right\}$. (Hint: Use the R function *contToDisc*.)
4. Generate sets of augmented binary data from the discretized random numbers.
5. Use the R package *VGAM* to estimate multinomial logistic competing risks models with constant baseline hazards.
6. For each of the three events fit a discrete single spell survival model with logistic link function.
7. For each correlation matrix calculate the squared deviations between the true survival functions and the estimated survival functions.
8. For each correlation matrix average the results across the observations and Monte Carlo samples.
9. Display and interpret the results by comparing the squared deviations from competing risks and single spell models.

Chapter 9
Frailty Models and Heterogeneity

In regression modeling one tries to include all relevant variables. But in empirical studies typically only a limited number of potentially influential variables are observed and one has to suspect that part of the heterogeneity in the population remains unobserved. In particular in survival modeling unobserved heterogeneity, when ignored, may cause severe artifacts.

A simple example illustrates the potential effects. Let the population be partitioned into M subpopulations, where in each subpopulation the hazard rate is constant over time. Thus, in the jth subpopulation the hazard rate is $\lambda_j(t) = \lambda_j$. One easily derives that for a randomly sampled individual the population hazard is given by

$$\lambda(t) = \frac{\sum_{j=1}^{M} \lambda_j(t)\tilde{S}_j(t)p(j)}{\sum_{j=1}^{M} \tilde{S}_j(t)p(j)},$$

where $\tilde{S}_j(t) = P_j(T \geq t)$ is the survival function and $p(j)$ the probability of sampling an individual from the jth subpopulation (Exercise 9.1). Although the hazard rates in subpopulations are constant, the hazard function $\lambda(t)$ varies over time unless $\lambda_1 = \cdots = \lambda_M$. Figure 9.1 shows this effect for two subpopulations with $\lambda_1 = 0.2, \lambda_2 = 0.6$ and $p(1) = p(2) = 0.5$. It is seen that the discrete hazard in the mixture population decreases over time. Thus, if heterogeneity is ignored one observes a time-dependent hazard function although the individual hazards are constant over time.

This chapter presents various approaches to account for unobserved heterogeneity in discrete time-to-event models. We start with the *discrete hazard frailty model*, which incorporates random intercept terms to account for subject-specific variations caused by unobserved covariate information (Sects. 9.1 and 9.2). In Sect. 9.3 discrete hazard frailty models are extended to the case where covariate effects are allowed

G. Tutz, M. Schmid, *Modeling Discrete Time-to-Event Data*,
Springer Series in Statistics, DOI 10.1007/978-3-319-28158-2_9

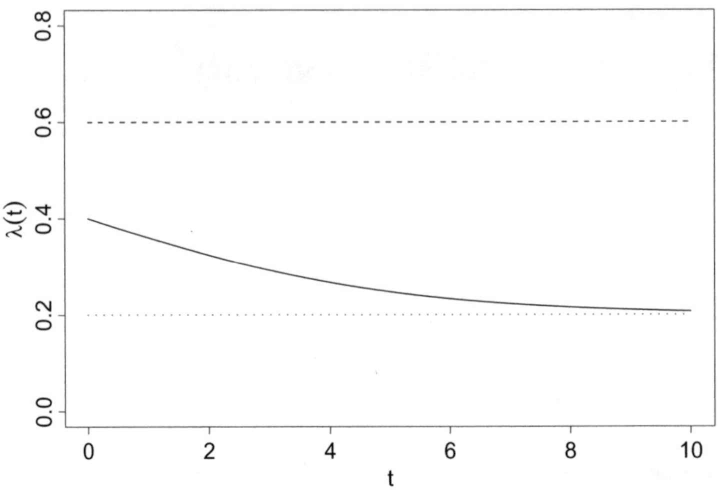

Fig. 9.1 Time-varying hazard resulting from a mixture of two subpopulations with time-constant hazard functions. The *solid line* shows the overall hazard function $\lambda(t)$ whereas the *dashed lines* refer to the time-constant hazards ($\lambda_1 = 0.2$, $\lambda_2 = 0.4$) of the subpopulations

to be smooth and nonlinear. The model class that is considered are *discrete additive hazard frailty models*. Because model misspecification is a critical issue in random effects models, Sect. 9.4 presents an efficient strategy to variable selection in discrete hazard frailty models. Alternative approaches to incorporate unobserved heterogeneity in discrete time-to-event models are presented in Sects. 9.5 and 9.6, which deal with penalized fixed-effects and finite mixture modeling, respectively. The final section of this chapter extends the basic discrete hazard frailty model to sequential models in item response theory (Sect. 9.7).

9.1 Discrete Hazard Frailty Model

Frailty models aim at the explicit modeling of the heterogeneity in a population. They allow for individual effects in the model, frequently in the form of so-called random effects.

9.1.1 Individual and Population Level Hazard

When modeling heterogeneity it is essential to distinguish between the hazard on the individual level and the hazard observed in the population. To illustrate the difference we use the mixture model considered by Aalen (1988). He considers the example where the probability of an event on the individual level is the same at all time points (within given time intervals) but may vary in the population. It can be seen as a demographic model for fecundability: A couple who wants to have a child has in each interval the same probability of succeeding, but the probabilities vary strongly over couples. Let the probability for one couple at each time point be given by λ. Thus, one assumes on the individual level of the couple a constant hazard function $\lambda(t) = \lambda$. For the probability of being successful at time t one obtains the geometric distribution with possible outcomes $\{1, 2, \dots\}$

$$P(T = t \,|\, \lambda) = \lambda\,(1 - \lambda)^{t-1}.$$

If one assumes for the distribution of λ a beta distribution with density $f(\lambda) = [\Gamma(\alpha + \beta)/(\Gamma(\alpha)\Gamma(\beta))]\ \lambda^{\alpha-1}(1 - \lambda)^{\beta-1}$, $\alpha, \beta > 0$, one obtains for the marginal distribution of T

$$P(T = t) = \int_0^1 P(T = t \,|\, \lambda) f(\lambda) d\lambda = \frac{B(\alpha + 1, \beta + k - 1)}{B(\alpha, \beta)},$$

where $B(\alpha, \beta) = \Gamma(\alpha)\Gamma(\beta)/\Gamma(\alpha + \beta)$. This distribution is a special case of the beta negative binomial distribution. For the *marginal hazard function* one obtains

$$\lambda_m(t) = P(T = t \,|\, T \geq t) = \frac{\alpha}{\alpha + \beta + t - 1}.$$

Thus for a couple *drawn at random from the population* the probability that an event occurs at time t given it has not occurred before is determined by $\lambda_m(t)$.

While one has a constant hazard, $\lambda(t) = \lambda$, on the *individual level*, the hazard on the *population level* is a decreasing function of t determined by the parameters α and β. What one observes are in fact realizations of T on the population level, not on the individual level. Therefore the (estimated) hazard function refers to the marginal hazard rate, not to the individual hazard rate which is not observed. It should be noted that even if the model for the marginal hazard fits the data well, this does not mean that the model on the individual level holds. This is because similar population models can be derived from quite different individual level models. Aalen (1988) demonstrated that the mixture model defined previously can be used to fit a data set referring to incidence rates of conception per months. But from this result one can hardly infer that the hazard is constant over time for single couples. Nevertheless, individual level models are a tool to derive models that may hold on the population level. In the following we will discuss various strategies to model individual effects.

9.1.2 Basic Frailty Model Including Covariates

The basic random effects model assumes that the hazard given covariates depends on the sum of the linear predictor $\boldsymbol{x}_i^T\boldsymbol{\gamma}$ and a subject-specific random effect b_i:

$$\lambda(t\,|\,\boldsymbol{x}_i, b_i) = h(b_i + \gamma_{0t} + \boldsymbol{x}_i^T\boldsymbol{\gamma}), \tag{9.1}$$

where b_i follows a mixing distribution with density $f(\cdot)$. A common distribution often used in random effects models is the normal distribution, i.e., $b_i \sim N(0, \sigma^2)$.

In the random effects model (9.1) it is assumed that each individual has its own hazard function. Individuals with large b_i live under higher risk and tend to live shorter; if b_i is small, the mean survival time is higher than for a randomly chosen individual. Therefore the distribution of the b_i's reflects the "frailty" in the population. It is implicitly assumed that the individual effects b_i are measured on the same scale as the linear predictor and remain constant over time. Thus the increase or decrease of the risk also holds over time. It should be noted that the model considered in the preceding section can be seen as the special case where $h(\cdot)$ is the identity function, $\gamma_{0t} = 0$, $\boldsymbol{\gamma}^T = (0, \ldots, 0)$, and the random effects b_i are drawn from a beta distribution.

The effects of the modeled heterogeneity are most easily seen in the clog-log and Gumbel models. The grouped Cox model (i.e., the clog-log model) uses the response function $h(\eta) = 1 - \exp(-\exp(\eta))$, and one obtains for the survival function of the ith individual

$$S(t\,|\,\boldsymbol{x}_i, b_i) = P(T > t\,|\,\boldsymbol{x}_i, b_i) = S(t\,|\,\boldsymbol{x}_i, b_i = 0)^{\exp(b_i)}$$

(Exercise 9.2). Therefore the survival function of an individual with random effect b_i is obtained as a power function of the survival function of the "reference" individual with $b_i = 0$. Figure 9.2 illustrates the modification of the reference survival function by individual effects. It is seen that the hazard rates show distinct variation over individuals. For the Gumbel model (log-log model) with response function $h(\eta) = \exp(-\exp(-\eta))$ one obtains a similar relation for the hazard function, i.e.,

$$\lambda(t\,|\,\boldsymbol{x}_i, b_i) = \lambda(t\,|\,\boldsymbol{x}_i, b_i = 0)^{\exp(b_i)}.$$

Typically there is no closed form for the corresponding marginal hazard function. Scheike and Jensen (1997) used the clog-log model and, for convenience, assumed that $\exp(b_i)$ is gamma distributed with mean 1 and variance ν. Then the marginal hazard has the form

$$\lambda(t|\boldsymbol{x}_i) = 1 - \left(\frac{1 - \nu \log S(t-1|\boldsymbol{x}_i)}{1 - \nu \log S(t|\boldsymbol{x}_i)}\right)^{1/\nu},$$

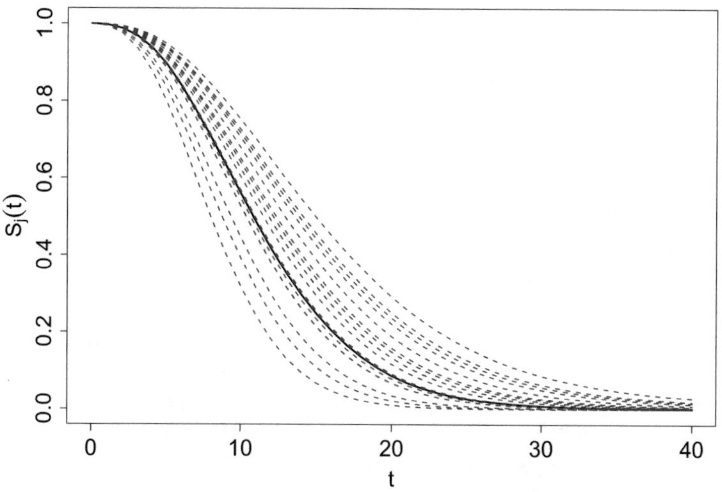

Fig. 9.2 Survival functions for individuals with varying random effects for the grouped proportional hazards model. The *bold line* refers to the survival function of the reference individual with $b_i = 0$

where $S(t|\boldsymbol{x}_i)$ is the marginal survival function of the clog-log model. However, in general, no closed form is available.

In the following we consider the general form with censoring, where δ_i denotes the censoring indicator. The unconditional probability of observing (t_i, δ_i) is given by

$$P(t_i, \delta_i|\boldsymbol{x}_i) = \int P(t_i, \delta_i|\boldsymbol{x}_i, b_i) f(b_i)\, db_i$$

and therefore by

$$P(t_i, \delta_i|\boldsymbol{x}_i) = c_i \int P(T_i = t_i\,|\,\boldsymbol{x}_i, b_i)^{\delta_i} P(T_i > t_i\,|\,\boldsymbol{x}_i, b_i)^{1-\delta_i} f(b_i)\, db_i,$$

where again it is assumed that censoring occurs at the end of the interval and that $c_i = P(C_i \geq t_i)^{\delta_i} P(C_i = t_i)^{1-\delta_i}$ does not depend on the parameters.

As shown in Chap. 3, the model can also be represented by binary observations as

$$P(t_i, \delta_i|\boldsymbol{x}_i) = c_i \int \prod_{s=1}^{t_i} \lambda(s|\boldsymbol{x}_i, b_i)^{y_{is}} (1 - \lambda(s|\boldsymbol{x}_i, b_i))^{1-y_{is}} f(b_i)\, db_i, \tag{9.2}$$

where $(y_{i1}, \ldots, y_{it_i}) = (0, \ldots, 0, 1)$ if $\delta_i = 1$ and $(y_{i1}, \ldots, y_{i,t_i}) = (0, \ldots, 0)$ if $\delta_i = 0$. The representation with binary dummy variables that code transitions helps to embed the estimation procedures into the framework of binary mixed-effects models. It also helps to investigate which estimates are to be expected if heterogeneity is ignored.

It is well known that in binary random effects models, where one assumes $P(y_{is}|\boldsymbol{x}_i, b_i) = h(b_i + \boldsymbol{x}_i^T \boldsymbol{\gamma})$ with random effect b_i, the marginal effects (i.e., the effects of covariates on the marginal probability $P(y_{is}|\boldsymbol{x}_i)$) are attenuated, see, for example, Tutz (2012, Sect. 14.2). In the case where the mixing distribution is normal, i.e. $b_i \sim N(0, \sigma^2)$, and the response function $h(.)$ is the standard normal distribution function, one can derive that the effect on the marginal probabilities is captured by the weights $\boldsymbol{\gamma}/(1 + \sigma^2)$. This implies that ignoring heterogeneity may lead to estimated effects that are much smaller than the effects on the individual level. In particular for large σ^2 the shrinkage can be rather strong. Similar effects occur for alternative link functions such as the logistic or clog-log link: If heterogeneity is ignored, the estimated parameter vectors tend to be too small. From the binary representation in (9.2) it is seen that this effect carries over from binary response models to discrete survival models: In the same way as in random effects models—and in contrast to marginal (or population-averaged) models—the effect of covariates is measured on the *individual level*. One models the effect of covariates given the random effect for single individuals, hence the conditioning $\lambda(t|\boldsymbol{x}_i, b_i)$ which explicitly contains b_i. In nonlinear models, which are commonly used in discrete survival, one should keep in mind that the effects on the individual level differ from the effects on the population level.

9.1.3 Modeling with Frailties

The inclusion of a frailty term accounts for the hidden heterogeneity in the population and should therefore be closer to the underlying data-generating process. On the other hand, adding a frailty term may also lead to model misspecification. While the link function and the predictor (which is assumed to be linear) may already be misspecified in models without subject-specific effects, now there is an additional risk of misspecifying the frailty term. Moreover, identifiability issues can arise.

The problem of misspecified distributions has been studied in particular for continuous survival models. The basic case of misspecified heterogeneity is *ignored heterogeneity*. Heckman and Singer (1984a) showed analytically that ignoring heterogeneity yields biased estimated hazards towards *negative duration dependence*, where negative duration dependence means that the hazard function decreases as in Fig. 9.1. The occurring estimation bias implies that the derivatives of the marginal hazard function tend to be smaller than the integrated derivatives of the individual hazards. The intuition is that individuals who have a high unobserved risk are more likely to have shorter survival times, such that the individuals who survive are those with small unobserved risk. These individuals form the selected sample that is considered at later time points. As a consequence the observed marginal hazard decreases. Nicoletti and Rondinelli (2010) referred to this phenomenon as "weeding out" or "sorting effect." Similar effects have been described by Lancaster (1992) and Van den Berg (2001). It has also been shown that parameter estimates can be inconsistent when heterogeneity is ignored. For example, Lancaster (1985) considered a Weibull distribution model without censoring and showed that parameter estimates are asymptotically biased towards zero. For an overview on results for continuous time models, see Van den Berg (2001).

Also the *wrong form of the mixing distribution* may have an impact on the estimation results. Heckman and Singer (1984a) investigated a Weibull duration model and found that estimates and inference varied greatly depending on the functional form selected for the mixing distribution. Since estimates also suffer from misspecified hazard functions, the findings of Heckman and Singer (1984a) could alternatively have been caused by a lack-of-fit of the Weibull model. But similar results were also reported by Baker and Melino (2000). To overcome this problem, Heckman and Singer (1984b) developed a consistent nonparametric maximum likelihood estimator for the mixing distribution. Further references, which also cover problems of identifiability, are found in Van den Berg (2001). An analytic result that supports the choice of the gamma distribution as mixing distribution in models for continuous time has been derived by Abbring and Van den Berg (2007). Specifically, the authors showed that for a large class of continuous hazard models the distribution of heterogeneity among survivors converges to a gamma distribution.

Misspecified mixing distributions in discrete survival have been considered in particular by Baker and Melino (2000) and Nicoletti and Rondinelli (2010). Baker and Melino (2000) examined the behavior of the nonparametric maximum likelihood estimator that assumes a discrete distribution for the mixing distribution and found severe bias concerning the estimation of duration dependence and unobserved heterogeneity. Nicoletti and Rondinelli (2010) found in their simulations that ignoring heterogeneity yields attenuated covariate coefficients for time-invariant covariates. In contrast, for covariates that vary over time attenuation was very weak. Also the effects did not strongly depend on the mixing distribution for the subject-specific effects. For negative duration dependence the baseline hazard was overestimated, which reflects the sorting effect. If the true duration dependence was positive, i.e. if the hazard increased, ignoring heterogeneity nevertheless tended to show spurious negative duration dependence. Misspecification of the mixing distribution was investigated by the authors by using a logistic model with discrete, gamma, and normal mixtures and by fitting a normal mixture model. It turned out that when fitting a logistic model estimates of covariate coefficients did not strongly depend on the type of heterogeneity that generated the data. When a probit and a clog-log model was fitted, results were similar to situations where one used appropriately rescaled parameter estimates. The reason is that parameters cannot be taken by their face value when comparing models like the logit model and the probit model because the response function is based on different means and/or variances (see Sect. 3.2.2). The required normalization seems to have been neglected by Baker and Melino (2000), with the consequence that they found severe biases. The results of Nicoletti and Rondinelli (2010) seem encouraging if one stays within the range of models considered by them. Nevertheless, in particular for single-spell duration, some caution seems warranted because of the effects found in continuous-time models. Van den Berg (2001) notes that "with single-spell data, minor changes in the assumed parametric specification of the mixed proportional hazards model, while leading to a similar overall fit, may produce very different parameter estimates. Also, very different models may generate similar data. Estimation results from single-spell data are sensitive to misspecification of the functional forms associated with the model determinants, and this sensitivity is stronger than usual in econometrics".

9.2 Estimation of Frailty Models

Let us consider the more general frailty model

$$\lambda(t\,|\,\boldsymbol{x}_{it}, \boldsymbol{b}_i) = h(\boldsymbol{w}_{it}^T\boldsymbol{\gamma} + \boldsymbol{z}_{it}^T\boldsymbol{b}_i) \tag{9.3}$$

with explanatory variables $\boldsymbol{w}_{it}, z_{it}$ and random effect vector $\boldsymbol{b}_i$. In Model (9.3) different sets of predictor variables are collected in the vectors $\boldsymbol{w}_{it}$ and z_{it}, referring to the fixed and random effects $\boldsymbol{\gamma}$ and $\boldsymbol{b}_i$, respectively. For example, the simple frailty model with random intercepts uses $\boldsymbol{w}_{it}^T = (0, \ldots, 1, \ldots, 0, \boldsymbol{x}_i^T)$ with parameters $\boldsymbol{\beta}^T = (\gamma_{01}, \ldots, \gamma_{0q}, \boldsymbol{\gamma}^T)$ and $z_{it} = 1$.

A common assumption for random effects is a normal distribution, $\boldsymbol{b}_i \sim N(\boldsymbol{0}, \boldsymbol{Q})$. The representation of the probability $P(t_i, \delta_i|\boldsymbol{x}_i, b_i)$ (see Eq. (9.2)) as a binary response model allows to use estimation concepts for generalized linear mixed models (GLMMs) for the binary responses $y_{i1}, \ldots, y_{it_i}$.

To estimate $\boldsymbol{\beta}$ and $\boldsymbol{Q}$ simultaneously, one can apply numerical integration techniques that solve the integral in (9.2). This can be done by maximizing the marginal log-likelihood

$$l(\boldsymbol{\beta}, \boldsymbol{Q}) = \sum_{i=1}^{n} \log\left(\int \prod_{s=1}^{t_i} \lambda(s|\boldsymbol{x}_i)^{y_{is}}(1 - \lambda(s|\boldsymbol{x}_i))^{1-y_{is}}\right) d\boldsymbol{b}_i\,. \tag{9.4}$$

Two popular approaches for numerical integration are the *Gauss–Hermite quadrature* and *Monte Carlo approximations*. The Gauss–Hermite procedure approximates the integral in (9.4) by using a pre-specified number of quadrature points. With increasing number of quadrature points the exactness of the approximation increases. Typically, for simple models with random intercept estimates are stable if 8–15 quadrature points are used. Gauss–Hermite has been considered by Hinde (1982), and Anderson and Aitkin (1985). A procedure that may reduce the number of quadrature points is the adaptive Gauss–Hermite quadrature (Liu and Pierce 1994; Pinheiro and Bates 1995; Hartzel et al. 2001).

An alternative way to estimate random effects models is *penalized quasi-likelihood estimation*, which uses the Laplace approximation (Breslow and Clayton 1993). It estimates the parameters $\boldsymbol{\beta}$ and $\boldsymbol{b}_1, \ldots, \boldsymbol{b}_n$ (collected together in the vector $\boldsymbol{\delta}$) and the mixture parameters separately, for example by using restricted maximum likelihood (REML) estimators. The essential tool is the approximation of the log-likelihood by the penalized log-likelihood

$$l_p(\boldsymbol{\delta}) = \sum_{i=1}^{n} \log\left(f(\boldsymbol{y}_i|\boldsymbol{b}_i, \boldsymbol{\beta})\right) - \frac{1}{2}\sum_{i=1}^{n} \boldsymbol{b}_i^T \boldsymbol{Q}^{-1}\boldsymbol{b}_i, \tag{9.5}$$

where $f(\boldsymbol{y}_i|\boldsymbol{b}_i, \boldsymbol{\beta}) = \prod_{s=1}^{t_i} \lambda(s|\boldsymbol{x}_i)^{y_{is}}(1-\lambda(s|\boldsymbol{x}_i))^{1-y_{is}}$. A disadvantage of this method is its tendency to underestimate the variance of the mixing distribution and therefore the true values of the random effects (see, for example, McCulloch 1997). However, this effect can be ameliorated by using the modifications proposed by Breslow and Lin (1995) and Lin and Breslow (1996). The penalized quasi-likelihood method can be justified in various ways (see also Schall 1991; Wolfinger 1994; McCulloch and Searle 2001).

Example 9.1 Family Dynamics
We illustrate parameter estimation in frailty models on data from Germany's current panel analysis of intimate relationships and family dynamics ("Pairfam") described in Example 1.5.

For each of the anchor women from the two age groups [24; 30] and [34; 40] it is known whether she has given birth to her first child within the year between two interview dates. Altogether, 137 events were observed. We consider years as the unit in our discrete survival model and start with 24 years, which is the age of the youngest woman in the sample. We consider a discrete hazard model with the covariates "relstat," "siblings," "yeduc," and "leisure" (see Table 9.1) and investigate whether the inclusion of a frailty term accounts for the heterogeneity among the anchor women. For the categorical variable "relstat" the reference level "cohabitation" was chosen. Table 9.2 contains the coefficient estimates that were obtained from fitting a continuation ratio model with person-specific random intercepts to the Pairfam data. For numerical optimization of the log-likelihood we applied the Gauss–Hermite quadrature with 20 quadrature points (first column of Table 9.2) using the R package *glmmML* (Broström 2013) and a penalized likelihood-based method implemented in the R package *mgcv* (*bs* = *"re"* option of the *gam* function, second column of Table 9.2). The last column of Table 9.2 contains the effects obtained from an ordinary continuation ratio model without frailty term. As expected, the coefficient estimates of the frailty models were larger in absolute size than the respective estimates of the discrete hazard model. The variance estimates for

Table 9.1 Pairfam data. Description of the variables that were used in Example 9.1

Variable	Description
age	Age of the anchor woman (in years)
relstat	status of relationship (categorical with three levels: "living apart together", "cohabitation", "married")
yeduc	Years of education ($\in [8, 20]$) of the anchor woman
siblings	number of siblings of the anchor woman
leisure	(approx.) yearly leisure time of the anchor woman (in hours) spent for the following five major categories: (1) bar/cafe/restaurant (2) sports; (3) internet/TV; (4) meet friends; (5) discotheque

Table 9.2 Pairfam data. The first two columns contain the coefficient estimates obtained from a frailty model (continuation ratio model with person-specific random intercepts) that was fitted to the complete data via Laplace approximation (first column) and via the penalized likelihood-based approach (second column). Column 3 contains the respective estimates of an ordinary continuation ration model without frailty term (lat = living apart together)

	Coefficient estimates		
	Frailty, Gauss–Hermite	Frailty, pen. log-lik	Discrete hazard
relstat = lat	−1.0741	−1.0460	−1.0440
relstat = married	0.9412	0.9001	0.8809
Siblings	0.0227	0.0215	0.0201
yeduc	−0.0462	−0.0445	−0.0440
Leisure	−0.0002	−0.0002	−0.0002
$\hat{\sigma}^2$	0.5563^2	0.5060^2	–

the random intercept were 0.5563^2 (Gauss–Hermite) and 0.5060^2 (penalized likelihood), implying a notable (yet non-significant, $p = 0.346$ and $p = 0.246$, respectively) heterogeneity among the anchor women. Note that, as expected, the variance estimate was smaller for the penalized likelihood-based fitting routine than for the Gauss–Hermite routine. □

Cautionary Remark Although the inclusion of frailty terms into discrete hazard models is a well-founded strategy to account for unobserved heterogeneity, maximization of the resulting log-likelihood function is often numerically problematic. This is especially true if there are many time-constant covariates in the model, and also if the baseline hazard is allowed to vary freely (e.g., if baseline parameters are modeled via dummy variables or splines). In these cases, the inclusion of a subject-specific random effect often results in an almost perfect model fit and hence in numerical problems associated with the various fitting routines. It is therefore recommended to use not only one but several of the routines for model fitting and to carefully inspect and compare the results. If convergence problems occur, a solution might be to restrict the functional form of the baseline hazard (for example, to a lower-order polynomial or to a time-constant function). Alternatively, adding a ridge penalty to the baseline parameters might increase the numerical stability of the fitting process.

9.3 Extensions to Additive Models Including Frailty

In the model considered previously the linear predictor had the form $\eta_{it} = \boldsymbol{x}_{it}^T\boldsymbol{\gamma} + \boldsymbol{z}_{it}^T\boldsymbol{b}_i$. For a more general additive predictor let the explanatory variables be given by $(\boldsymbol{x}_{it}, \boldsymbol{u}_{it}, \boldsymbol{z}_{it})$, $i = 1, \ldots, n$, $t = 1, \ldots, t_i$, with $\boldsymbol{x}_{it}^T = (x_{it1}, \ldots, x_{itp})$, $\boldsymbol{u}_{it}^T = (u_{it1}, \ldots, u_{itm})$, $\boldsymbol{z}_{it}^T = (z_{it1}, \ldots, z_{its})$ denoting vectors of covariates, which may vary across individuals and observations. The components in $\boldsymbol{u}_{it}$ are assumed to represent continuous variables which do not necessarily have a linear effect within the model. The corresponding additive semiparametric mixed model has the predictor

$$\eta_{it} = \boldsymbol{x}_{it}^T \boldsymbol{\gamma} + \sum_{j=1}^{m} \alpha_{(j)}(u_{itj}) + \boldsymbol{z}_{it}^T \boldsymbol{b}_i,$$

whereas in the generalized linear mixed model $\boldsymbol{b}_i$ is a random vector for which it is typically assumed that $\boldsymbol{b}_i \sim N(\boldsymbol{0}, \boldsymbol{Q})$. The new terms in the predictor are the unknown functions $\alpha_{(1)}(\cdot), \dots, \alpha_{(m)}(\cdot)$. Let these functions be expanded in basis functions, that is,

$$\alpha_{(j)}(u) = \sum_{s=1}^{m_j} \alpha_s^{(j)} \phi_s^{(j)}(u) = \boldsymbol{\alpha}_j^T \boldsymbol{\phi}_j(u),$$

where $\phi_1^{(j)}(u), \dots, \phi_{m_j}^{(j)}(u)$ are appropriately chosen basis functions for variable u_{itj}. Defining $\boldsymbol{\alpha}^T := (\boldsymbol{\alpha}_1^T, \dots, \boldsymbol{\alpha}_m^T)$ and $\boldsymbol{\phi}_{it}^T := (\boldsymbol{\phi}_1(u_{it1})^T, \dots, \boldsymbol{\phi}_m(u_{itm})^T)$, one obtains the linear predictor

$$\eta_{it} = \boldsymbol{x}_{it}^T \boldsymbol{\gamma} + \boldsymbol{\phi}_{it}^T \boldsymbol{\alpha} + \boldsymbol{z}_{it}^T \boldsymbol{b}_i,$$

which contains fixed parameters $\boldsymbol{\gamma}, \boldsymbol{\alpha}$ and random effects $\boldsymbol{b}_i$.

If the number of basis functions is small one, can use maximum likelihood (ML) estimation. More flexibility is obtained by using a large number of basis functions and by applying penalized ML estimation. Let the parameters $\boldsymbol{\gamma}, \boldsymbol{\alpha}$ and $\boldsymbol{b}_1, \dots, \boldsymbol{b}_n$ be collected in $\boldsymbol{\delta}$. Then for given covariance matrix one maximizes

$$l_p(\boldsymbol{\delta}) = \sum_{i=1}^{n} \log\,(f(\boldsymbol{y}_i|\boldsymbol{b}_i)) - \frac{1}{2} \sum_{i=1}^{n} \boldsymbol{b}_i^T \boldsymbol{Q}^{-1} \boldsymbol{b}_i - \sum_{j=1}^{m} \lambda_j \sum_{s} (\alpha_{j,s+1} - \alpha_{j,s})^2,$$

which, when compared to (9.5), contains an additional penalty that smooths the differences between adjacent weights on basis functions $\alpha_{j,s}, \alpha_{j,s+1}$. The parameters $\lambda_1, \dots, \lambda_m$ are tuning parameters that have to be chosen appropriately.

The tuning parameters can be chosen by applying cross-validation or by maximizing some information criterion, but alternative ways are available as well. In particular, models with additive terms and random effects can be embedded into the mixed modeling representation of smoothing where tuning parameters are estimated as variance components (see, e.g., Lin and Zhang 1999; Ruppert et al. 2003; Wood 2006). The versatile R package *mgcv* contains the function *gamm* that allows one to fit generalized additive mixed models. Alternatively, the *bs* = *"re"* option for smooth fits can be used in combination with the *gam* function of *mgcv*.

Example 9.2 Time Between Cohabitation and First Childbirth
In Example 5.2 we analyzed the data collected for the Second National Survey on Fertility and showed that the predictor variable "age at the beginning of cohabitation" (measured in years) had a significant nonlinear effect on the time between the beginning of cohabitation and first childbirth (see Fig. 5.5). We now investigate whether there is unobserved heterogeneity in the data. To this purpose, we extended the additive model of Example 5.2 to include a subject-specific random intercept term. This was done by using the *gam* function in R package *mgcv* with option *bs* = *"re"*. The coefficient estimates for the covariates with linear effects are shown in Table 9.3. As expected, most of the estimates of the model with random intercept are larger in absolute value than the respective estimates of the original additive model in Example 5.2. The estimated standard deviation of the random effect was $\hat{\sigma} = 0.536$ ($p < 0.001$), suggesting that there is considerable unobserved heterogeneity in the data.

The estimated smooth effect of the covariate "age at the beginning of cohabitation" is shown in Fig. 9.3. It has a very similar structure as the corresponding effect of the original additive model without random intercept (cf. Fig. 5.5). Especially in the time range between 18 and 32 years (which contains the majority of the data values) the two estimates are almost identical. □

Table 9.3 Years between cohabitation to first childbirth. The table shows the estimates of the linear effects and the respective estimated standard deviations that were obtained from fitting a logistic discrete hazard model to the data (edu = educational attainment, area = geographic area, cohort = cohort of birth, occ = occupational status, sibl = number of siblings). In contrast to Table 5.1, an additional random intercept term was added to the model in order to account for unobserved heterogeneity. Columns 4 and 5 contain the estimates of the original additive model without random intercept (see also Table 5.1)

	Model with random intercept		Model without random intercept	
Covariate	Parameter estimate	Est. std. error	Parameter estimate	Est. std. error
edu First stage basic (ref. category)				
edu Second stage basic	0.0153	0.0825	0.0351	0.0747
edu Upper secondary	−0.2423	0.0876	−0.1960	0.0793
edu Degree	−0.3261	0.1218	−0.2787	0.1099
cohort 1946–1950 (ref. category)				
cohort 1951–1955	−0.0477	0.0850	−0.0421	0.0767
cohort 1956–1960	−0.2949	0.0871	−0.2638	0.0787
cohort 1961–1965	−0.3532	0.0877	−0.3112	0.0794
cohort 1966–1975	−0.8268	0.0992	−0.7682	0.0908
area North (ref. category)				
area Center	0.3245	0.0692	0.2957	0.0626
area South	0.7407	0.0684	0.6784	0.0621
occ Worker (ref. category)				
occ Non-worker	0.2499	0.0584	0.2272	0.0529
sibl	0.0634	0.0296	0.0548	0.0269

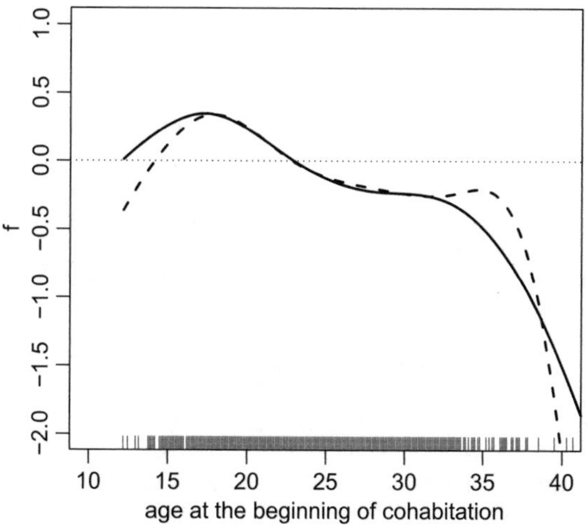

Fig. 9.3 Time between cohabitation and first childbirth. The *solid line* shows the P-spline estimate of the effect of the covariate "age at beginning of cohabitation" that was obtained from a proportional continuation ratio model with random intercept term. The *dashed line* corresponds to the respective estimate that was obtained from the original model without random intercept (cf. Fig. 5.5). Both effect estimates were centered such that the fitted values had zero mean

9.4 Variable Selection in Frailty Models

Selection of predictors in frailty models is a sensible topic because the number of included variables is typically linked to the frailty. The mixing distribution in a frailty model accounts for the heterogeneity that is left after the available predictors have been included. Therefore the mixing distribution will be more important if one has few predictors in the model. For example, if the mixing distribution is specified as a normal distribution, $N(0, \sigma^2)$, the variance σ^2 tends to be larger for few predictors and smaller if many predictors are in the model. Nevertheless one wants only predictors in the model that are relevant. If the full model that contains all available predictors can be fitted, it is possible to use test statistics from random effects models to exclude irrelevant terms. If there are too many predictors available to be included in one model, and if variable selection is of importance, one can use forward/backward selection strategies. An alternative approach, which is considered in the following and which is much more stable than forward/backward selection, is to use regularization methods to extract the relevant features. In our approach an additional penalty is included in the penalized log-likelihood (9.5), yielding

$$l_{\text{lasso}}(\boldsymbol{\delta}) = l_p(\boldsymbol{\delta}) - \sum_{j=1}^{p} |\gamma_j|. \tag{9.6}$$

The additional lasso-type penalty $\sum_j |\gamma_j|$ enforces variable selection. For details on the maximization of $l_{\text{lasso}}(\boldsymbol{\delta})$ see Groll and Tutz (2014).

Example 9.3 Family Dynamics
We illustrate variable selection in frailty models using the Pairfam data. Again we consider years as the unit of discrete survival and start with 24 years. The baseline hazard, which corresponds to the effect of age, is now included in the form of a penalized smooth effect. Similarly, we allow for a nonlinear effect of the male partner's age by including polynomial terms of this covariate. For the categorical variables *relstat*, *casprim*, and *pcasprim* the reference levels "living apart together" and "non-working," respectively, are chosen. It should be noted that all variables can vary over time and are included as time-varying.

A frailty model with smooth effect of age and with variable selection based on the lasso penalty was performed by use of the package *glmmLasso* (Groll 2015). To demonstrate the difference between AIC and BIC with regard to model sparsity, we used both criteria to select the tuning parameter λ. The results of the estimation of fixed effects and the amount of heterogeneity (measured by the estimated variance $\hat{\sigma}^2$) are given in Table 9.4. Figure 9.4 shows the estimated smooth effect(s) of age. As expected, the estimated functions are nonlinear and bell-shaped with a maximum in the mid-twenties (gray line: AIC, black line: BIC). For more details on the modeling of family dynamics with frailty models, see Groll and Tutz (2016). □

Table 9.4 Estimated effects and standard deviation of the random intercept for the pairfam data (standard errors in brackets)

	glmmLasso (AIC)	*glmmLasso* (BIC)
Intercept	−2.41 (0.14)	−2.32 (0.13)
Page	0.39 (4.96)	.
Page^2	−0.25 (10.19)	.
Page^3	−0.48 (5.57)	.
Page^4	.	.
hlt7	.	.
sat6	.	.
$\text{reldur}^{(1/3)}$	−0.06 (0.14)	.
Siblings	.	.
relstat:cohab	0.53 (0.18)	0.52 (0.15)
relstat:married	0.87 (0.17)	0.80 (0.14)
yeduc	.	.
pyeduc	−0.24 (0.11)	.
$\text{Leisure}^{(1/3)}$	−0.07 (0.11)	.
Leisure.partner	0.06 (0.12)	.
Holiday	0.26 (0.10)	.
casprim:educ	0.38 (0.50)	.
casprim:fulltime	0.72 (0.54)	.
casprim:parttime	0.37 (0.28)	.
casprim:other	0.19 (0.22)	.
pcasprim:educ	−0.31 (0.18)	.
pcasprim:fulltime	−0.32 (0.18)	.
pcasprim:parttime	−0.23 (0.15)	.
pcasprim:other	−0.07 (0.12)	.
$\hat{\sigma}$	1.13	1.04

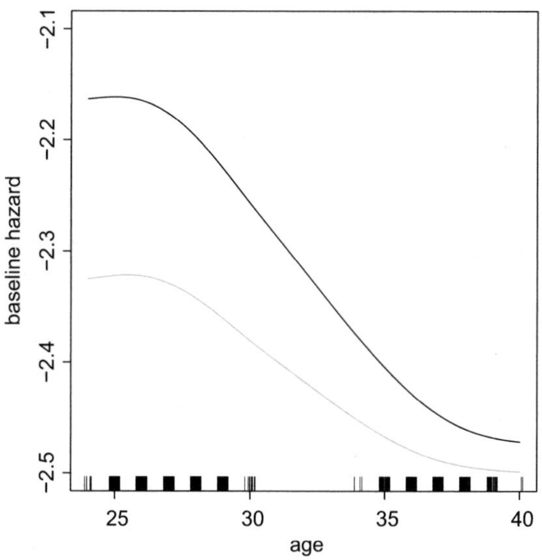

Fig. 9.4 Estimates of the smoothed hazard as a function of age for the pairfam data (*gray line*: tuning parameter selection based on AIC, *black line*: tuning parameter selection based on BIC)

9.5 Fixed-Effects Model

Random effects models are a strong tool to model heterogeneity. However, the approach has also drawbacks. One is that inference on the unknown distributional assumption is hard to obtain and that the choice of the distribution may affect the results, see, for example, Heagerty and Kurland (2001), Agresti et al. (2004), and McCulloch and Neuhaus (2011).

Alternatives to random effects models that do not assume a specific distribution are *fixed effects models*. In discrete survival one assumes that the hazard function has the form

$$\lambda(t|\boldsymbol{x}_i, b_i) = h(\beta_i + \gamma_{0t} + \boldsymbol{x}_i^T \boldsymbol{\gamma}), \tag{9.7}$$

where β_i is not a random but a *fixed parameter* that characterizes the ith individual. Fixed effects models have several advantages. One advantage of the models is that they do not assume that the individual parameters are independent of the explanatory variables. In particular in econometrics this is regarded as a disadvantage of the random effects model that also concerns the frailty model (9.1). The reason is that correlation between random effects and covariates leads to biases and inconsistent estimators, as demonstrated, for example, by Neuhaus and McCulloch (2006). In special cases, it is possible to use alternative estimators that are consistent. For example, conditional likelihood methods (Diggle et al. 2002) can be used for canonical links. Also mixed-effects models that decompose covariates into between- and within-cluster components (Neuhaus and McCulloch 2006) can alleviate the problem of biased estimates in specific settings.

Of course, model (9.7) contains many parameters, and estimation tends to fail if there are many individuals relative to the sample size. However, if one assumes that the variation of the individual parameters is not overly large (so that many of the individuals share parameters of similar size), estimates can be nevertheless obtained. One strategy to fit the model is to use penalized likelihood methods. In particular one can include into the log-likelihood the penalty

$$\lambda J := \lambda \sum_{r<s} (\beta_r - \beta_s)^2, \tag{9.8}$$

where λ is a tuning parameter. For large λ most of the parameters β_r will be estimated as being very similar. Fusion penalty terms of this form have been considered, for example, by Bondell and Reich (2009), Gertheiss and Tutz (2010), and Tutz and Oelker (2015).

Example 9.4 Breast Cancer
We reconsider the breast cancer data of Example 7.2 and investigate the effects of the clinical covariates "tumor diameter," "number of affected lymph nodes," "estrogen receptor status," "tumor grade," and "age at diagnosis" on survival. Survival times were grouped into three-month intervals (with the last interval being defined as "$>$ 15 months").

In Example 7.2, the lasso method selected 15 of the 70 genes in addition to the clinical covariates. This result indicated that the gene expression data contain relevant information about the individual survival times. Therefore, if one wants to evaluate the effect of clinical covariates when no genetic information is available, it seems warranted to include patient-specific effects to allow for the heterogeneity in the gene expression levels.

Table 9.5 contains the coefficient estimates that were obtained from fitting a continuation ratio model with patient-specific intercepts to the breast cancer data (column 1 of Table 9.5). All intercept terms were regarded as fixed, but their variation was restricted by the quadratic difference penalty in (9.8). The *gam* function in the R package *mgcv* was used for parameter estimation. For comparison, we also fitted a mixed-effects model with patient-specific random intercepts and time-constant baseline hazard to the data, as well as an ordinary continuation ratio model without frailty term (columns 2 and 3 of Table 9.5, respectively). As expected, most of the coefficient estimates of the fixed-effects model were larger in absolute size than the respective estimates of the discrete hazard model. This indicates that there was indeed unobserved heterogeneity among the patients in the clinical model, which could be due to differences in the individual gene expression levels. Estimates of the fixed-effects model differ from the respective estimates of the random-effects model, which could be the result of correlations between the covariates and the patient-specific effects. □

Table 9.5 Breast cancer data. The first column contains the coefficient estimates obtained from a continuation ratio model with fixed patient-specific intercept terms (clinical model, $n = 144$). The variation of the intercepts was restricted by the penalty in (9.8) (*paraPen* argument in the *gam* function of R package *mgcv*). The second column contains the estimates of a frailty model with patient-specific random effects and time-constant baseline hazard (fitted via the Gauss–Hermite quadrature with 20 quadrature points, as implemented in the R package *glmmML*, Broström 2013). Column 3 contains the effect estimates obtained from an ordinary continuation ratio model without frailty term. Abbreviations of covariates are as follows: Diam = tumor diameter, N = number of affected lymph nodes, ER = estrogen receptor status

	Coefficient estimates		
	Frailty, fixed effects	Frailty, random effects	Discrete hazard
Diam $\leq$ 2 cm	0.0000	0.0000	0.0000
Diam > 2 cm	0.4027	0.5375	0.3979
$N \geq 4$	0.0000	0.0000	0.0000
$N1-3$	−0.9086	−1.1704	−0.8485
ER negative	0.0000	0.0000	0.0000
ER positive	−0.5145	−0.6543	−0.5266
Grade poorly diff.	0.0000	0.0000	0.0000
Grade intermediate	−0.7248	−0.9839	−0.6066
Grade well diff.	−0.2132	−0.2574	−0.2533
Age	−0.0726	−0.0988	−0.0585

9.6 Finite Mixture Models

An alternative way to account for heterogeneity in the population is to assume that the observed survival time is determined by a finite mixture of hazard functions. The basic idea of finite mixtures is that the population is not homogeneous. It is divided into subpopulations that have their own hazard functions. Each of these functions involves parameters that are specific for the respective subpopulation. What is observed is a mixture of the subpopulations since the membership to the subpopulation itself is not observable. Mixtures occur in particular when relevant categorical predictors are omitted or not observable. Then the subpopulations are considered as *latent classes*.

Let the mixture consist of m latent classes, with the hazard function in the jth subpopulation or class determined by

$$\lambda_j(t\,|\,\boldsymbol{x}, \gamma_{otj}, \boldsymbol{\gamma}_j) = h(\gamma_{otj} + \boldsymbol{x}^T\boldsymbol{\gamma}_j).$$

The probability of discrete survival in the mixture is given by

$$P(T = t\,|\,\boldsymbol{x}) = \sum_{j=1}^{m} \pi_j P_j(T = t\,|\,\boldsymbol{x}),$$

where $P_j(T = t\,|\,\boldsymbol{x})$ denotes the probability of survival in the jth component of the mixture and the unknown weights $\pi_j, j = 1, \dots, m$, denote the proportions in the population, which fulfill $\sum_{j=1}^{m} \pi_j = 1, \pi_j > 0, j = 1, \dots, m$. A similar mixture holds for the survival function $S(t|\boldsymbol{x}) = P(T > t\,|\,\boldsymbol{x})$. One obtains

$$S(t|\boldsymbol{x}) = \sum_{j=1}^{m} \pi_j S_j(t|\boldsymbol{x}), \tag{9.9}$$

where $S_j(t|\boldsymbol{x})$ is the survival time in the jth component. The *population level hazard* can be directly derived from $\lambda(t|\boldsymbol{x}) = P(T = t\,|\,\boldsymbol{x})/P(T \geq t\,|\,\boldsymbol{x})$.

The simplest mixture, which in the following is mostly used for illustration, contains just two components. With

$$S(t|\boldsymbol{x}) = \pi\, S_1(t\,|\,\boldsymbol{x}, \gamma_{ot1}, \boldsymbol{\gamma}_1) + (1 - \pi)\, S_2(t\,|\,\boldsymbol{x}, \gamma_{ot2}, \boldsymbol{\gamma}_2) \tag{9.10}$$

it involves two populations, where π and $1 - \pi$ represent the probabilities of occurrence in the whole population. It can be used to build structured models that assume specific hazard functions in subpopulations. For example, in survival analysis there is the concept of *long-time survivors*, that means, a subpopulation that does not seem to be at risk. The corresponding mixture model assumes for the subpopulation of individuals at risk

$$\lambda_1(t\,|\,\boldsymbol{x}, \gamma_{0t}, \boldsymbol{\gamma}_1) = h(\gamma_{0t} + \boldsymbol{x}^T\boldsymbol{\gamma})$$

and for the long-time survivors

$$\lambda_2(t|\boldsymbol{x}) = 0,$$

yielding the survival function

$$S(t|\boldsymbol{x}) = \pi S_1(t|\boldsymbol{x}) + (1 - \pi),$$

where $S_1(t|\boldsymbol{x})$ is the survival function for the population at risk. The model has been used by Muthén and Masyn (2005) in discrete survival modeling. In continuous survival modeling the concept of long-time survivors has been used much earlier, for an overview see Maller and Zhou (1996). Similar models have been considered under the name *cure model*. Cure models were originally developed for use in biomedical applications because for some severe diseases patients often react differently on a treatment. In particular, a class of patients who respond to treatment and are free of symptoms may be considered cured (and therefore as long-time survivors). An example of modeling unobserved heterogeneity by finite mixtures of hazard functions is given in Exercise 9.4.

9.6.1 Extensions to Covariate-Dependent Mixture Probabilities

The mixture model can be extended by letting the mixture be determined by covariates. Then the membership to class j is determined by a multinomial response model, typically the multinomial logit model. The probability π_j is replaced in this model by

$$P(C=j\,|\,z) = \frac{\exp(\alpha_{0j} + z^T \boldsymbol{\alpha}_j)}{1+\sum_{s=1}^{m-1}\exp(\alpha_{0s} + z^T \boldsymbol{\alpha}_s)}, \qquad j = 1, \ldots, m-1,$$

where C denotes the class membership and z is a vector of covariates.

Some care should be taken when interpreting the effects of covariates on the mixture probability and the hazard: The parameters $\boldsymbol{\alpha}_j$ determine the membership to the latent class. Consequently they show which variables are important to distinguish the classes. The corresponding intercept parameters α_{0j} indicate the basic probabilities of class membership. If no covariates are included in the multinomial model, the latter just represent a reparameterization of the probabilities π_j. The parameters $\boldsymbol{\gamma}_j$, which are used in the hazard functions, have a quite different meaning; they determine the effect of covariates on the hazard function, that is, they specify if the hazard function increases or decreases as covariates change their values. The corresponding intercept parameters γ_{otj} specify the functional form of the baseline hazard as a function of time within class j.

One extreme case is the model (9.10), which contains no effects of covariates on the mixture probabilities. The other extreme is the model without covariate effects on the hazard function, where the hazard within classes is given by

$$\lambda_j(t|\gamma_{0j}) = h(\gamma_{0j}).$$

This model assumes that the hazards are constant within classes, that is, the hazard is low or high but does not vary over time. The effect of covariates captured in $\boldsymbol{\alpha}_j$ has a simple interpretation, because it indicates which variables are responsible for being in a high or low risk group. The model imposes a very simple structure but profits from good and simple interpretation.

It is tempting to allow the vector z to be identical to the vector $\boldsymbol{x}$, which determines the effect of covariates on the hazard within classes. But then it is hard to separate the effects because both relate to the risk. For example, let us consider the simple case of two classes with constant baseline hazards, $\lambda_j(t\,|\,\boldsymbol{x}, \gamma_{0j}, \boldsymbol{\gamma}_j) = h(\gamma_{0j} + \boldsymbol{x}^T \boldsymbol{\gamma}_j)$. Then the survival function has the form

$$\begin{aligned} S(t|\boldsymbol{x}, z) = {} & \frac{\exp(\alpha_0 + z^T \boldsymbol{\alpha})}{1+\exp(\alpha_0 + z^T \boldsymbol{\alpha}))} \left(1 - h(\gamma_{01} + \boldsymbol{x}^T \boldsymbol{\gamma}_1)\right)^{t-1} \\ & + \frac{1}{1+\exp(\alpha_0 + z^T \boldsymbol{\alpha}))} \left(1 - h(\gamma_{02} + \boldsymbol{x}^T \boldsymbol{\gamma}_2)\right)^{t-1}. \end{aligned}$$

Let $\boldsymbol{x}$ and $\boldsymbol{z}$ represent the same variable, for example, gender in 0–1 coding (with 1 indicating males) and let us focus on the first class. If $\boldsymbol{\alpha}$ is positive, men tend to be in the first class. If class 1 is the group with higher risk ($\gamma_{01} > \gamma_{02}$), males show an increased risk. But there is an additional effect: If γ_1 is positive, the risk in class 1 is higher for males than for females; if γ_1 is negative, the risk for males is smaller than for females. In particular for negative γ_1 the effect within the class contradicts the effect in the membership probability. Thus interpretation has to refer to both parameters and, moreover, also has to include the intercepts, which makes interpretation tricky.

It therefore seems advisable to include a covariate either in the membership probability or in the hazard function, but not in both terms. But there still remains a choice to be made. One strategy is to either include all variables in the hazard and to let membership probabilities be fixed, or to let the membership probability be determined by covariates and assume constant hazards.

A simple model for m classes with constant hazard within classes and effects on membership only is

$$S(t|\boldsymbol{x}) = \sum_{j=1}^{m} P(C = j\,|\,\boldsymbol{z})\,(1 - h(\gamma_{0j}))^{t-1},$$

which in the classes assumes a geometrical distribution of survival time. Even then a multinomial logistic model for the membership parameters $P(C = j\,|\,\boldsymbol{z})$ can yield a complicated interpretation of parameters. This can be simplified by ordering the hazards such that $\gamma_{01} < \ldots < \gamma_{0m}$ (that is, class 1 has the lowest and class m the highest hazard) and by assuming for $P(C = j\,|\,\boldsymbol{z})$ an ordered model, for example, the cumulative hazard model $P(C \le j\,|\,\boldsymbol{z}) = F(\alpha_{0j} + \boldsymbol{z}^T\boldsymbol{\alpha})$. Then the effect of a predictor is contained in just one parameter (see Agresti 2009). A weaker model is obtained by assuming time-varying hazard functions $h(\gamma_{0tj})$ with the restriction $\gamma_{0t1} < \ldots < \gamma_{0tm}$ for all t, such that classes are still ordered.

9.6.2 The Cure Model

The *long-time survivor* or *cure* model has the advantage that the mixture components are more structured. By assuming for the long-time survivors the hazard $\lambda_2(t|\boldsymbol{x}) = 0$ and for individuals in the susceptible group who will eventually experience the event of interest if followed for long enough the survival function $S_1(t|\boldsymbol{x})$, one obtains the model

$$S(t|\boldsymbol{x}) = P(C = 1\,|\,\boldsymbol{z})\,S_1(t|\boldsymbol{x}) + (1 - P(C = 1\,|\,\boldsymbol{z})),$$

with $S_1(t|\boldsymbol{x})$ determined by

$$S_1(t|\boldsymbol{x}) = \prod_{s=1}^{t-1}(1 - h(\gamma_{0t} + \boldsymbol{x}^T\boldsymbol{\gamma})).$$

If $\boldsymbol{\gamma}$ is set to zero, the hazard depends on time but covariates determine the mixture probabilities only.

As in all mixture models the problem of identifiability arises, that is, one has to ensure that the parameters that describe a specific response structure are unique. The cure model is certainly not identifiable if both the survival function $S_1(t|\boldsymbol{x})$ and the mixture probabilities $P(C = 1 \mid z)$ do not depend on covariates. The same holds if the survival function does not depend on $\boldsymbol{x}$ and a single binary covariate determines the mixture probabilities. This results from the identifiability conditions given by Li et al. (2001). The authors investigate cure models for continuous time and show in particular that even for continuous time the cure model is not identified in these cases. However, they also show that models are identified if the mixture probability is specified as a logistic function depending on continuous covariate z although the survival function does not depend on covariates. They also investigate the case of proportional hazards models with covariates and show that the corresponding cure model is identifiable under weak conditions.

Example 9.5 SEER Breast Cancer Data

For illustration of the cure model we analyze data from the Surveillance, Epidemiology, and End Results (SEER) Program of the U.S. National Cancer Institute (http://seer.cancer.gov), which collects information on cancer incidences and survival from various locations throughout the USA. Here we consider a random sample of 6000 breast cancer patients that entered the SEER database between 1997 and 2011 (SEER 1973–2011 Research Data, version of November 2013). Discrete-time survival models are used to analyze the time from diagnosis to death from breast cancer in years. Tables 9.6 and 9.7 show the variables that are used for statistical analysis. Categorical predictor variables include tumor grade (I–III), estrogen receptor (ER) status, progesterone receptor (PR) status, and number of positive lymph nodes. In addition, we consider the age at diagnosis and the tumor size; for details on the predictors, we refer to the SEER text data file description at http://seer.cancer.gov. We included all variables from Tables 9.6 and 9.7 in the mixture component and in the hazard function. For the hazards of the subpopulation at risk we use the continuation ratio model. The mixture is determined by a logit model. Table 9.8 shows the coefficient estimates together with bootstrap-based standard errors and confidence intervals (500 bootstrap samples). It is seen that most of the covariates show no significant effect on the probability of being cured. Exceptions are the size of the tumor and age. With the exception of the PR status all variables seem to have an effect on survival in the subpopulation at risk that cannot be neglected.

The estimated survival functions for different grades and different tumor sizes are presented in Fig. 9.5. Tumor sizes for which survival functions are shown correspond to the minimum value and the quartiles in the sample; the respective values are 1, 10, 16, 21, and 25 mm. The curves refer

Table 9.6 Quantitative explanatory variables for the SEER breast cancer data

	Minimum	First Quantile	Median	Mean	Third Quantile	Maximum
Age (years)	18	48	56	56	64	75
Tumor size (mm)	1	10	16	21	25	230

Table 9.7 Categorical explanatory variables for the SEER breast cancer data

	Category	Observations	Proportions (%)
Grade	I	1300	22
	II	2569	43
	III	2131	35
No of pos. nodes	0	4018	67
	1–3	1416	24
	> 3	566	9
ER status	Positive	4760	79
	Negative	1240	21
PR status	Positive	4241	71
	Negative	1759	29

Table 9.8 Estimates for the cure model (SEER breast cancer data). The upper part of the table contains the mixture coefficients, in the lower part the coefficients for the hazard of the population at risk are given

	Estimates	BS SE	0.95 confidence intervals
Constant	−0.0224	0.0176	[−0.0694, −0.0062]
Age	−0.0170	0.0067	[−0.0274, −0.0008]
Grade II	0.0115	0.0189	[−0.0120, 0.0612]
Grade III	−0.0297	0.0330	[−0.1198, 0.0009]
No of pos. nodes 1–3	−0.0650	0.0550	[−0.1895, −0.0011]
No of pos. nodes > 3	0.0714	0.0736	[0.0013, 0.2534]
Size of tumor	0.0202	0.0120	[0.0033, 0.0520]
ER status (negative)	−0.0544	0.0509	[−0.1712, −0.0007]
PR status (negative)	−0.0349	0.0400	[−0.1401, 0.0007]
Age	0.0180	0.0066	[0.0053, 0.0298]
Grade II	0.6330	0.2205	[0.2498, 1.0708]
Grade III	1.4980	0.2345	[1.0622, 1.9777]
No of pos. nodes 1–3	1.0990	0.1960	[0.7034, 1.4466]
No of pos. nodes > 3	1.8510	0.1929	[1.4018, 2.1525]
Size of tumor	0.0060	0.0046	[−0.0006, 0.0165]
ER status (negative)	0.7430	0.1911	[0.3719, 1.1253]
PR status (negative)	0.1210	0.1724	[−0.2165, 0.4438]

to a person who is 56 years old with ER and PR status positive and no positive nodes. In the plot for different grades the tumor size was 16 mm, whereas in the plot for different tumor sizes the grade was one. The left column shows the mixture survival functions, that is, the survival functions in the total population. The right column shows the survival functions for the population at risk. It is seen that the grade has a strong effect on survival, yielding quite different functions for both populations. Since the effect of grade on the mixture is weak and the probability of being at risk is large for the person under consideration the curves found for different grades are very similar in the total population and the population at risk. In contrast, the curves for different tumor sizes found for the mixture are quite different from the curves found for the population at risk. While the curves for tumor sizes between 1 and 25 are not so far apart in the population at risk, the curves differ much more strongly in the mixture population, because in these curves the strong effect of the tumor size on the mixture is included and the other variables have almost no effect on the mixture. □

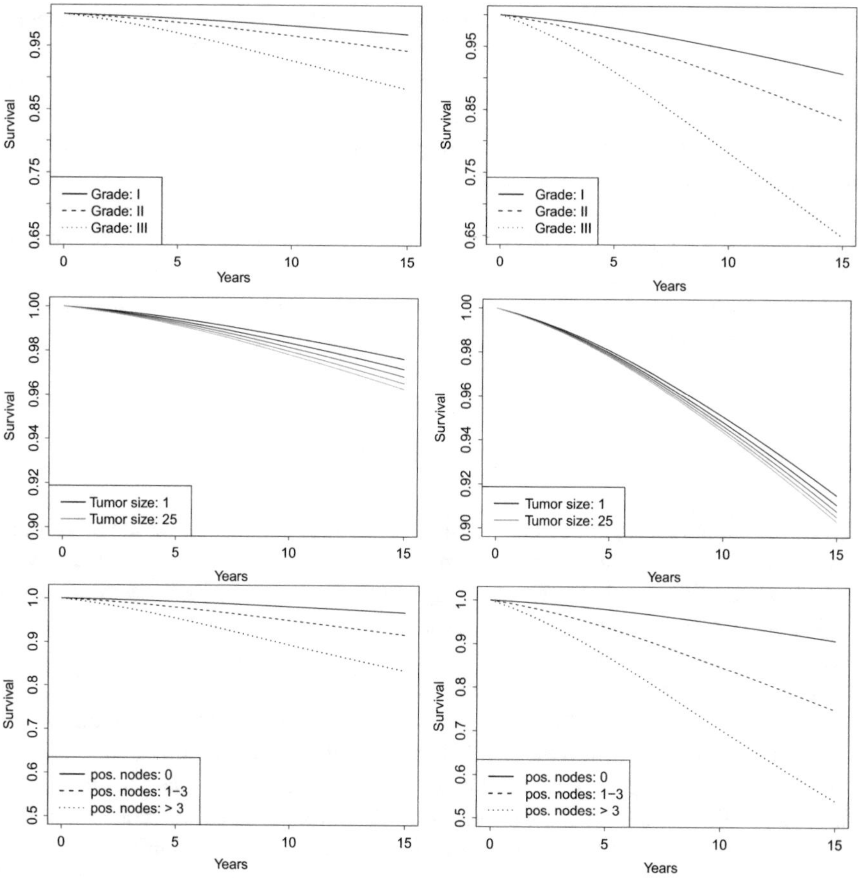

Fig. 9.5 Survival functions for the SEER breast cancer data. The *left column* shows the mixture survival functions, whereas the *right column* shows the survival functions for the population at risk

9.6.3 *Estimation for Finite Mixtures*

The basic assumption in finite mixtures is that the probability of survival time is given by $P(T = t \mid \boldsymbol{x}) = \sum_{j=1}^{m} \pi_j P_j(T = t \mid \boldsymbol{x})$. For random censoring one derives in a similar way as in Sect. 3.4 that the probability of an observation (t_i, δ_i) is given by

$$P(t_i, \delta_i|\boldsymbol{x}_i) = c_i \left(\sum_{j=1}^{m} \pi_j P_j(T_i = t_i \mid \boldsymbol{x}_i) \right)^{\delta_i} \left(\sum_{j=1}^{m} \pi_j S_j(t_i|\boldsymbol{x}_i) \right)^{1-\delta_i}$$

$$= c_i \sum_{j=1}^{m} \pi_j \prod_{s=1}^{t_i} \lambda_j(s|\boldsymbol{x}_i)^{y_{is}} (1 - \lambda_j(s|\boldsymbol{x}_i))^{1-y_{is}}, \tag{9.11}$$

where $c_i = P(C_i \geq t_i)^{\delta_i} P(C_i = t_i)^{1-\delta_i}$ is assumed not to depend on the parameters and $(y_{i1}, \ldots, y_{it_i}) = (0, \ldots, 0, 1)$ if $\delta_i = 1$, $(y_{i1}, \ldots, y_{i,t_i}) = (0, \ldots, 0)$ if $\delta_i = 0$ (Exercise 9.3). The last formula contains a product of binomial terms for the probability of failure within classes. Although this representation does not help to construct a likelihood for a binary mixture model, it can be used to construct an EM algorithm for binary response models.

Mixture models in general were considered, for example, by Follmann and Lambert (1989) and Aitkin (1999). An extensive treatment was given by Frühwirth-Schnatter (2006). Follmann and Lambert (1989) investigated the identifiability of finite mixtures of binomial regression models and gave sufficient identifiability conditions for mixing at the binary and the binomial level.

9.7 Sequential Models in Item Response Theory

In regression modeling as considered in the previous sections one wants to account for heterogeneity but one is not interested in the individual effects themselves. This is quite different in psychometrics, where the individual effects contain the ability of persons. If one wants to evaluate a specific ability of a person as, for example, the mathematical intelligence, a standard procedure is to let persons try to solve a number of items, which are assumed to be sensitive to the latent trait under investigation. From the obtained answers one wants to learn about the ability of a person. Probabilistic latent trait theory for item responses assumes that the probability of solving an item is determined by the ability of the person and the difficulty of the item. For simple binary items the classical model is the Rasch model (Rasch 1961), which assumes that person i solves item j with probability

$$P(R_{ij} = 1) = \frac{\exp(\beta_i - \delta_j)}{1 + \exp(\beta_i - \delta_j)},$$

where $R_{ij} \in \{0, 1\}$ indicates that item j is not solved or solved, β_i is the ability of the person, and δ_j is the difficulty of the item. The Rasch model is simply a logistic regression model with latent traits as regressors. With $F(\eta) = \exp(\eta)/(1 + \exp(\eta))$ denoting the logistic distribution function, it has the form $P(R_{ij} = 1) = F(\beta_i - \delta_j)$. Therefore, if the ability of the person, β_i, equals the difficulty of the item, δ_j, the probability of solving the item is 0.5. If the ability is larger than the difficulty of the item, the probability of solving the item is accordingly increased.

In modern item response theory one frequently uses items that have more than two categories. Then one has graded response categories that reflect to what extent an item is solved. More specifically, the responses for item j take values from $\{1, \ldots k_j\}$, where larger numbers indicate better performance. Of particular interest are items that contain several steps and are solved in a consecutive manner. A simple example is the item $\sqrt{9.0/0.3 - 5}$ considered by Masters (1982). Three levels of performance may be distinguished: No sub-problem solved (level 1), $9.0/0.3 = 30$ solved (level 2), $30 - 5 = 25$ solved (level 3), $\sqrt{25} = 5$ (level 4). The important feature is that each level in a solution to the problem can be reached only if the previous level is reached. A latent trait model for items of this sort is the *sequential model* or *step model* (Tutz 1990; Verhelst et al. 1997), which has the form

$$P(R_{ij} > r \,|\, R_{ij} \geq r) = F(\beta_i - \delta_{jr}), \quad r = 0, \ldots, k_j - 1,$$

where $F(.)$ again is the logistic distribution function, β_i is the ability of the person, and δ_{jr} is the difficulty of solving the rth step. Thus the transition to the next level of performance is determined by a binary Rasch model determined by the ability of the person and the corresponding difficulty of the transition. The alternative form of the model,

$$P(R_{ij} = r \,|\, R_{ij} \geq r) = F(\delta_{jr} - \beta_i), \quad r = 0, \ldots, k_j - 1, \tag{9.12}$$

shows that it is a discrete hazard model with latent traits as regressors. The response in categories (denoted here by the random variable R_{ij}) can also be a genuine time, for example, if several trials at solving an item are allowed in answer-until-correct test administrations. For an application to this type of data, see Culpepper (2014).

The sequential item response model (9.12) has the structure of a discrete survival model but with repeated measurements since each person tries to solve all the items. Estimation refers to the item difficulties as well as the person abilities. An estimation strategy that uses the Rasch model structure for single transitions was given by Tutz (1990). Better estimates for the item difficulties, which are of special importance when designing an assessment test, were given by De Boeck et al. (2011). Effectively they use a random effects representation of the model. Overviews on item response theory were given by van der Linden and Hambleton (1997) and De Boeck and Wilson (2004). Further details on the sequential model are found in Rijmen et al. (2003) and Tutz (2015).

9.8 Literature and Further Reading

Frailty in Duration Models Vaupel et al. (1979), Elbers and Ridder (1982), and Vaupel and Yashin (1985) were among the first to investigate the impact of heterogeneity on survival. Heckman and Singer (1984a) and Heckman and Singer (1984b) investigated it from an econometric perspective. Hougaard (1984) and Aalen (1988) considered survival from a biostatistical perspective.

Random Effects in Discrete Survival Ham and Rea Jr. (1987) used a logistic model to analyze unemployment duration. Vermunt (1996) proposed a modified loglinear model, which is restricted to categorical covariates. Land et al. (2001) extended the model to allow for metric covariates. McDonald and Rosina (2001) investigated a mixture model for recurrent event times and gave an analysis of Hutterite birth histories. Nicoletti and Rondinelli (2010) focused on the misspecification of discrete survival models; applications are found in Hedeker et al. (2000). Xue and Brookmeyer (1997) avoided the specification of the frailty distribution by using a marginal model where regression coefficients have population-averaged interpretation. Frederiksen et al. (2007) considered the modeling of group level heterogeneity.

Cure Models Proportional hazards cure models were proposed by Kuk and Chen (1992) and Sy and Taylor (2000). Yu et al. (2004) considered cure models for grouped survival times with fixed distributions of survival time. A cure model for interval-censored data was considered by Kim and Jhun (2008).

Discrete Mixture Models A standard reference for finite mixture models is the book by McLachlan and Peel (2000), which also contains a chapter on continuous survival mixtures. Almansa et al. (2014) considered a factor mixture model for multivariate survival data. Muthén and Masyn (2005) proposed a latent variable approach to mixture models.

9.9 Software

Generalized Linear Mixed Models The function *glmmML* that is contained in the R package *glmmML* allows one to fit GLMs with random intercepts by maximum likelihood estimation with numerical integration via a Gauss–Hermite quadrature. The function *glmer* contained in the package *lme4* offers the adaptive Gauss–Hermite approximation proposed by Liu and Pierce (1994). *glmmML* and *glmer* also allow to use the Laplace approximation. Another function that fits GLMMs by using penalized quasi-likelihood methods is *glmmPQL* from the package *MASS*.

Variable Selection Variable selection for generalized mixed models is implemented in the R package *glmmLasso* (Groll 2015).

Generalized Additive Mixed Models The package *mgcv* contains the function *gamm*, which allows one to fit GLMMs that contain smooth functions. Alternatively, the *bs = "re"* option for smooth fits can be used in combination with the *gam* function of *mgcv*.

Mixture Models The package *flexmix* (Grün and Leisch 2008) provides a flexible tool to estimate discrete mixtures.

9.10 Exercises

9.1 Let the population be partitioned into m subpopulations. Further denote by $\lambda_j(t)$ the hazard rate and by $P_j(T \geq t)$ the survival function in the jth subpopulation. Show that for a randomly sampled individual the hazard rate is given by

$$\lambda(t) = \frac{\sum_{j=1}^{M} \lambda_j(t) P_j(T \geq t)\, p(j)}{\sum_{j=1}^{M} P_j(T \geq t)\, p(j)}.$$

9.2 Show that for the random effects clog-log model

$$\lambda(t|\boldsymbol{x}_i, b_i) = 1 - \exp(-\exp(b_i + \gamma_{0t} + \boldsymbol{x}_i^T \boldsymbol{\gamma}))$$

the survival function is given by

$$S(t|\boldsymbol{x}_i, b_i) = S(t|\boldsymbol{x}_i, b_i = 0)^{\exp(b_i)}.$$

9.3 Show that under the assumption of random censoring the probability of an observation (t_i, δ_i) is given by

$$P(t_i, \delta_i|\boldsymbol{x}_i) = c_i \sum_{j=1}^{m} \prod_{s=1}^{t_i} \lambda_j(t_i|\boldsymbol{x}_i)^{y_{is}} (1 - \lambda_j(t_i|\boldsymbol{x}_i))^{y_{is}}$$

with a term c_i that depends on censoring only and dummy variables y_{is}.

9.4 Reconsider the clinical model for the breast cancer data of Example 9.4. The analysis of these data in Sect. 9.5 suggested considerable heterogeneity among the patients, so that fixed and random effects modeling was appropriate to account for the heterogeneity. The aim of this exercise is to investigate whether unobserved heterogeneity can also be modeled using finite mixtures of hazard functions, as presented in Sect. 9.6.

(a) Fit finite mixture models with varying numbers of components to the breast cancer data. (Hint: Use the *stepFlexmix* function of the R package *flexmix* (Grün and Leisch 2008) for model fitting. Use the *fixed* argument of *stepFlexmix* to guarantee that the estimates of covariate effects do not vary across the components.)
(b) For each of the models calculate Akaike's information criterion (AIC). (Hint: use the *AIC* function in R package *flexmix*.) What is the optimum number of components according to the AIC criterion?
(c) Compare the coefficient estimates of the optimal model to the estimates obtained from random and fixed effects modeling (as presented in Table 9.5). Which of the models performs best according to the AIC criterion?

Chapter 10
Multiple-Spell Analysis

In the previous chapters only single spells of duration have been considered. This is an appropriate modeling strategy in many applications; for example, if in biostatistics the transition to an absorbing state like death is modeled, only single spells matter. But in many areas like economics and the social sciences subjects can experience a sequence of events as time elapses. For instance, subjects can have a first spell of unemployment, then be employed for some time, then have a second spell of employment, etc. Thus a person's history can be divided into spells with transitions between various states.

The term *event history*, which is used in particular in sociology, refers to the modeling of duration and transition between states of interest. For example, Willett and Singer (1995) illustrated their method using longitudinal data on exit from, and re-entry into, the teaching profession. Johnson (2006) modeled the enrolment history of students, which was divided into periods of enrolment and non-enrolment. Hamerle and Tutz (1989) considered breast cancer data with competing risks occurrence of metastases and death.

In the following we briefly consider basic concepts in discrete-time multiple-spell modeling.

10.1 Multiple Spells

Let the duration times for the consecutive spells be denoted by $T_0 = 0 \leq T_1 \leq T_2 \leq \ldots$ and $Y_0, Y_1, Y_2, \ldots$ represent the corresponding state variable with $Y_k \in \{1, \ldots, m\}$. An individual starts at $T_0 = 0$ in state y_0. The first transition occurs at time t_1 to state y_1, which is followed by the next transition to state y_2 at time t_2 (with $t_2 > t_1$), etc. In discrete models it is again assumed that $t \in \{1, 2, \ldots\}$.

G. Tutz, M. Schmid, *Modeling Discrete Time-to-Event Data*,
Springer Series in Statistics, DOI 10.1007/978-3-319-28158-2_10

Let the *cause-specific hazard function* for spell or episode k be defined by

$$\lambda_r^{(k)}(t \mid H_{k-1}, \boldsymbol{x}_k) = P(T_k = t, Y_k = r \mid T_k \geq t, H_{k-1}, \boldsymbol{x}_k),$$

where $\boldsymbol{x}_k$ is a vector of covariates that determines duration in spell k and H_{k-1} contains the history of the process up till t_{k-1}, that is, $H_{k-1} = \{y_0, t_1, y_1, \boldsymbol{x}_1, \ldots, t_{k-1}, y_{k-1}, \boldsymbol{x}_{k-1}\}$. It should be noted that the cause-specific hazard is defined for the kth spell. For $t \leq t_{k-1}$ it is set to zero, that is, $\lambda_r^{(k)}(t|H_{k-1}, \boldsymbol{x}_k) = 0$. Moreover, since measurements are on a discrete scale, for example, in months, it is assumed that at a fixed time point only one transition can occur. As a consequence the hazard rate of the kth spell is informative only for $t_{k-1} + 1, t_{k-1} + 2, \ldots$.

The overall hazard in the kth spell is given by

$$\lambda^{(k)}(t \mid H_{k-1}, \boldsymbol{x}_k) = \sum_{r \neq y_{k-1}} \lambda_r^{(k)}(t \mid H_{k-1}, \boldsymbol{x}_k) = P(T_k = t \mid T_k \geq t, H_{k-1}, \boldsymbol{x}_k).$$

It is the conditional probability of leaving the state y_{k-1} within the kth spell conditional on $T_k \geq t$. Thus, given $T_k \geq t$ the conditional probabilities are

$$\lambda_r^{(k)}(t \mid H_{k-1}, \boldsymbol{x}_k), r \neq y_{k-1}, \;\; 1 - \lambda^{(k)}(t \mid H_{k-1}, \boldsymbol{x}_k),$$

where $1 - \lambda^{(k)}(t \mid H_{k-1}, \boldsymbol{x}_k)$ is the conditional probability that no transition occurs. The corresponding survival function in the kth spell is

$$S^{(k)}(t \mid H_{k-1}, \boldsymbol{x}_k) = P(T_k > t \mid H_{k-1}, \boldsymbol{x}_k) = \prod_{i=t_{k-1}+1}^{t} (1 - \lambda^{(k)}(i \mid H_{k-1}, \boldsymbol{x}_k)).$$

Parametric models for the kth spell have the familiar form

$$\lambda_r^{(k)}(t \mid H_{k-1}, \boldsymbol{x}_k) = h(\gamma_{otr}^{(k)} + \boldsymbol{x}_k^T \boldsymbol{\gamma}_r^{(k)}), \tag{10.1}$$

where for simplicity the history H_{k-1} is included in the predictor $\boldsymbol{x}_k$.

10.1.1 Estimation

Let us first consider the case of uncensored data, with observed data given by $y_{i0}, (t_{ik}, y_{ik}, \boldsymbol{x}_{ik}), i = 1, \ldots, n, k = 1, \ldots, k_i$. The likelihood contribution of the ith observation is

$$L_i = P(T_{k_i} = t_{k_i}, Y_{k_i} = y_{k_i}, \boldsymbol{x}_k, \ldots, T_1 = t_1, Y_1 = y_1, \boldsymbol{x}_1 \mid y_0),$$

where the subscript i is suppressed on the right-hand side. Since duration times are consecutive, the contribution is given by

$$L_i = \prod_{k=1}^{k_i} P(T_k = t_k, Y_k = y_k, \boldsymbol{x}_k \mid H_{k-1}),$$

where $H_{k-1} = \{y_0, t_1, y_1, \boldsymbol{x}_1, \ldots, t_{k-1}, y_{k-1}, \boldsymbol{x}_{k-1}\}$ and $H_0 = y_0$. One obtains

$$L_i = \prod_{k=1}^{k_i} P(T_k = t_k, Y_k = y_k \mid T_k \geq t_k, H_{k-1}, \boldsymbol{x}_k)\; P(T_k \geq t_k \mid H_{k-1}, \boldsymbol{x}_k)\; P(\boldsymbol{x}_k \mid H_{k-1})$$

$$= \prod_{k=1}^{k_i} \lambda_{y_k}^{(k)}(t_k \mid H_{k-1}, \boldsymbol{x}_k) \prod_{s=t_{k-1}+1}^{t_k-1} (1 - \lambda^{(k)}(s \mid H_{k-1}, \boldsymbol{x}_k))\; P(\boldsymbol{x}_k \mid H_{k-1}),$$

where $P(\boldsymbol{x}_k \mid H_{k-1})$ represents the conditional density of the covariate in spell k given the history. If it is not informative, the likelihood contribution is determined by the hazards. If censoring occurs in the last spell, one has

$$L_i = \prod_{k=1}^{k_i} [\lambda_{y_k}^{(k)}(t_k \mid H_{k-1}, \boldsymbol{x}_k)]^{\delta_k} \prod_{s=t_{k-1}+1}^{t_k-1} (1 - \lambda^{(k)}(s \mid H_{k-1}, \boldsymbol{x}_k))\; P(\boldsymbol{x}_k \mid H_{k-1}),$$

where $\delta_k = 1$ (for $k = 1, \ldots, k_i - 1$), $\delta_{k_i} = 1$ if in the last spell failure is observed, and $\delta_{k_i} = 0$ if in the last spell censoring occurs.

In closed form the total likelihood is

$$L = \prod_{i=1}^{n} \prod_{k=1}^{k_i} \prod_{r=1}^{m} [\lambda_{y_k}^{(k)}(t_{ik} \mid H_{k-1}, \boldsymbol{x}_{ik})]^{\delta_{ikr}} \prod_{s=t_{i,k-1}+1}^{t_k-1} (1-\lambda^{(k)}(s \mid H_{k-1}, \boldsymbol{x}_{ik}))\; P(\boldsymbol{x}_k \mid H_{k-1})^{\epsilon_{ik}},$$

where

$$\delta_{ikr} = \begin{cases} 1, & i\text{th individual ends at } t_{ik} \text{ in state } r, \\ 0, & \text{otherwise}, \end{cases}$$

$$\epsilon_{ik} = \begin{cases} 1, & i\text{th individual survives spell } k, \\ 0, & \text{otherwise}. \end{cases}$$

If the parameters are specific for the spell (as in Model (10.1)), the likelihood can be maximized separately for the spells by considering only those individuals who were observed for the specific spell. Similar forms of the likelihood can be derived by assuming that the covariate process $\boldsymbol{x}_{it}, t = 1, 2, \ldots$ is linked to discrete time rather than being fixed within spells. But for time-varying covariates the counting process approach provides a much more general framework, and estimation should be embedded into this framework (see, for example, Fleming and Harrington 2011).

10.2 Multiple Spells as Repeated Measurements

In many applications the objective is less ambitious than described in the previous section. One does not aim at modeling all transitions between various states over time but focusses on one specific recurrent transition. For example, in studies on unemployment duration, one person can be unemployed several times during the time of the study. The main interest is often on the duration of unemployment, whereas the duration of employment serves as a predictor but is not itself modeled. For the ith individual, the corresponding simplified model uses the hazard function

$$\lambda^{(k)}(t \,|\, \boldsymbol{x}_{ik}) = P(T_{ik} = t \,|\, T_{ik} \geq t, \boldsymbol{x}_{ik}),$$

which determines the duration of the kth spell given covariates $\boldsymbol{x}_{ik}$.

Since $T_{i1}, \ldots, T_{ik_i}$ are measurements on the same individual, the model should include a subject-specific effect as in frailty models. The basic model for the hazard of the ith individual in the kth spell is

$$\lambda^{(k)}(t \,|\, \boldsymbol{x}_{ik}, b_i) = P(T_{ik} = t \,|\, T_{ik} \geq t, \boldsymbol{x}_{ik}, b_i) = h(b_i + \gamma_{0t} + \boldsymbol{x}_{ik}^T \boldsymbol{\gamma}), \tag{10.2}$$

where b_i is the individual effect and it is assumed that the spell durations are independent drawings from the common distribution of the frailty. For example, one often assumes $b_i \sim N(0, \sigma^2)$.

Let the data for the survival times $T_{i1}, \ldots, T_{ik_i}$ of the spells be given by $t_{i1}, \ldots, t_{ik_i}, \delta_i$, where $\delta_i = 0$ denotes censoring in the last spell. The kth spell is again represented as a sequence of binary variables $y_{ik1}, \ldots, y_{ikt_{ik}}$, where

$$y_{ikt} = \begin{cases} 1, & i\text{th individual fails at } t \text{ in spell } k \text{ given it reaches } t, \\ 0, & \text{otherwise}. \end{cases}$$

The corresponding marginal log-likelihood is given by

$$l(\boldsymbol{\gamma}, \sigma^2) = \sum_{i=1}^{n} \log \left(\int \prod_{k=1}^{k_i} \prod_{s=1}^{t_i-(1-\delta_{ik})} \lambda(s|\boldsymbol{x}_i)^{y_{iks}} (1 - \lambda(s|\boldsymbol{x}_i))^{1-y_{iks}} db_i \right),$$

where $\delta_{ik} = 1$ for $k = 1, \ldots, k_i - 1$, $\delta_{ik_i} = \delta_i$.

The representation with binary variables implies that the model can be estimated in the same way as a binary mixed-effects model for repeated measurements. The repeated measurements now refer to the separate spells and time points.

Example 10.1 Unemployment Spells

We analyze the duration of unemployment spells using data from the German socio-economic panel. Here we consider the time of unemployment (measured in 1-month intervals) with terminating event "full-time job." This is a typical example of multiple spells, since each person in the socio-economic panel can have several unemployment spells during the study period. For statistical analysis we use a subsample of 1693 persons who live in the German region of North Rhine-Westphalia. For these persons data were collected between January 1990 and December 2011. Altogether, the data comprised 2512 unemployment spells; the overall number of events was 1010. Using a continuation ratio model with subject-specific random effects (*bs* = *"re"* option in the *gam* function of R package *mgcv*), we investigate the effects of the covariates "age" (in years), "gender" (male/female), and "status" (married/married but separated/single/divorced/widowed/husband/wife abroad) on the time to employment at full-time job. In addition to the main effects of the covariates, we include an interaction term between gender and status in the model. The baseline hazard is modeled by a penalized regression spline, as described in Chap. 5.

Coefficient estimates are presented in Table 10.1. Judged by the main effects, men had a higher chance of getting re-employed at full-time job than women. The results presented in Table 10.1

Table 10.1 German socio-economic panel. The table contains the coefficient estimates that were obtained from a multiple-spell continuation ratio model with subject-specific random intercept terms. Estimation was based on data from a subsample of 1693 persons that live in the German region of North Rhine-Westphalia. The response variable was the time to re-employment at full-time job (measured in months)

Variable name	Coef. estimate	Standard dev.	*z* value	*p*-value
Intercept	−2.8262	0.1584	−17.841	<0.0001
Gender female (ref. category)	0.0000			
Gender male	1.1075	0.1083	10.218	<0.0001
Age	−0.0396	0.0031	−12.660	<0.0001
Status married (ref. category)	0.0000			
Status married but separated	0.3514	0.2516	1.396	0.1625
Status single	0.4978	0.1346	3.698	0.0002
Status divorced	−0.3235	0.2496	−1.296	0.1948
Status widowed	−0.5645	1.0088	−0.560	0.5757
Status husband/wife abroad	1.8210	0.6236	2.920	0.0035
Gender male: status married (ref. category)	0.0000			
Gender male: status married but separated	−0.2015	0.3592	−0.561	0.5747
Gender male: status single	−0.8586	0.1537	−5.585	<0.0001
Gender male: status divorced	0.1261	0.2959	0.426	0.6698
Gender male: status widowed	0.5682	1.1068	0.513	0.6076
Gender male: status husband/wife abroad	−2.4181	0.8590	−2.815	0.0048

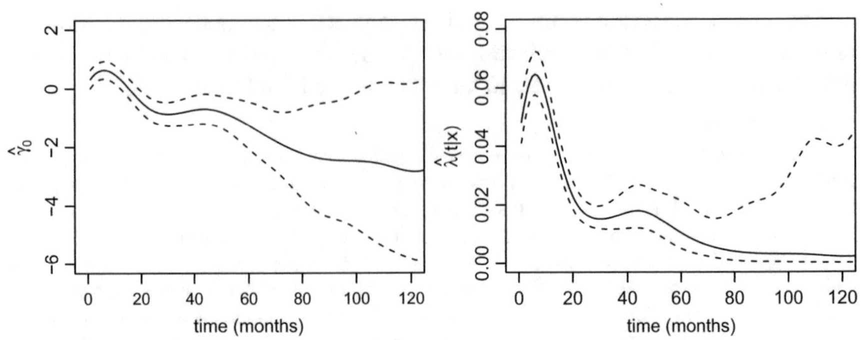

Fig. 10.1 German socio-economic panel. The *left panel* shows the estimated smooth function $\hat{\gamma}_0(t)$ for the baseline hazard in Example 10.1. The *right panel* shows the respective hazard estimate $\hat{\lambda}(t|\boldsymbol{x})$ for a 40-year-old male person with "status = married"

Table 10.2 German socio-economic panel. The table contains the hazard estimates for a 40-year-old person at $t = 10$ months. Estimates were obtained from the multiple-spell continuation ratio model in Example 10.1. They reflect the chance of getting re-employed at full-time job given a 10-month unemployment spell. Numbers in brackets are 95 % confidence intervals

	Hazard (= chance of getting re-employed)	
Status	Male	Female
Married	0.056 (0.050, 0.064)	0.019 (0.016, 0.023)
Married but separated	0.065 (0.040, 0.103)	0.027 (0.017, 0.043)
Single	0.040 (0.034, 0.047)	0.031 (0.025, 0.038)
Divorced	0.047 (0.035, 0.063)	0.014 (0.009, 0.022)
Widowed	0.057 (0.024, 0.129)	0.011 (0.001, 0.075)
Husband/wife abroad	0.032 (0.010, 0.095)	0.109 (0.035, 0.292)

also show the well-known effect of age on the (conditional) probability of getting re-employed: The older the persons, the smaller the probability of getting re-employed (coefficient estimate = −0.04 per year, p-value < 0.0001). Figure 10.1 shows the estimated smooth function $\hat{\gamma}_0(t)$ for the baseline hazard. It is seen that the baseline hazard increases in the time interval (0, 10], reflecting short-term unemployment. After 10 months, the baseline hazard starts to decrease indicating that the probability of re-employment decreases with the duration of unemployment. Figure 10.1 also shows the corresponding hazard function for a 40-year-old male person with "status = married." It is seen that for an unemployment duration longer than 5 years the probability of reemployment becomes very small. The variance of the subject-specific random effect is significantly different from zero (p-value = 0.0228) but small in magnitude ($\hat{\sigma} = 1.1524 \cdot 10^{-8}$), suggesting that not much heterogeneity is left when the explanatory variables are included.

The interaction effects between gender and status are summarized in Table 10.2. It is seen that the probability of getting re-employed is higher for men than for women in all status categories, with the only exception being the category "husband/wife abroad." For some categories of "status," the relation between effects is similar within the male and female groups. For example, for both male and female subjects chances of getting re-employed are higher in the "married but separated" group than in the "married" group. However, there are also notable differences between male and female subjects. In particular, women have a higher chance of getting re-employed if they are single instead of married, whereas for male subjects the respective coefficient estimates suggest an opposite trend. It should be noted that the results in Tables 10.1 and 10.2 do not provide information on whether subjects were actively looking for a full-time job during the study period. For this reason the hazard estimates of the continuation ratio model do not only reflect unequal opportunities for the various subgroups in the labor market, but also the family situation(s) of the study participants and transitions to part-time employment. □

10.3 Generalized Estimation Approach to Repeated Measurements

As in the preceding section we consider the simplified model for repeated failure times, which for the ith person uses the hazard function

$$\lambda^{(k)}(t \mid \boldsymbol{x}_{ik}) = P(T_{ik} = t \mid T_{ik} \geq t, \boldsymbol{x}_{ik}).$$

In estimation one should be aware that $T_{i1}, \ldots, T_{ik_i}$ are measurements on the same person and therefore cannot be assumed to be independent. For example, persons with many job opportunities (large values in the hazard) tend to have shorter unemployment spells during the whole observation period. In contrast, less qualified persons with high values in the hazard tend to have longer spells. Model (10.2) accounts for this potential dependence by including a subject-specific random effect. Alternatively, one can consider

$$\lambda^{(k)}(t \mid \boldsymbol{x}_{ik}) = h(\gamma_{0t}^{(k)} + \boldsymbol{x}_{ik}^T \boldsymbol{\gamma}^{(k)}) \tag{10.3}$$

as a model for the *marginal* responses T_{ik}. Model (10.3) does not specify the association between components of the vector $(T_{i1}, \ldots, T_{ik_i})$. Since each component follows a multinomial distribution, the vector $(T_{i1}, \ldots, T_{ik_i})$ itself is multinomially distributed. Maximum likelihood estimation for marginal models with multinomially distributed components is a rather advanced topic, and most approaches are limited to binary responses (McCullagh and Nelder 1989, Fitzmaurice and Laird 1993, Lang and Agresti 1994, Glonek and McCullagh 1995, and Bergsma et al. 2009). A more easily accessible approach is the estimation of Model (10.3) by generalized estimation equations (GEEs), which is sketched in the following.

Let us consider one component, T_{ik}, of the multiple response vector $(T_{i1}, \ldots, T_{ik_i})$. It can again be represented as a sequence of binary variables $y_{ik1}, \ldots, y_{ikt_{ik}}$, where

$$y_{ikt} = \begin{cases} 1, & i\text{th individual fails at } t \text{ in spell } k \text{ given it reaches } t \\ 0, & \text{otherwise}\,. \end{cases}$$

The model for the binary variables is determined by $P(y_{ikt} = 1) = \lambda^{(k)}(t \mid \boldsymbol{x}_{ik})$. It is marginal in the sense that only one spell is modeled, but conditional on previous responses within one spell because only sequences of the form $(0, 0, \ldots, 1)$ can occur. The corresponding variance is $\text{var}(y_{ikt} = 1) = \lambda^{(k)}(t|\boldsymbol{x}_{ik})(1-\lambda^{(k)}(t|\boldsymbol{x}_{ik}))$. The strength of generalized estimation equations (GEEs) is that the covariance matrix of the responses does not have to be specified correctly. Instead one works with a so-called working covariance structure. A simple working covariance structure for the whole sequence

$$\boldsymbol{y}_i^T = (y_{i11}, \ldots, y_{i1t_{i1}}, \ldots y_{ik_i1}, \ldots, y_{ik_it_{ik_i}})$$

is given by

$$\widetilde{\text{cov}}(y_{ikr}, y_{iks}) = -\lambda^{(k)}(r|\boldsymbol{x}_{ik})\lambda^{(k)}(s|\boldsymbol{x}_{ik}), \; r \neq s$$

and

$$\widetilde{\text{cov}}(y_{ikr}, y_{i\tilde{k}s}) = 0, \; k \neq \tilde{k}.$$

The first equation specifies the working covariance within spells as the usual covariance of the multinomial distribution, and the second equation uses independence as working covariance for components that refer to distinct spells. Let $\boldsymbol{W}$ contain the working variances and covariances in correspondence to the vector $\boldsymbol{y}_i$. Then the GEE that has to be solved to obtain an estimate of the coefficients is

$$\sum_{i=1}^{n} \boldsymbol{X}_i^T \boldsymbol{D}_i(\boldsymbol{\beta}) \boldsymbol{W}_i^{-1}(\boldsymbol{\beta}, \boldsymbol{\alpha})(\boldsymbol{y}_i - \boldsymbol{\mu}_i(\boldsymbol{\beta})) = \boldsymbol{0}, \tag{10.4}$$

where $\boldsymbol{D}_i(\boldsymbol{\beta}) = \text{diag}(\partial h(\eta_{i11})/\partial\eta, \ldots, \partial h(\eta_{ik_it_{ik_i}})/\partial\eta)$ contains the derivatives at the values of the linear predictors $\eta_{ikt} = \gamma_{0t}^{(k)} + \boldsymbol{x}_k^T \boldsymbol{\gamma}^{(k)}$. The matrix $\boldsymbol{X}_i$ contains the values of the explanatory variables, where each row of $\boldsymbol{X}_i$ contains the covariate values to the corresponding response in $\boldsymbol{y}_i$. Although the working covariance is not assumed to be the true covariance matrix, one obtains asymptotically normally distributed estimates under weak regularity conditions and can compute standard errors by the sandwich estimator

$$\widehat{\text{cov}}(\boldsymbol{\gamma}) = \boldsymbol{V}_W^{-1} \boldsymbol{V}_{\Sigma} \boldsymbol{V}_W^{-1},$$

where $\boldsymbol{V}_W = \sum_{i=1}^n \boldsymbol{X}_i^T \boldsymbol{D}_i \boldsymbol{W}_i^{-1} \boldsymbol{D}_i \boldsymbol{X}_i$, $\boldsymbol{V}_{\Sigma} = \sum_{i=1}^n \boldsymbol{X}_i^T \boldsymbol{D}_i \boldsymbol{W}_i^{-1} \boldsymbol{\Sigma}_i \boldsymbol{W}_i^{-1} \boldsymbol{D}_i \boldsymbol{X}_i$, and $\boldsymbol{\Sigma}_i$ is the true covariance matrix.

For the theory of GEEs, see in particular Liang and Zeger (1986), Prentice (1988), Liang et al. (1992), Liang and Zeger (1993), Xie and Yang (2003), and Wang (2011).

The estimation procedure described above uses the representation of the duration times by binary variables that code transitions. If censoring occurs in the last spell, the vector of observations $\boldsymbol{y}_i$ is shortened by omitting the last component. If no censoring occurs, one can also use the framework of multinomially distributed marginal responses T_{ik}. Then the marginal model is represented by the probabilities $P(T_{ik} = t_{ik})$ instead of the hazard rates, and one obtains a multivariate marginal model. A short introduction to multivariate GEEs is given in Tutz (2012).

10.4 Literature and Further Reading

Multi-spell Models in Continuous Time The mixed proportional hazards model has been used to model continuous-time recurrent events. For example, Ham and Rea Jr. (1987) and Hamerle (1989) used this type of model to estimate unemployment duration. Lillard and Panis (1996) considered marriage duration with multi-spell data, and Van den Berg (2001) investigated the identifiability of the mixed proportional hazards model.

Discrete-Time Modeling Johnson (2006) modeled student's enrolment history by dividing observation times into periods of enrolment and nonenrolment. Ondrich and Rhody (1999) extended the grouped proportional hazards model to multiple-spell data. Callens and Croux (2009) used multilevel recurrent discrete-time hazard analysis to model poverty entry and exit. General frameworks for discrete multi-spell data have been provided by Hamerle and Tutz (1989) and Willett and Singer (1995).

10.5 Software

The estimation of binary mixed-effects models for repeated measurements can be carried out with the same software packages as those mentioned in Sect. 9.9. Software for GEEs is available in the R packages *gee* (Ripley 2015) and *geepack* (Hojsgaard et al. 2014).

10.6 Exercises

10.1 Reconsider the data from the German socio-economic panel that were analyzed in Example 10.1. Figure 10.2 and Tables 10.3 and 10.4 contain the results obtained from a continuation ratio model with subject-specific random effects that was fitted to a subsample of 995 persons living in the German region of Baden–Wuerttemberg. This subsample comprised 1489 unemployment spells; the overall number of events was 652.

(a) Interpret the results and compare them to the results obtained from the region of North Rhine-Westphalia shown in Fig. 10.1 and Tables 10.1 and 10.2.

(b) Compare the numbers of events and analyzed persons in the two German regions and discuss the results in Fig. 10.2 and Tables 10.3 and 10.4 in the light of the remark on page 194.

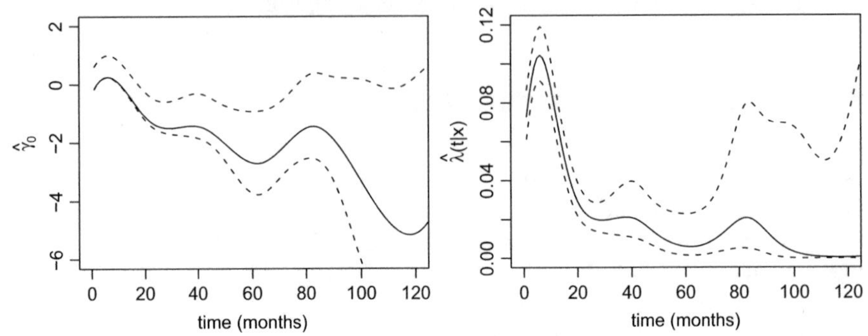

Fig. 10.2 German socio-economic panel. The *left panel* shows the estimated smooth function $\hat{\gamma}_0(t)$ for the baseline hazard in Exercise 10.1. The *right panel* shows the respective hazard estimate $\hat{\lambda}(t|\boldsymbol{x})$ for a 40-year-old male person with "status = married"

Table 10.3 German socio-economic panel. The table contains the coefficient estimates that were obtained from a multiple-spell continuation ratio model with subject-specific random intercept terms. Estimation was based on data from a subsample of 995 persons who live in the German region of Baden–Wuerttemberg. The response variable was the time to re-employment at full-time job (measured in months)

Variable name	Coef. estimate	Standard dev.	*z* value	*p*-value
Intercept	−2.323	0.201	−11.556	< 0.001
Gender female (ref. category)	0.000			
Gender male	0.906	0.135	6.714	< 0.001
Age	−0.044	0.004	−10.573	< 0.001
Status married (ref. category)	0.000			
Status married but separated	0.169	0.376	0.449	0.653
Status single	0.596	0.158	3.762	< 0.001
Status divorced	0.268	0.244	1.099	0.271
Status widowed	−1.067	1.010	−1.057	0.290
Status husband/wife abroad	−15.06	1669.0	−0.009	0.992
Gender male: status married (ref. category)	0.000			
Gender male: status married but separated	−1.099	0.635	−1.729	0.083
Gender male: status single	−0.835	0.181	−4.591	< 0.001
Gender male: status divorced	0.106	0.343	0.309	0.757
Gender male: status widowed	1.474	1.095	1.347	0.178
Gender male: status husband/wife abroad	0.000	1833.0	0.000	1.000

Table 10.4 German socio-economic panel. The table contains the hazard estimates for a 40-year-old person at $t = 10$ months. Estimates were obtained from the multiple-spell continuation ratio model in Exercise 10.1. They reflect the chance of getting re-employed at full-time job given a 10-month unemployment spell. Numbers in brackets are 95 % confidence intervals

	Hazard (= chance of getting re-employed)	
Status	Male	Female
Married	0.046 (0.040, 0.053)	0.019 (0.015, 0.023)
Married but separated	0.018 (0.007, 0.049)	0.022 (0.011, 0.044)
Single	0.036 (0.030, 0.043)	0.034 (0.027, 0.042)
Divorced	0.065 (0.042, 0.099)	0.024 (0.016, 0.037)
Widowed	0.067 (0.030, 0.141)	0.006 (0.001, 0.045)
Husband/wife abroad	0.000 (0.000, 1.000)	0.000 (0.000, 1.000)

10.2 Investigate the behavior of the binary mixed effects and GEE procedures by generating simulated data as follows:

(a) Specify the number of subjects and generate values of a binary covariate x_1 and a three-level covariate x_2 by using the following probability table:

		x_1	
		0	1
x_2	0	0.26	0.30
	1	0.15	0.14
	2	0.09	0.06

(b) Generate a set of subject-specific intercepts by drawing random numbers from a normal distribution with zero mean and variance σ^2.
(c) Compute the subject-specific hazard and survival functions by using a continuation ratio model with coefficients 0.3 (if $x_1 = 1$), 0.1 (if $x_2 = 1$), 0.2 (if $x_2 = 2$) and constant baseline hazard $\gamma_{0t} = -0.5$.
(d) Generate five duration times ("spells") per subject and convert the data into an augmented data set with binary outcome variable.
(e) Fit a binary mixed-effects model (using the *bs* = *"re"* option of the *gam* function in R package *mgcv*) and a GEE model (using the *id* argument of the *gee* function in R package *gee*) to the data.

Compare the estimated coefficients of the mixed-effects and GEE procedures for various numbers of subjects and different values of the subject-specific variance σ^2.

References

Aalen, O. O. (1988). Heterogeneity in survival analysis. *Statistics in Medicine, 7*, 1121–1137.
Abbring, J. H., & Van den Berg, G. J. (2007). The unobserved heterogeneity distribution in duration analysis. *Biometrika, 94*, 87–99.
Abrahamowicz, M., & MacKenzie, T. A. (2007). Joint estimation of time-dependent and non-linear effects of continuous covariates on survival. *Statistics in Medicine, 26*, 392–408.
Agresti, A. (2009). *Analysis of ordinal categorical data* (2nd ed.). New York: Wiley.
Agresti, A. (2013). *Categorical data analysis* (3rd ed.). New York: Wiley.
Agresti, A., Caffo, B., & Ohman-Strickland, P. (2004). Examples in which misspecification of a random effects distribution reduces efficiency, and possible remedies. *Computational Statistics & Data Analysis, 47*, 639–653.
Aitkin, M. (1999). A general maximum likelihood analysis of variance components in generalized linear models. *Biometrics, 55*, 117–128.
Allison, P. D. (1995). *Survival analysis using the SAS system: A practical guide*. Cary, NC: SAS Institute.
Almansa, J., Vermunt, J. K., Forero, C. G., & Alonso, J. (2014). A factor mixture model for multivariate survival data: An application to the analysis of lifetime mental disorders. *Journal of the Royal Statistical Society, Series C, 63*, 85–102.
Amemiya, T. (1981). Qualitative response models: A survey. *Journal of Economic Literature, XIX*, 1483–1536.
Andersen, P. K., Borgan, O., Gill, R., & Keiding, N. (1993). *Statistical models based on counting processes*. New York/Berlin: Springer.
Anderson, D. A., & Aitkin, M. (1985). Variance component models with binary response: Interviewer variability. *Journal of the Royal Statistical Society, Series B, 47*, 203–210.
Aranda-Ordaz, F. J. (1983). An extension of the proportional-hazard-model for grouped data. *Biometrics, 39*, 109–118.
Baker, M., & Melino, A. (2000). Duration dependence and nonparametric heterogeneity: A monte carlo study. *Journal of Econometrics, 96*, 357–393.
Barrier, A., Boelle, P.-Y., Roser, F., Gregg, J., Tse, C., Brault, D., et al. (2006). Stage II colon cancer prognosis prediction by tumor gene expression profiling. *Journal of Clinical Oncology, 24*, 4685–4691.
Bender, H., & Schumacher, M. (2008). Allowing for mandatory covariates in boosting estimation of sparse high-dimensional survival models. *BMC Bioinformatics, 9*, 14.
Bergsma, W., Croon, M., & Hagenaars, J. (2009). *Marginal models*. New York: Springer.
Besedes, T., & Prusa, T. J. (2006). Product differentiation and duration of US import trade. *Journal of International Economics, 70*, 339–358.

G. Tutz, M. Schmid, *Modeling Discrete Time-to-Event Data*, Springer Series in Statistics, DOI 10.1007/978-3-319-28158-2

Betensky, R. A., Rabinowitz, D., & Tsiatis, A. A. (2001). Computationally simple accelerated failure time regression for interval censored data. *Biometrika, 88*, 703–711.

Beyersmann, J., Allignol, A., & Schumacher, M. (2011). *Competing risks and multistate models with R*. New York: Springer.

Bojesen Christensen, R. H. (2015). *Ordinal: Regression models for ordinal data.* R package version 2015.6-28. http://cran.r-project.org/web/packages/ordinal/

Bonde, J., Hjollund, N., Jensen, T., Ernst, E., Kolstad, H., Henriksen, T., et al. (1998). A follow-up study of environmental and biologic determinants of fertility among 430 danish first-pregnancy planners: Design and methods. *Reproductive Toxicology, 12*, 19–27.

Bondell, H. D., & Reich, B. J. (2009). Simultaneous factor selection and collapsing levels in anova. *Biometrics, 65*, 169–177.

Bou-Hamad, I., Larocque, D., & Ben-Ameur, H. (2011a). Discrete-time survival trees and forests with time-varying covariates: Application to bankruptcy data. *Statistical Modelling, 11*, 429–446.

Bou-Hamad, I., Larocque, D., & Ben-Ameur, H. (2011b). A review of survival trees. *Statistics Surveys, 5*, 44–71.

Bou-Hamad, I., Larocque, D., Ben-Ameur, H., Masse, L., Vitaro, F., & Tremblay, R. (2009). Discrete-time survival trees. *Canadian Journal of Statistics, 37*, 17–32.

Boulesteix, A.-L., & Hothorn, T. (2010). Testing the additional predictive value of high-dimensional data. *BMC Bioinformatics, 11*, 78.

Boulesteix, A.-L., & Sauerbrei, W. (2011). Added predictive value of high-throughput molecular data to clinical data and its validation. *Briefings in Bioinformatics, 12*, 215–229.

Box-Steffensmeier, J. M., & Jones, B. S. (2004). *Event history modeling: A guide for social scientists*. New York: Cambridge University Press.

Breheny, P. (2015). *grpreg: Regularization paths for regression models with grouped covariates*. R package version 2.8-1. http://cran.r-project.org/web/packages/grpreg/index.html

Breiman, L. (1996). Bagging predictors. *Machine Learning, 24*, 123–140.

Breiman, L. (2001). Random forests. *Machine Learning, 45*, 5–32.

Breiman, L., Cutler, A., Liaw, A., & Wiener, M. (2015). *randomForest: Breiman and Cutler's random forests for classification and regression*. R package version 4.6-12. http://cran.r-project.org/web/packages/randomForest

Breiman, L., Friedman, J. H., Olshen, R. A., & Stone, J. C. (1984). *Classification and regression trees*. Monterey, CA: Wadsworth.

Breslow, N., & Crowley, J. (1974). A large sample study of the life table and product limit estimates under random censorship. *The Annals of Statistics, 2*, 437–453.

Breslow, N. E., & Clayton, D. G. (1993). Approximate inference in generalized linear mixed model. *Journal of the American Statistical Association, 88*, 9–25.

Breslow, N. E., & Lin, X. (1995). Bias correction in generalized linear mixed models with a single component of dispersion. *Biometrika, 82*, 81–91.

Brier, G. W. (1950). Verification of forecasts expressed in terms of probability. *Monthly Weather Review, 78*, 1–3.

Broström, G. (2013). *glmmML: Generalized linear models with clustering*. R package version 1.0. http://cran.r-project.org/web/packages/glmmML

Boström, H. (2007). Estimating class probabilities in random forests. In *ICMLA '07: Proceedings of the 6th International Conference on Machine Learning and Applications* (pp. 211–216). Washington, DC: IEEE Computer Society.

Brouhns, N., Denuit, M., & Vermunt, J. K. (2002). A Poisson log-bilinear regression approach to the construction of projected lifetables. *Insurance: Mathematics and Economics, 31*, 373–393.

Brown, C. (1975). On the use of indicator variables for studying the time-dependence of parameters in a response-time model. *Biometrics, 31*, 863–872.

Brüderl, J., Preisendörfer, P., & Ziegler, R. (1992). Survival chances of newly founded business organizations. *American Sociological Review, 57*, 227–242.

Bühlmann, P. (2006). Boosting for high-dimensional linear models. *Annals of Statistics, 34*, 559–583.

Bühlmann, P., Gertheiss, J., Hieke, S., Kneib, T., Ma, S., Schumacher, M., et al. (2014). Discussion of "The evolution of boosting algorithms" and "Extending statistical boosting". *Methods of Information in Medicine, 53*, 436–445.

Bühlmann, P., & Hothorn, T. (2007). Boosting algorithms: Regularization, prediction and model fitting (with discussion). *Statistical Science, 22*, 477–505.

Bühlmann, P., & Yu, B. (2003). Boosting with the L2 loss: Regression and classification. *Journal of the American Statistical Association, 98*, 324–339.

Cai, T., & Betensky, R. A. (2003). Hazard regression for interval-censored data with penalized spline. *Biometrics, 59*, 570–579.

Callens, M., & Croux, C. (2009). Poverty dynamics in Europe: A multilevel recurrent discrete-time hazard analysis. *International Sociology, 24*, 368–396.

Cameron, A. C., & Trivedi, P. K. (2005). *Microeconometrics: Methods and applications*. Cambridge: Cambridge University Press.

Candes, E., & Tao, T. (2007). The Dantzig selector: Statistical estimation when p is much larger than n. *Annals of Statistics, 35*, 2313–2351.

Cantoni, E., Flemming, J. M., & Ronchetti, E. (2011). Variable selection in additive models by non-negative garrote. *Statistical modelling, 11*, 237–252.

Capaldi, D. M., Crosby, L., & Stoolmiller, M. (1996). Predicting the timing of first sexual intercourse for adolescent males. *Child Development, 67*, 344–359.

Chamberlain, G. (1980). Analysis of covariance with qualitative data. *The Review of Economic Studies, 47*, 225–238.

Chen, D., Sun, J., & Peace, K. E. (2012). *Interval-censored time-to-event data: Methods and applications*. New York: Chapman & Hall/CRC.

Chiang, C. L. (1972). On constructing current life tables. *Journal of the American Statistical Association, 67*, 538–541.

Chiang, C. L. (1984). *The life table and its applications*. Malabar, FL: Robert E. Krieger Publishing.

Claeskens, G., Krivobokova, T., & Opsomer, J. D. (2009). Asymptotic properties of penalized spline estimators. *Biometrika, 96*, 529–544.

Cleveland, W. S. (1979). Robust locally weighted regression and smoothing scatterplots. *Journal of the American Statistical Association, 74*, 829–836.

Cox, D. R. (1972). Regression models and life tables (with discussion). *Journal of the Royal Statistical Society, Series B, 34*, 187–220.

Croissant, Y. (2015). *Ecdat: Data sets for econometrics*. R package version 0.2-9. http://cran.r-project.org/web/packages/Ecdat/index.html

Culpepper, S. A. (2014). If at first you don't succeed, try, try again – applications of sequential IRT models to cognitive assessments. *Applied Psychological Measurement, 38*, 632–644.

Currie, I. D., Durban, M., & Eilers, P. H. C. (2004). Smoothing and forecasting mortality rates. *Statistical Modelling, 4*, 279–298.

Czado, C. (1992). On link selection in generalized linear models. In *Advances in GLIM and statistical modelling. Springer lecture notes in statistics* (Vol. 78, pp. 60–65). New York: Springer.

Czado, C. (1997). On selecting parametric link transformation families in generalized linear models. *Journal of Statistical Planning and Inference, 61*, 125–139.

De Boeck, P., Bakker, M., Zwitser, R., Nivard, M., Hofman, A., Tuerlinckx, F., et al. (2011). The estimation of item response models with the lmer function from the lme4 package in R. *Journal of Statistical Software, 39*(12), 1–28.

De Boeck, P., & Wilson, M. (2004). *A framework for item response models*. New York: Springer.

De Boor, C. (1978). *A practical guide to splines*. New York: Springer.

Delwarde, A., Denuit, M., & Eilers, P. (2007). Smoothing the Lee–Carter and Poisson log-bilinear models for mortality forecasting – a penalized log-likelihood approach. *Statistical Modelling, 7*, 29–48.

Diggle, P. J., Heagerty, P., Liang, K.-Y., & Zeger, S. L. (2002). *Analysis of longitudinal data* (2nd ed.). New York: Oxford University Press.

Efron, B. (1988). Logistic regression, survival analysis, and the Kaplan-Meier-curve. *Journal of the American Statistical Association, 83*, 414–425.

Eilers, P. H. C., & Marx, B. D. (1996). Flexible smoothing with B-splines and Penalties. *Statistical Science, 11*, 89–121.

Eilers, P. H. C., & Marx, B. D. (2003). Multivariate calibration with temperature interaction using two-dimensional penalized signal regression. *Chemometrics and Intelligent Laboratory Systems, 66*, 159–174.

Elbers, C., & Ridder, G. (1982). True and spurious duration dependence: The identifiability of the proportional hazard model. *The Review of Economic Studies, 49*, 403–409.

Enberg, J., Gottschalk, P., & Wolf, D. (1990). A random-effects logit model of work-welfare transitions. *Journal of Econometrics, 43*, 63–75.

Fahrmeir, L. (1994). Dynamic modelling and penalized likelihood estimation for discrete time survival data. *Biometrika, 81*, 317–330.

Fahrmeir, L. (1998). Discrete survival-time models. In P. Armitage & T. Colton (Eds.), *Encyclopedia of biostatistics* (Vol. 2). Chichester: Wiley.

Fahrmeir, L., Hamerle, A., & Tutz, G. (1996). Regressionsmodelle zur Analyse von Verweildauern. In L. Fahrmeir, A. Hamerle, & G. Tutz (Eds.), *Multivariate statistische Verfahren*. Berlin: De Gruyter.

Fahrmeir, L., & Kneib, T. (2011). *Bayesian smoothing and regression for longitudinal, spatial and event history data*. Oxford: Oxford University Press.

Fahrmeir, L., & Knorr-Held, L. (1997). Dynamic discrete-time duration models: Estimation via Markov Chain Monte Carlo. *Sociological Methodology, 27*, 417–452.

Fahrmeir, L., & Tutz, G. (2001). *Multivariate statistical modelling based on generalized linear models*. New York: Springer.

Fahrmeir, L., & Wagenpfeil, S. (1996). Smoothing hazard functions and time-varying effects in discrete duration and competing risks models. *Journal of the American Statistical Association, 91*, 1584–1594.

Fan, J., & Gijbels, I. (1996). *Local polynomial modelling and its applications*. London: Chapman & Hall.

Fan, J., & Li, R. (2001). Variable selection via nonconcave penalized likelihood and its oracle properties. *Journal of the American Statistical Association, 96*, 1348–1360.

Ferri, C., Flach, P. A., & Hernandez-Orallo, J. (2003). Improving the AUC of probabilistic estimation trees. In *Proceedings of the 14th European Conference on Artifical Intelligence* (Vol. 2837, pp. 121–132). Berlin: Springer.

Finkelstein, D. M. (1986). A proportional hazards model for interval-censored failure time data. *Biometrics, 42*, 845–854.

Fitzmaurice, G. M., & Laird, N. M. (1993). A likelihood-based method for analysing longitudinal binary responses. *Biometrika, 80*, 141–151.

Fleming, T. R., & Harrington, D. P. (2011). *Counting processes and survival analysis*. New York: Wiley.

Follmann, D., & Lambert, D. (1989). Generalizing logistic regression by non-parametric mixing. *Journal of the American Statistical Association, 84*, 295–300.

Fox, J., & Weisberg, S. (2015). *car: Companion to applied regression*. R package version 2.1-0. http://cran.r-project.org/web/packages/car

Frank, I. E., & Friedman, J. H. (1993). A statistical view of some chemometrics regression tools (with discussion). *Technometrics, 35*, 109–148.

Frederiksen, A., Honoré, B. E., & Hu, L. (2007). Discrete time duration models with group-level heterogeneity. *Journal of Econometrics, 141*, 1014–1043.

Freund, Y., & Schapire, R. E. (1996). Experiments with a new boosting algorithm. In *Proceedings of the Thirteenth International Conference on Medicine Learning* (pp. 148–156). San Francisco: Morgan Kaufmann.

Friedman, J., Hastie, T., & Tibshirani, R. (2015). *glmnet: Lasso and elastic-net regularized generalized linear models*. R package version 2.0-2. http://cran.r-project.org/web/packages/glmnet/

Friedman, J. H. (2001). Greedy function approximation: A gradient boosting machine. *The Annals of Statistics, 29*, 1189–1232.

Friedman, J. H., Hastie, T., & Tibshirani, R. (2000). Additive logistic regression: A statistical view of boosting. *Annals of Statistics, 28*, 337–407.

Frühwirth-Schnatter, S. (2006). *Finite mixture and Markov switching models*. New York: Springer.

Gerds, T. A. (2015). *pec: Prediction error curves for survival models*. R package version 2.4.7. http://cran.r-project.org/web/packages/pec/

Gerds, T. A., & Schumacher, M. (2006). Consistent estimation of the expected Brier score in general survival models with right-censored event times. *Biometrical Journal, 48*, 1029–1040.

Gertheiss, J., & Tutz, G. (2010). Sparse modeling of categorial explanatory variables. *Annals of Applied Statistics, 4*, 2150–2180.

Glonek, G. F. V., & McCullagh, P. (1995). Multivariate logistic models. *Journal of the Royal Statistical Society, Series B, 57*, 533–546.

Gneiting, T., & Raftery, A. (2007). Strictly proper scoring rules, prediction, and estimation. *Journal of the American Statistical Association, 102*, 359–376.

Goeman, J., Meijer, R., & Chaturvedi, N. (2014). *penalized: L1 (lasso and fused lasso) and L2 (ridge) penalized estimation in GLMs and in the Cox model*. R package version 0.9-45. http://cran.r-project.org/web/packages/penalized/index.html

Graf, E., Schmoor, C., Sauerbrei, W., & Schumacher, M. (1999). Assessment and comparison of prognostic classification schemes for survival data. *Statistics in Medicine, 18*, 2529–2545.

Greenwood, M. (1926). The natural duration of cancer. Reports of Public Health and Medical Subjects 33, His Majesty's Stationary Office, London.

Groll, A. (2015). *glmmLasso: Variable selection for generalized linear mixed models by L1-penalized estimation*. R package version 1.3.6. http://cran.r-project.org/web/packages/glmmLasso

Groll, A., & Tutz, G. (2014). Variable selection for generalized linear mixed models by L_1-penalized estimation. *Statistics and Computing, 24*, 137–154.

Groll, A., & Tutz, G. (2016). Variable selection in discrete survival models including heterogeneity. *Lifetime Data Analysis* [published online].

Grün, B., & Leisch, F. (2008). FlexMix version 2: Finite mixtures with concomitant variables and varying and constant parameters. *Journal of Statistical Software, 28*(4), 1–35.

Gu, C. (2002). *Smoothing splines ANOVA models*. New York: Springer.

Gu, C., & Wahba, G. (1993). Semiparametric analysis of variance with tensor product thin plate splines. *Journal of the Royal Statistical Society, Series B, 55*, 353–368.

Ham, J. C., & Rea, S. A., Jr. (1987). Unemployment insurance and male unemployment duration in Canada. *Journal of Labor Economics, 5*, 325–353.

Hamerle, A. (1989). Multiple-spell regression models for duration data. *Applied Statistics, 38*, 127–138.

Hamerle, A., & Tutz, G. (1989). *Diskrete Modelle zur Analyse von Verweildauern und Lebenszeiten*. Frankfurt/New York: Campus Verlag.

Han, A., & Hausman, J. A. (1990). Flexible parametric estimation of duration and competing risk models. *Journal of Applied Econometrics, 5*, 1–28.

Harrell, F. E., Jr., Lee, K. L., & Mark, D. B. (1996). Multivariable prognostic models: Issues in developing models, evaluating assumptions and adequacy, and measuring and reducing errors. *Statistics in Medicine, 15*, 361–387.

Hartzel, J., Liu, I., & Agresti, A. (2001). Describing heterogenous effects in stratified ordinal contingency tables, with applications to multi-center clinical trials. *Computational Statistics & Data Analysis, 35*, 429–449.

Hastie, T., & Loader, C. (1993). Local regression: Automatic kernel carpentry. *Statistical Science, 8*, 120–143.

Hastie, T., & Tibshirani, R. (1990). *Generalized additive models*. London: Chapman & Hall.

Hastie, T., Tibshirani, R., & Friedman, J. H. (2009). *The elements of statistical learning* (2nd ed.). New York: Springer.

Heagerty, P. J., & Kurland, B. F. (2001). Misspecified maximum likelihood estimates and generalised linear mixed models. *Biometrika, 88*, 973–984.

Heagerty, P. J., Lumley, T., & Pepe, M. S. (2000). Time-dependent ROC curves for censored survival data and a diagnostic marker. *Biometrics, 56*, 337–344.

Heagerty, P. J., & Zheng, Y. (2005). Survival model predictive accuracy and ROC curves. *Biometrics, 61*, 92–105.

Heckman, J. J., & Singer, B. (1984a). Econometric duration analysis. *Journal of Econometrics, 24*, 63–132.

Heckman, J. J., & Singer, B. (1984b). A method for minimizing the impact of distributional assumptions in econometric models of duration. *Econometrica, 52*, 271–320.

Hedeker, D., Siddiqui, O., & Hu, F. B. (2000). Random-effects regression analysis of correlated grouped-time survival data. *Statistical Methods in Medical Research, 9*, 161–179.

Hess, W. (2009). A flexible hazard rate model for grouped duration data. Working Paper No. 2009:18, Department of Economics, Lund University.

Hess, W., & Persson, M. (2012). The duration of trade revisited – continuous-time vs. discrete-time hazards. *Empirical Economics, 43*, 1083–1107.

Hess, W., Tutz, G., & Gertheiss, J. (2014). A flexible link function for discrete-time duration models. Technical Report 155, Department of Statistics, University of Munich.

Hinde, J. (1982). Compound Poisson regression models. In R. Gilchrist (Ed.), *GLIM 1982 International Conference on Generalized Linear Models* (pp. 109–121). New York: Springer.

Hofner, B., Mayr, A., Robinzonov, N., & Schmid, M. (2014). Model-based boosting in R: A hands-on tutorial using the R package mboost. *Computational Statistics, 29*, 3–35.

Hojsgaard, S., Halekoh, U., & Yan, J. (2014). *geepack: Generalized estimating equation package*. R package version 1.2-0. http://cran.r-project.org/web/packages/geepack/index.html

Hothorn, T., Bühlmann, P., Kneib, T., Schmid, M., & Hofner, B. (2015). *mboost: Model-based boosting*. R package version 2.5-0. http://cran.r-project.org/web/packages/mboost/

Hothorn, T., Hornik, K., & Zeileis, A. (2006). Unbiased recursive partitioning: A conditional inference framework. *Journal of Computational and Graphical Statistics, 15*, 651–674.

Hothorn, T., Lausen, B., Benner, A., & Radespiel-Tröger, M. (2004). Bagging survival trees. *Statistics in Medicine, 23*, 77–91.

Hougaard, P. (1984). Life table methods for heterogeneous populations: Distributions describing the heterogeneity. *Biometrika, 71*, 75–83.

Huinink, J., Brüderl, J., Nauck, B., Walper, S., Castiglioni, L., & Feldhaus, M. (2011). Panel analysis of intimate relationships and family dynamics (pairfam): Conceptual framework and design. *Journal of Family Research, 23*, 77–101.

Ishwaran, H., Kogalur, U. B., Blackstone, E. H., & Lauer, M. S. (2008). Random survival forests. *Annals of Applied Statistics, 2*, 841–860.

Ishwaran, H., Kogalur, U. B., Chen, X., & Minn, A. J. (2011). Random survival forests for high-dimensional data. *Statistical Analysis and Data Mining, 4*, 115–132.

Jackman, S. (2015). *pscl: Political science computational laboratory*, Stanford University. R package version 1.4.9. http://cran.r-project.org/web/packages/pscl

James, G. M., & Radchenko, P. (2009). A generalized Dantzig selector with shrinkage tuning. *Biometrika, 96*, 323–337.

Jenkins, S. P. (2004). *Survival analysis*. Unpublished manuscript, Institute for Social and Economic Research, University of Essex. http://www.iser.essex.ac.uk/teaching/degree/stephenj/ec968/pdfs/ec968lnotesv6.pdf

Joergensen, H. S., Nakayama, H., Reith, J., Raaschou, H. O., & Olsen, T. S. (1996). Acute stroke with atrial fibrillation - the Copenhagen Stroke Study. *Stroke, 27*, 1765–1769.

Johnson, I. Y. (2006). Analysis of stopout behavior at a public research university: The multi-spell discrete-time approach. *Research in Higher Education, 47*, 905–934.

Jones, B. (1994). *A Longitudinal Perspective on Congressional Elections*. Ph.D. thesis, State University of New York at Stony Brook.

Kalbfleisch, J. D., & Prentice, R. L. (2002). *The statistical analysis of failure time data* (2nd ed.). New York: Wiley.

Kaplan, E. L., & Meier, P. (1958). Nonparametric estimation from incomplete observations. *Journal of the American Statistical Association, 53*, 457–481.

Kauermann, G., Krivobokova, T., & Fahrmeir, L. (2009). Some asymptotic results on generalized penalized spline smoothing. *Journal of the Royal Statistical Society, Series B, 71*, 487–503.

Kauermann, G., Tutz, G., & Brüderl, J. (2005). The survival of newly founded firms: A case-study into varying-coefficient models. *Journal of the Royal Statistical Society, Series A, 168*, 145–158.

Kim, J.-H. (2009). Estimating classification error rate: Repeated cross-validation, repeated hold-out and bootstrap. *Computational Statistics and Data Analysis, 53*, 3735–3745.

Kim, Y.-J., & Jhun, M. (2008). Cure rate model with interval censored data. *Statistics in Medicine, 27*, 3–14.

Klein, J. P., & Moeschberger, M. L. (2003). *Survival analysis: Statistical methods for censored and truncated data* (2nd ed.). New York: Springer.

Klein, J. P., Moeschberger, M. L., & J. Yan (2012). *KMsurv: Data sets from Klein and Moeschberger (1997), survival analysis*. R package version 0.1-5. http://cran.r-project.org/web/packages/KMsurv

Kleinbaum, D. G., & Klein, M. (2013). *Survival analysis: A self-learning text* (3rd ed.). New York: Springer.

Koenker, R., & Yoon, J. (2009). Parametric links for binary choice models: A Fisherian–Bayesian colloquy. *Journal of Econometrics, 152*, 120–130.

Kooperberg, C., Stone, C. J., & Truong, Y. K. (1995). Hazard regression. *Journal of the American Statistical Association, 90*, 78–94.

Kruskal, W. H. (1958). Ordinal measures of association. *Journal of the American Statistical Association, 53*, 814–861.

Kuk, A. Y., & Chen, C.-H. (1992). A mixture model combining logistic regression with proportional hazards regression. *Biometrika, 79*, 531–541.

Laird, N., & Olivier, D. (1981). Covariance analysis of censored survival data using log-linear analysis techniques. *Journal of the American Statistical Association, 76*, 231–240.

Lancaster, T. (1985). Generalised residuals and heterogeneous duration models: With applications to the Weibull model. *Journal of Econometrics, 28*, 155–169.

Lancaster, T. (1992). *The econometric analysis of transition data*. Cambridge: Cambridge University Press.

Land, K. C., Nagin, D. S., & McCall, P. L. (2001). Discrete-time hazard regression models with hidden heterogeneity: The semiparametric mixed Poisson regression approach. *Sociological Methods & Research, 29*, 342–373.

Lang, J. B., & Agresti, A. (1994). Simultaneous modelling joint and marginal distributions of multivariate categorical responses. *Journal of the American Statistical Association, 89*, 625–632.

Lawless, J. F. (1982). *Statistical models and methods for lifetime data*. New York: Wiley.

LeBlanc, M., & Crowley, J. (1993). Survival trees by goodness of split. *Journal of the American Statistical Association, 88*, 457–467.

LeBlanc, M., & Crowley, J. (1995). A review of tree-based prognostic models. *Journal of Cancer Treatment and Research, 75*, 113–124.

Lee, R. (2000). The Lee-Carter method for forecasting mortality, with various extensions and applications. *North American Actuarial Journal, 4*, 80–91.

Lee, R. D., & Carter, L. R. (1992). Modeling and forecasting US mortality. *Journal of the American Statistical Association, 87*, 659–671.

Leitenstorfer, F., & Tutz, G. (2011). Estimation of single-index models based on boosting techniques. *Statistical Modelling, 11*, 183–197.

Li, C.-S., Taylor, J. M., & Sy, J. P. (2001). Identifiability of cure models. *Statistics & Probability Letters, 54*, 389–395.

Li, Y., & Ruppert, D. (2008). On the asymptotics of penalized splines. *Biometrika, 95*, 415–436.

Liang, K.-Y., & Zeger, S. (1986). Longitudinal data analysis using generalized linear models. *Biometrika, 73*, 13–22.

Liang, K.-Y., & Zeger, S. (1993). Regression analysis for correlated data. *Annual Review of Public Health, 14*, 43–68.

Liang, K.-Y., Zeger, S., & Qaqish, B. (1992). Multivariate regression analysis for categorical data (with discussion). *Journal of the Royal Statistical Society, Series B, 54*, 3–40.

Lichman, M. (2013). UCI machine learning repository. School of Information and Computer Sciences, University of California, Irvine. http://archive.ics.uci.edu/ml

Lillard, L. A., & Panis, C. W. (1996). Marital status and mortality: The role of health. *Demography, 33*, 313–327.

Lin, X., & Breslow, N. E. (1996). Bias correction in generalized linear mixed models with multiple components of dispersion. *Journal of the American Statistical Association, 91*, 1007–1016.

Lin, X., & Zhang, D. (1999). Inference in generalized additive mixed models by using smoothing splines. *Journal of the Royal Statistical Society, Series B, 61*, 381–400.

Lindsey, J. C., & Ryan, L. M. (1998). Methods for interval-censored data. *Statistics in Medicine, 17*, 219–238.

Liu, Q., & Pierce, D. A. (1994). A note on Gauss-Hermite quadrature. *Biometrika, 81*, 624–629.

Loader, C. (1999). *Local regression and likelihood*. New York: Springer.

Maller, R. A., & Zhou, X. (1996). *Survival analysis with long-term survivors*. New York: Wiley.

Mantel, N., & Hankey, B. F. (1978). A logistic regression analysis of response time data where the hazard function is time dependent. *Communications in Statistics – Theory and Methods, A7*, 333–347.

Marra, G., & Wood, S. N. (2011). Practical variable selection for generalized additive models. *Computational Statistics & Data Analysis, 55*, 2372–2387.

Marx, B. D., & Eilers, P. H. C. (1998). Direct generalized additive modelling with penalized likelihood. *Computational Statistics & Data Analysis, 28*, 193–209.

Masters, G. N. (1982). A Rasch model for partial credit scoring. *Psychometrika, 47*, 149–174.

Mayer, P., Larocque, D., & Schmid, M. (2014). *DStree: Recursive partitioning for discrete-time survival trees*. R package version 1.0. http://cran.r-project.org/web/packages/DStree/index.html

Mayr, A., Binder, H., Gefeller, O., & Schmid, M. (2014a). The evolution of boosting algorithms (with discussion). *Methods of Information in Medicine, 53*, 419–427.

Mayr, A., Binder, H., Gefeller, O., & Schmid, M. (2014b). Extending statistical boosting (with discussion). *Methods of Information in Medicine, 53*, 428–435.

Mayr, A., & Schmid, M. (2014). Boosting the concordance index for survival data – a unified framework to derive and evaluate biomarker combinations. *PLoS One, 9*(1), e84483.

McCullagh, P. (1980). Regression model for ordinal data (with discussion). *Journal of the Royal Statistical Society, Series B, 42*, 109–127.

McCullagh, P., & Nelder, J. A. (1989). *Generalized linear models* (2nd ed.). New York: Chapman & Hall.

McCulloch, C. E. (1997). Maximum likelihood algorithms for generalized linear mixed models. *Journal of the American Statistical Association, 92*, 162–170.

McCulloch, C. E., & Neuhaus, J. M. (2011). Misspecifying the shape of a random effects distribution: Why getting it wrong may not matter. *Statistical Science, 26*, 388–402.

McCulloch, C. E., & Searle, S. (2001). *Generalized, linear, and mixed models*. New York: Wiley.

McDonald, J. W., & Rosina, A. (2001). Mixture modelling of recurrent event times with long-term survivors: Analysis of Hutterite birth intervals. *Statistical Methods and Applications, 10*, 257–272.

McLachlan, G. J., & Peel, D. (2000). *Finite mixture models*. New York: Wiley.

McCall, B. P. (1996). Unemployment insurance rules, joblessness, and part-time work. *Econometrica, 64*, 647–682.

Meier, L. (2015). *grplasso: Fitting user specified models with Group Lasso penalty*. R package version 0.4-5. http://cran.r-project.org/web/packages/grplasso/index.html

Meier, L., van de Geer, S., & Bühlmann, P. (2008). The group lasso for logistic regression. *Journal of the Royal Statistical Society, Series B, 70*, 53–71.

Molinaro, A., Simon, R., & Pfeiffer, R. M. (2005). Predition error estimation: A comparison of resampling methods. *Bioinformatics, 21*, 3301–3307.

Morgan, B. J. T. (1985). The cubic logistic model for quantal assay data. *Applied Statistics, 34*, 105–113.

Morgan, J. N., & Sonquist, J. A. (1963). Problems in the analysis of survey data, and a proposal. *Journal of the American Statistical Association, 58*, 415–435.

Möst, S. (2014). *Regularization in Discrete Survival Models*. Ph.D. Thesis, Department of Statistics, University of Munich.

Möst, S., Pößnecker, W., & Tutz, G. (2015). Variable selection for discrete competing risks models. *Quality & Quantity*. doi:10.1007/s11135-015-0222-0.

Muggeo, V. M., Attanasio, M., & Porcu, M. (2009). A segmented regression model for event history data: An application to the fertility patterns in Italy. *Journal of Applied Statistics, 36*, 973–988.

Muggeo, V. M., & Ferrara, G. (2008). Fitting generalized linear models with unspecified link function: A P-spline approach. *Computational Statistics & Data Analysis, 52*, 2529–2537.

Muthén, B., & Masyn, K. (2005). Discrete-time survival mixture analysis. *Journal of Educational and Behavioral Statistics, 30*, 27–58.

Nagelkerke, N. J. D. (1991). A note on a general definition of the coefficient of determination. *Biometrika, 78*, 691–692.

Nakazawa, M. (2015). *fmsb: Functions for medical statistics book with some demographic data*. R package version 0.5.2. http://cran.r-project.org/web/packages/fmsb

Narendranathan, W., & Stewart, M. B. (1993). Modelling the probability of leaving unemployment: Competing risks models with flexible base-line hazards. *Applied Statistics, 42*, 63–83.

Nauck, B., Brüderl, J., Huinink, J., & Walper, S. (2013). The German Family Panel (pairfam). GESIS Data Archive, Cologne. ZA5678 Data file Version 4.0.0. doi:10.4232/pairfam.5678.4.0.0.

Neuhaus, J. M., & McCulloch, C. E. (2006). Separating between- and within-cluster covariate effects by using conditional and partitioning methods. *Journal of the Royal Statistical Society, Series B, 68*, 859–872.

Nicoletti, C., & Rondinelli, C. (2010). The (mis)specification of discrete duration models with unobserved heterogeneity: A Monte Carlo study. *Journal of Econometrics, 159*, 1–13.

Ondrich, J., & Rhody, S. E. (1999). Multiple spells in the Prentice-Gloeckler-Meyer likelihood with unobserved heterogeneity. *Economics Letters, 63*, 139–144.

Patil, P. N., & Bagkavos, D. (2012). Semiparametric smoothing of discrete failure time data. *Biometrical Journal, 54*, 5–19.

Pepe, M. S. (2003). *The statistical evaluation of medical tests for classification and prediction*. New York: Chapman & Hall.

Pinheiro, J. C., & Bates, D. M. (1995). Approximations to the log-likelihood function in the nonlinear mixed-effects model. *Journal of Computational and Graphical Statistics, 4*, 12–35.

Pregibon, D. (1980). Goodness of link tests for generalized linear models. *Applied Statistics, 29*, 15–24.

Prentice, R. L. (1975). Discrimination among some parametric models. *Biometrika, 62*, 607–614.

Prentice, R. L. (1976). A generalization of the probit and logit methods for dose response curves. *Biometrics, 32*, 761–768.

Prentice, R. L. (1988). Correlated binary regression with covariates specific to each binary observation. *Biometrics, 44*, 1033–1084.

Prentice, R. L., & Gloeckler, L. A. (1978). Regression analysis of grouped survival data with application to breast cancer data. *Biometrics, 34*, 57–67.

Preston, S., Heuveline, P., & Guillot, M. (2000). *Demography: Measuring and modeling population processes*. Chichester: Wiley-Blackwell.

Provost, F., & Domingos, P. (2003). Tree induction for probability-based ranking. *Machine Learning, 52*, 199–215.

Quinlan, J. R. (1993). *C4.5: Programs for machine learning*. San Francisco, CA: Morgan Kaufmann.

R Core Team. (2015). *R: A language and environment for statistical computing*. Vienna, Austria: R Foundation for Statistical Computing. Software version 3.2.2, http://www.R-project.org

Rabinowitz, D., Tsiatis, A., & Aragon, J. (1995). Regression with interval-censored data. *Biometrika, 82*, 501–513.

Rasch, G. (1961). On general laws and the meaning of measurement in psychology. In J. Neyman (Ed.), *Proceedings of the Fourth Berkeley Symposium on Mathematical Statistics and Probability*. Berkeley: University of California Press.

Rijmen, F., Tuerlinckx, F., De Boeck, P., & Kuppens, P. (2003). A nonlinear mixed model framework for item response theory. *Psychological Methods, 8*, 185–205.

Ripley, B. (2015). *gee: Generalized estimation equation solver*. R package version 4.13-19. http://cran.r-project.org/web/packages/gee/index.html

Ripley, B. D. (1996). *Pattern recognition and neural networks*. Cambridge: Cambridge University Press.

Ruckstuhl, A., & Welsh, A. (1999). Reference bands for nonparametrically estimated link functions. *Journal of Computational and Graphical Statistics, 8*, 699–714.

Ruppert, D., Wand, M. P., & Carroll, R. J. (2003). *Semiparametric regression*. Cambridge: Cambridge University Press.

Schall, R. (1991). Estimation in generalised linear models with random effects. *Biometrika, 78*, 719–727.

Scheike, T., & Jensen, T. (1997). A discrete survival model with random effects: An application to time to pregnancy. *Biometrics, 53*, 318–329.

Scheike, T., & Keiding, N. (2006). Design and analysis of time-to-pregnancy. *Statistical Methods in Medical Research, 15*, 127–140.

Schmid, M., & Hothorn, T. (2008). Boosting additive models using component-wise P-splines. *Computational Statistics & Data Analysis, 53*, 298–311.

Schmid, M., Hothorn, T., Maloney, K. O., Weller, D. E., & Potapov, S. (2011). Geoadditive regression modeling of stream biological condition. *Environmental and Ecological Statistics, 18*, 709–733.

Schmid, M., Kestler, H. A., & Potapov, S. (2015). On the validity of time-dependent AUC estimators. *Briefings in Bioinformatics, 16*, 153–168.

Schmid, M., Küchenhoff, H., Hoerauf, A., & Tutz, G. (2016). A survival tree method for the analysis of discrete event times in clinical and epidemiological studies. *Statistics in Medicine, 35*, 734–751.

Schmid, M., & Potapov, S. (2012). A comparison of estimators to evaluate the discriminatory power of time-to-event models. *Statistics in Medicine, 31*, 2588–2609.

Singer, J. D., & Willett, J. B. (2003). *Applied longitudinal data analysis: Modeling change and event occurrence*. Oxford: Oxford University Press.

Steele, F., Goldstein, H., & Browne, W. (2004). A general multilevel multistate competing risks model for event history data, with an application to a study of contraceptive use dynamics. *Statistical Modelling, 4*, 145–159.

Strobl, C., Malley, J., & Tutz, G. (2009). An introduction to recursive partitioning: Rationale, application and characteristics of classification and regression trees, bagging and random forests. *Psychological Methods, 14*, 323–348.

Stukel, T. A. (1988). Generalized logistic models. *Journal of the American Statistical Association, 83*, 426–431.

Sun, J. (2006). *The statistical analysis of interval-censored failure time data*. New York/Heidelberg: Springer.

Sy, J. P., & Taylor, J. M. (2000). Estimation in a Cox proportional hazards cure model. *Biometrics, 56*, 227–236.

Therneau, T., Atkinson, B., & Ripley, B. (2015). *rpart: Recursive partitioning*. R package version 4.1-9. http://cran.r-project.org/web/packages/rpart

Thompson, W. A. (1977). On the treatment of grouped observations in life studies. *Biometrics, 33*, 463–470.

Tibshirani, R. (1996). Regression shrinkage and selection via the lasso. *Journal of the Royal Statistical Society, Series B, 58*, 267–288.

Tibshirani, R., & Ciampi, A. (1983). A family of proportional- and additive-hazards models for survival data. *Biometrics, 39*, 141–147.

Tutz, G. (1990). Sequential item response models with an ordered response. *British Journal of Statistical and Mathematical Psychology, 43*, 39–55.

Tutz, G. (1995). Competing risks models in discrete time with nominal or ordinal categories of response. *Quality & Quantity, 29*, 405–420.

Tutz, G. (2012). *Regression for categorical data*. Cambridge: Cambridge University Press.

Tutz, G. (2015). Sequential models for ordered responses. In W. van der Linden & R. Hambleton (Eds.), *Handbook of modern item response theory*. New York: Springer.

Tutz, G., & Binder, H. (2004). Flexible modelling of discrete failure time including time-varying smooth effects. *Statistics in Medicine, 23*, 2445–2461.

Tutz, G., & Binder, H. (2006). Generalized additive modeling with implicit variable selection by likelihood-based boosting. *Biometrics, 62*, 961–971.

Tutz, G., & Oelker, M. (2015). Modeling clustered heterogeneity: Fixed effects, random effects and mixtures. *International Statistical Review* (to appear).

Tutz, G., & Petry, S. (2012). Nonparametric estimation of the link function including variable selection. *Statistics and Computing, 21*, 545–561.

Tutz, G., Pößnecker, W., & Uhlmann, L. (2015). Variable selection in general multinomial logit models. *Computational Statistics & Data Analysis, 82*, 207–222.

Tutz, G., & Pritscher, L. (1996). Nonparametric estimation of discrete hazard functions. *Lifetime Data Analysis, 2*, 291–308.

Uno, H., Cai, T., Pencina, M. J., D'Agostino, R. B., & Wei, L. J. (2011). On the C-statistics for evaluating overall adequacy of risk prediction procedures with censored survival data. *Statistics in Medicine, 30*, 1105–1117.

Uno, H., Cai, T., Tian, L., & Wei, L. J. (2007). Evaluating prediction rules for t-year survivors with censored regression models. *Journal of the American Statistical Association, 102*, 527–537.

van de Vijver, M. J., He, Y. D., van't Veer, L. J., Dai, H., Hart, A. A. M., Voskuil, D. W., et al. (2002). A gene-expression signature as a predictor of survival in breast cancer. *New England Journal of Medicine, 347*, 1999–2009.

Van den Berg, G. J. (2001). Duration models: Specification, identification and multiple durations. In J. J. Heckman & E. Leamer (Eds.), *Handbook of econometrics* (Vol. V, pp. 3381–3460). Amsterdam: North Holland.

van der Laan, M. J., & Robins, J. M. (2003). *Unified methods for censored longitudinal data and causality*. New York: Springer.

van der Linden, W., & Hambleton, R. K. (1997). *Handbook of modern item response theory*. New York: Springer.

Vaupel, J. W., Manton, K. G., & Stallard, E. (1979). The impact of heterogeneity in individual frailty on the dynamics of mortality. *Demography, 16*, 439–454.

Vaupel, J. W., & Yashin, A. I. (1985). Heterogeneity's ruses: Some surprising effects of selection on population dynamics. *The American Statistician, 39*, 176–185.

Verhelst, N. D., Glas, C., & De Vries, H. (1997). A steps model to analyze partial credit. In W. van der Linden & R. K. Hambleton (Eds.), *Handbook of modern item response theory* (pp. 123–138). New York: Springer.

Vermunt, J. K. (1996). *Log-linear event history analysis: A general approach with missing data, latent variables, and unobserved heterogeneity*. Tilburg: Tilburg University Press.

Wand, M. P. (2000). A comparison of regression spline smoothing procedures. *Computational Statistics, 15*, 443–462.

Wang, H., & Leng, C. (2008). A note on adaptive group lasso. *Computational Statistics & Data Analysis, 52*, 5277–5286.

Wang, L. (2011). GEE analysis of clustered binary data with diverging number of covariates. *The Annals of Statistics, 39*, 389–417.

Wang, L., Sun, J., & Tong, X. (2010). Regression analysis of case II interval-censored failure time data with the additive hazards model. *Statistica Sinica, 20*, 1709–1723.

Weinberg, C., & Gladen, B. (1986). The beta-geometric distribution applied to comparative fecundability studies. *Biometrics, 42*, 547–560.

Weisberg, S., & Welsh, A. H. (1994). Adapting for the missing link. *The Annals of Statistics, 22*, 1674–1700.

Welchowski, T., & Schmid, M. (2015). *discSurv: Discrete time survival analysis*. R package version 1.1.1. http://cran.r-project.org/web/packages/discSurv

Willett, J. B., & Singer, J. D. (1995). It's déja vu all over again: Using multiple-spell discrete-time survival analysis. *Journal of Educational and Behavioral Statistics, 20*, 41–67.

Wolfinger, R. W. (1994). Laplace's approximation for nonlinear mixed models. *Biometrika, 80*, 791–795.

Wood, S. (2015). *mgcv: Mixed GAM Computation Vehicle with GCV/AIC/REML smoothness estimation*. R package version 1.8-9. http://cran.r-project.org/web/packages/mgcv

Wood, S. N. (2006). *Generalized additive models: An introduction with R*. London: Chapman & Hall/CRC.

Xie, M., & Yang, Y. (2003). Asymptotics for generalized estimating equations with large cluster sizes. *The Annals of Statistics, 31*, 310–347.

Xue, X., & Brookmeyer, R. (1997). Regression analysis of discrete time survival data under heterogeneity. *Statistics in Medicine, 16*, 1983–1993.

Yee, T. (2010). The VGAM package for categorical data analysis. *Journal of Statistical Software, 32*(10), 1–34.

Yu, B., Tiwari, R. C., Cronin, K. A., & Feuer, E. J. (2004). Cure fraction estimation from the mixture cure models for grouped survival data. *Statistics in Medicine, 23*, 1733–1747.

Yu, Y., & Ruppert, D. (2002). Penalized spline estimation for partially linear single-index models. *Journal of the American Statistical Association, 97*, 1042–1054.

Yuan, M., & Lin, Y. (2006). Model selection and estimation in regression with grouped variables. *Journal of the Royal Statistical Society, Series B, 68*, 49–67.

Zeng, D., Cai, J., & Shen, Y. (2006). Semiparametric additive risks model for interval-censored data. *Statistica Sinica, 16*, 287–302.

Zou, H. (2006). The adaptive lasso and its oracle properties. *Journal of the American Statistical Association, 101*, 1418–1429.

Zou, H., & Hastie, T. (2005). Regularization and variable selection via the elastic net. *Journal of the Royal Statistical Society, Series B, 67*, 301–320.

List of Examples

G. Tutz, M. Schmid, *Modeling Discrete Time-to-Event Data*,
Springer Series in Statistics, DOI 10.1007/978-3-319-28158-2

Subject Index

G. Tutz, M. Schmid, *Modeling Discrete Time-to-Event Data*,
Springer Series in Statistics, DOI 10.1007/978-3-319-28158-2

Author Index

G. Tutz, M. Schmid, *Modeling Discrete Time-to-Event Data*,
Springer Series in Statistics, DOI 10.1007/978-3-319-28158-2

Printed in the United States
By Bookmasters